Looking and Acting
Vision and eye movements in natural behaviour

Looking and Acting
Vision and eye movements in natural behaviour

Michael F. Land
Department of Biology and Environmental Science,
University of Sussex, UK

Benjamin W. Tatler
School of Psychology,
University of Dundee, UK

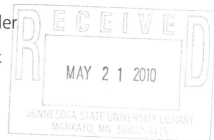
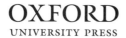
OXFORD
UNIVERSITY PRESS

OXFORD

UNIVERSITY PRESS

Great Clarendon Street, Oxford ox2 6dp

Oxford University Press is a department of the University of Oxford.
It furthers the University's objective of excellence in research, scholarship,
and education by publishing worldwide in

Oxford New York

Auckland Cape Town Dar es Salaam Hong Kong Karachi
Kuala Lumpur Madrid Melbourne Mexico City Nairobi
New Delhi Shanghai Taipei Toronto

With offices in

Argentina Austria Brazil Chile Czech Republic France Greece
Guatemala Hungary Italy Japan Poland Portugal Singapore
South Korea Switzerland Thailand Turkey Ukraine Vietnam

Oxford is a registered trade mark of Oxford University Press
in the UK and in certain other countries

Published in the United States
by Oxford University Press Inc., New York

© Oxford University Press, 2009

British Library Cataloguing in Publication Data
Data available

Library of Congress Cataloging in Publication Data
Data available

Typeset in Minion by Cepha Imaging Private Ltd., Banglore, India
Printed in Great Britain
on acid-free paper by
the MPG Books Group, Bodmin and King's Lynn

ISBN 978-0-19-857094-3 (Pbk)

10 9 8 7 6 5 4 3 2 1

For Rosemary and Sarah

Preface

This book could have been called 'A Natural History of Gaze'. Our intention has been to document the way people use their eyes when performing natural tasks in real settings, and we are particularly interested in the ways that vision is used to find the information needed to initiate and control actions. Although eye movement recordings have been made since the late years of the nineteenth century, for about 90 years these were essentially confined to viewing static images or text, usually with head and body movements prevented. It was simply not possible to study how the eyes behaved during purposeful action. This changed in the 1980s when head-mounted eye movement recording cameras became commercially available, and it became possible to record the direction of gaze during real behaviour. Our objective in this book is to outline the results of these recent studies, based on our own researches and those of others, and to discuss what they mean in terms of the ways that the vision and action systems of the brain interact.

We both came to this subject from a somewhat unusual direction. MFL spent most of his academic life working on vision in everything from scallops to snakes and seriously took up the study of human vision only in the late 1980s. MFL retained his observational approach to human vision from his zoological background. BWT trained as a neurophysiologist and started out in academic life by working briefly on flies' eyes before moving to human eye movements. Although BWT has recently been distracted by computer-based viewing paradigms, he also retains the naturalistic and observational approaches from his biological training. We have never truly understood psychologists' passion for removing all trace of the natural environment from experiments.

It is still true that the majority of eye movement research involves the interrogation of a static image, usually on a computer monitor screen. However, action control is very different from viewing an image. The latter is principally a perceptual and cognitive task, involving those parts of the brain involved in detecting and recognizing objects and making verbal reports: the 'ventral stream' of Milner and Goodale (1995). Action, on the other hand, also involves the 'dorsal stream': those regions of the cortex, particularly the parietal complex, concerned with the translation of visual information into a form suitable for the control of the body and limbs. In addition to the perceptual system, action control involves two other brain systems: one concerned with directing gaze to the location of particular objects or other informative places and the other capable of providing the motor system with the information needed by the limbs during object manipulation. Action control places quite different demands on the visual system from purely perceptual tasks, and uses different cortical hardware.

For these reasons, we have taken the view that the role of vision during action can usefully be studied only during the performance of action itself, preferably in conditions that are as unconstrained as possible. This is rather different from the approach in most psychological research, where it is usual to reduce the number of variables involved to a minimum so that the experiment will provide an either/or outcome. It may be useful to go down this reductionist route once natural gaze behaviour has been adequately described, but at this relatively early stage in the development of the subject it seems more profitable to adopt the minimal interference methods of ethology and allow the systems we wish to study to show what they are good for on their own terms. In selecting the research we discuss in this book we have emphasized naturalistic studies, and in general avoided those that just involve subjects looking at screens, or watching videos of action, on the grounds that these do not engage the brain systems relevant to action control.

Contents

Acknowledgements

Thanks are due to the following project students at the University of Sussex, whose work contributed directly to some of the studies in this book: Clare Isbell, Matt Armstrong, Heloise Tsang and Joella Tucknott (walking; Chapter 6), Mark Lynch and Robert Weston (table tennis; Chapter 8), Lynette Owen and Sam Walker (jigsaw puzzle; Chapter 4), Genevieve Baker and Louis Jackson (portrait drawing; Chapter 4).

We are very grateful to the following for reading and commenting on parts of the text: Mary Hayhoe (Austin, Texas) (Chapter 5 and parts of Chapter 8), Jenny Rusted and Sam Hutton (Sussex) (Chapter 12), Graham Hole (Sussex) (Chapter 7), Bruce Abernethy (Queensland) (Chapter 8), John Tchalenko (Camberwell School of Arts) (Chapter 4), and Alan Kennedy (Dundee) (Chapter 4). We are happy to acknowledge many fruitful discussions with Dana Ballard and Mary Hayhoe (Austin, Texas).

Iain Gilchrist (Bristol) and Ron Rensink (British Columbia) kindly allowed us to use their original illustrations (Figs 3.1 and 10.2).

The following publishers have given permission to reproduce copyright material. University of Chicago Press (Figs 1.3, 3.9, 3.12, and 4.4); Wiley Interscience (Figs 2.4 and 2.8); Plenum Press/Springer-Verlag (Figs 3.3, 3.4, 3.10, and 9.1); American Association for the Advancement of Science (Fig. 3.13); Elsevier (Fig. 4.15); Society for Neuroscience (Figs 5.5, 12.1); and MPTV.net (Fig. 9.5). Thanks are also due to to the American Psychological Association for their liberal policy on allowing reproduction from their many titles. Figure authors are referred to in the captions, and full citations appear in the reference list.

Videos of a number of the original eye-tracker recordings described in this book can be found on *www.scanpaths.org* and *www.activevisionlab.org*.

Part 1

Preliminaries

Chapter 1

Introduction

This introductory chapter is in three sections. First, we consider in very broad outline the relations between vision and action, and the role played by the gaze control system in directing the eyes to places from which information is required. Second, we give a brief history of the development of gaze recording techniques, from static laboratory methods to modern head-mounted devices that allow complete freedom of movement. Finally, we describe the scope of the book and give outlines of the chapter contents.

The relations of vision, gaze control, and action

For our neolithic ancestors, in the time before vision had become domesticated by writing and computers, the primary role of vision would have been to provide the information needed to carry out the tasks of everyday life. Perception, in the sense of discerning the relations of sensations to the external world, has a part to play in this, but of greater importance would have been the guidance of action: steering the individual through the environment and guiding the limbs in the execution of the activities required for survival.

Four interacting systems

Any action, for example picking up a mug, requires the cooperation of several systems in the brain, each of which has a different role in the execution of the action. When thirst or habit triggers an intention to find something to drink, the first job is likely to be to locate a cup, mug, or glass, and finding it is the function of the gaze control system. Objects are nearly always fixated by the foveae of the eyes before any action occurs (for reasons discussed in Chapter 2), and this may involve movements not just of the eyes, but of the head and body as well, as discussed in Chapter 6. (We use 'gaze direction' here in preference to 'eye direction' to distinguish where the fovea is pointing in space from where it is pointing relative to the head; the two are the same only if the head is fixed in space). If the mug is visible in peripheral vision it may be targeted directly, but if it is initially out of sight, the gaze system will need to access remembered information about where the mug is likely to be before it can be located. Once the mug has been imaged on the fovea, the motor system can set about the task of grasping it and lifting it. To do that it requires information supplied by the image processing regions of the visual system. Vision has to first confirm that the object is indeed a mug, and then determine the direction and distance the arm and hand must travel. For the efficient performance of the grasp, the orientation of the handle must be worked out, so that the hand can be shaped appropriately during the extension of the arm. Thus the whole task requires the gaze system to locate objects, the motor system to operate on them, and the visual system to supply the information that makes this possible (Fig. 1.1a).

Although the three systems just described may seem adequate for the simple action of grasping a mug it is clear that there has to be fourth system that selects what task to perform. Suppose our subject, having had his or her cup of tea, decides to read a book. The gaze system needs to locate the bookshelf and the books, the visual system has to be primed to recognize the correct title, and then to provide the motor system with information to guide the hands in extracting the book from the row. Although the overall locating, acting, and information-supplying functions are the same as they were in dealing with the mug, the details are very different, and they depend crucially on the task. Each system has to be primed with information from some supervisory body that knows the task and its requirements. Here we have referred to this as the schema control system. The word 'schema' has had many incarnations in psychology, but in this context we use it to mean the internal representation of a task and the instructions that go with it. This system can probably be formally identified with the 'Supervisory Attention System' of Norman and Shallice (1986) or the 'Central Executive' in the

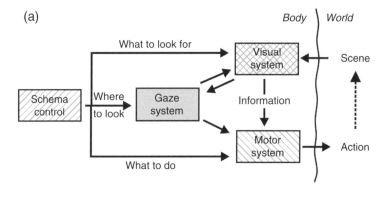

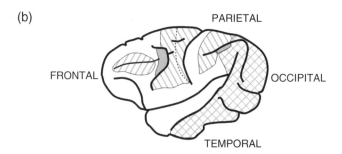

Fig. 1.1 (a) Diagram showing the four systems involved in the control of a motor action and the flow of information between them. (b) Parts of the macaque cortex identified with the four systems in (a).

working memory system of Baddeley (2007). In this context, its job is to both select the next task to be performed and inform the other three systems of their respective duties: where to look, what to do, and what to look for.

The distinction between these four roles is not just theoretical: they are performed by different regions of the brain (Fig. 1.1b). These will be discussed in some detail in Chapter 11. It is enough here to say that in the cortex, both the gaze and motor control systems are identified with separate areas in both the frontal and parietal regions, the visual system occupies the occipital lobe and parts of the parietal and temporal lobes, and the generally accepted centre of the schema control system is in the dorsolateral pre-frontal cortex (e.g. Jeannerod, 1997; Fuster, 2002). Most of these regions are reciprocally connected. Of course the cerebral cortex contains only the most accessible parts of the systems involved. There are many sub-cortical regions of the brain whose contributions to the initiation and control of action are every bit as important.

What gaze records tell us

A principal objective of this book is to provide an account of the gaze strategies we use in everyday life; however, it will be clear from the foregoing remarks that there is no point in it trying to study gaze in isolation from tasks being performed. We assert that where we look is determined primarily by where information that is needed for the next action is likely to be found: that is, where the visual system needs to be directed to guide and inform the motor system during the execution of the act. Consequently, a record of the places our gaze system decides to visit during a task provides us with what amounts to a running commentary on the changing information requirements of the motor system as the task unfolds. Consider the record of fixations shown in Fig. 1.2, which documents the fixations made by one of us (MFL) while filling a kettle prior to making a cup of tea (taken from Land et al., 1999, and discussed in detail in Chapter 5). These involve first the inspection and lifting of the kettle (11 fixations – it was a complicated electric kettle), then three fixations guiding

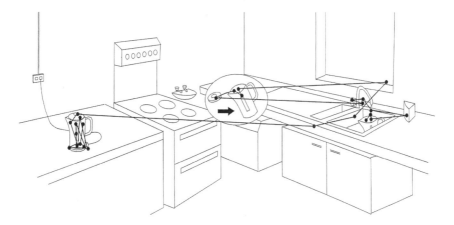

Fig. 1.2 Fixations made during a 10 s period when one author (MFL) was filling a kettle prior to making a cup of tea.

the few steps to the sink. During this walk the lid was removed from the kettle (four fixations). Gaze then transferred to the taps, where one was selected (three fixations) and then turned on while the kettle was set down in the sink. There are then four fixations on the water stream that began to fill the kettle and one to the sink tidy to the right.

It is very striking that gaze is directed almost exclusively to objects or places from which information is needed at the time. The kettle, the lid, and the taps are all objects that are to be either moved or manipulated. The three fixations on the sink are for guidance, and the fixations on the water stream monitor the progress of the filling. There is only a single fixation, on the sink tidy, that can be classified as irrelevant to the task; all others are directly concerned with the implementation of the successive actions. This last observation, that there are virtually no task-irrelevant fixations, is important because, since the well-known study by Itti and Koch (2000), it has been popular to model the destination of eye movements in terms of the visual 'salience' of objects in the field of view: that is, the constellation of image features (colour, brightness, spatial scale, motion, etc.) that seem to capture visual attention. We see no evidence here that the eyes are entrapped by the salience of objects not involved in the task. There are plenty of other features in the kitchen that are at least as salient as those fixated, but these are ignored. We will discuss this further in Chapter 3, but the conclusion at this stage is that, for most of the actions we will be dealing with in this book, it is the tasks themselves – represented by the top-down instructions from the schema control system – that determine where to look next.

The hidden knowledge of the gaze control system

Although the form of the fixation sequence, or scan path, shown in Fig. 1.2 is not particularly surprising once one knows the events in the task, it would have been very difficult to predict it in any detail. In general we have little or no knowledge of the scan paths that our eyes take and cannot even say where we were looking during the fixation before the present one (Tatler, 2001). The gaze movement system and the instructions it receives seem to be beyond conscious scrutiny. Often we cannot even guess what the gaze control system is trying to do on our behalf. We can illustrate this by asking three questions. How do skilled pianists use their eyes to sample the notes on the stave? (see Fig. 4.6). Where do motorists look to get the information that enables them to steer round the next bend? (see Fig. 7.3). Where do batsmen look when the ball leaves the bowler's hand? (see Fig. 8.9). We have found that our participants themselves do *not* know the answers to these questions, implying that introspection cannot allow us to answer these questions. We can, however, answer these questions by making objective recordings of gaze direction during these tasks. This tells us things we cannot find out any other way; in particular it provides insights into the instructions that the schema control system sends to the gaze control system about where to look (Fig. 1.1a). It turns out that these systems hold a great deal of often surprising knowledge: for example, the answers to the three questions above were available to the gaze control systems of the participants, although not their conscious minds.

Following from this, one of the attractions of studying gaze and fixation patterns is the surprise element. Often, finding out where gaze is directed tells us what information is particularly important for the execution of a task. So, for example, in table tennis or cricket, gaze moves rapidly (i.e. with a saccade, see Chapter 2) to a location near the bounce point of an approaching ball, up to 100 ms before the ball itself gets there (Chapter 8). This anticipatory saccade, which players are unaware of, means that the exact location and timing of the bounce can be observed accurately, and this turns out to be crucial for the ball to be struck effectively. Given that the alternative strategy of making smooth pursuit eye movements takes up to 200 ms to initiate, by which time a short fast ball would have already bounced, the anticipatory saccade strategy is very much more effective. Coaches tell us to keep our eyes on the ball; but players, or at least their gaze control systems, know better.

Eye movements, perception, and action

Throughout the twentieth and into the present century there has been a huge amount of physiological and psychological work on eye movements, but nearly all of this has been confined to the laboratory, and in most of it eye movements were studied as more or less isolated sub-systems – saccades, smooth-tracking, vergence movements, and vestibulo-ocular and optokinetic reflex adjustments. These are described in Carpenter (1988, 1991) and briefly in Chapter 2 of this book. We consider these sub-systems as the components that make up the strategies concerned with obtaining the information needed for action. It is these broader strategies, which nearly always involve a succession of gaze movements, that we will be dealing with in this book.

Part of vision is concerned with perception – the extraction of information from consciously available images for the discrimination and identification of objects – and these aspects of vision have been studied extensively by psychologists. We argue here, however, that the more fundamental function of vision is to provide the information needed for task execution, much of which is not readily available to conscious scrutiny. This lack of accessibility possibly accounts for the relative neglect of these 'action control' aspects of vision in the past. Perception has an important role in action tasks – it is important to verify what we are looking at, for example. However, that is not our primary concern here; our main focus will be on those aspects of vision that enable task performance and their inextricable link to the control of gaze.

A brief history of recording methods

Recording patterns of gaze in natural tasks: early studies

Eye movement recordings have been made for well over a century, Dodge and Cline making the first photographic records in 1901 (for a history of early eye movement studies see Wade and Tatler, 2005). However, until comparatively recently such recordings were confined to laboratory tasks in which the head had to be held more or less stationary (Fig. 1.3). These early studies are discussed in Chapter 4 and included tasks such as reading aloud (Buswell, 1920), typing (Butsch, 1932), viewing pictures (Buswell, 1935), and even playing the piano (Weaver, 1943). An important outcome of all these investigations was that fixations typically lead actions, usually by about a second. Vision is thus in the vanguard of action and not just summoned up as specific information is required. A further important advance was made by the Russian physiologist Alfred Yarbus in the 1950s, also using a head-fixed recording technique (Yarbus, 1967). He established that eye movements are not simply determined by the characteristics of the image, but their pattern could be changed radically by asking the subject different questions about the picture they are looking at (see Chapter 3). The idea of 'top-down' control had been hinted at earlier by Guy Buswell (1935), but Yarbus' work left no doubt about its importance. Eye movements could no longer be thought of as reflex responses to image features.

The studies just cited all used bench-mounted devices of various kinds to record the eye movements of restrained subjects (Fig. 1.3). For tasks involving active movements

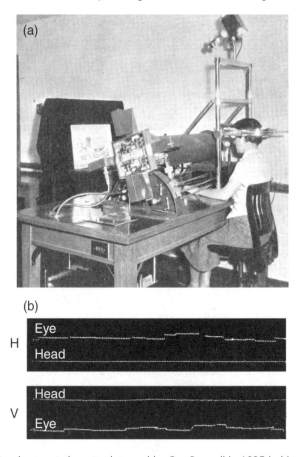

Fig. 1.3 (a) Bench-mounted eye tracker used by Guy Buswell in 1935 in his study of picture viewing. The subject, with head restrained, views the picture on the screen to the left. (b) Vertical and horizontal eye movements are recorded separately by imaging the reflection from the cornea onto moving film, seen at the near end of the horizontal tube in (a). Dots on the records are every 33 ms. The scan path is then reconstructed from these records, examples of which can be seen in Figs. 3.9 and 3.12. From Buswell (1935).

of participants a different system is required, and all the devices that have been used successfully for such recordings over the past 50 years have been mounted on the head rather than the bench. The first of these mobile eye trackers was made by Norman Mackworth in the 1950s (Thomas, 1968). His device consisted of a head-mounted ciné camera that made a film of the view from the subject's head, onto which was projected, via a periscope, an image of the corneal reflex magnified optically in such a way as to correspond with the direction the visual axis. Mackworth and Thomas (1962) used a TV camera version of the device to study the eye movements of drivers. These cameras were quite bulky and difficult to operate, and further advances had to wait for the development of more user-friendly devices in the 1980s, when video cameras became smaller and computers could be enlisted to assist the analysis of the image from the eye. It is only since about 1990 that it has become realistic to study what people do outside the laboratory – in the kitchen or workshop, on the road, or on the sports field.

Recent methods for recording eye movements

Most modern mobile eye trackers typically use two cameras, or one with a split field (Fig. 1.4). One camera images the view ahead and because the camera is attached to the head its field of view rotates with the head. The second camera, also attached to the head, images the eye and measures foveal direction by determining the position of the

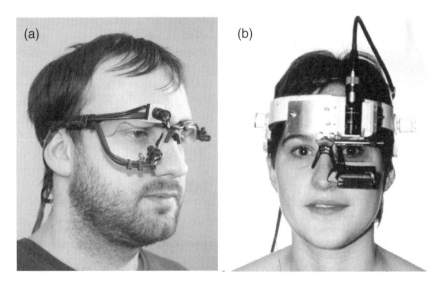

Fig. 1.4 Recent head-mounted eye movement cameras. (a) Spectacle-frame mounted camera which uses infra-red light to produce a 'white pupil' that is tracked by software and added to the image from the small forward-pointing scene camera above the eye. (b) Split-image eye camera in which the scene and an image of the eye are recorded onto the same video frame. Foveal direction is determined from the position of the iris. This camera was used for many of the recordings in this book.

pupil or the iris in head coordinates. This is usually done online by computer-aided tracking software, and often the pupil is illuminated with infra-red light to give a 'white' pupil that is easier to track. The coordinates are then used to position a spot or cross on the image from the scene camera, which, with suitable calibration, shows the location of the direction of the fovea on the scene. These devices are typically accurate to about 1°, or slightly better (i.e. roughly the angular width of the fovea). A review of the methodologies currently employed is given by Duchowski (2003).

Head and body movements

In freely behaving humans the direction of gaze is the result of movements of the eyes in the head, the head on the trunk, and the trunk in the world. In relation to the direction of regard in the surroundings, head-mounted eye trackers bypass the need to measure all three variables as the scene camera's field of view moves with the head just as the eyes do. However, it is often useful to have independent records of eye, head, and body movements. The interrelations of the different components are quite complex. For example, head movements usually augment eye movements during gaze shifts, but during fixations the effects of head movement are cancelled out by the vestibulo-ocular reflex that rotates the eye with a velocity equal and opposite to the head movement (Guitton and Volle, 1987; see Chapter 2). A similar reciprocity exists for head and trunk rotations, mediated by the vestibulo-collic reflex (Land, 2004). Head and body movements can be measured using various dedicated arrangements in which reflecting strips are attached to the head and other parts of the body and filmed from above or by using magnetic detectors. However, head-in-space measurements can be obtained directly from the scene camera of an eye tracker, by measuring the movement of background objects, relative to the stationary image frame. If the subject does not shift body position, this gives an accurate record of head rotation. During translational body movement, in walking or driving, for example, this can still give an accurate head rotation record provided distant objects are chosen that are in line with the subject's trajectory (without these precautions there is confusion between translation and rotation). This method has been used for a number of the studies in this book. Rotations of the trunk can similarly be determined by video methods. One technique used here is to match the orientation of the subject's body to a rotatable model of a person of similar physique. This method has an accuracy of about 3°, and we have used it in Chapter 6 to measure body rotations during turns accompanying large eye saccades.

Scope of the book

The book is in three parts: an introductory section (I, Preliminaries: Chapters 1–3), a main section dealing with gaze strategies involved in different types of natural task (II, Observations: Chapters 4–9), and a final section (III, Commentaries: Chapters 10–12) discussing the cognitive machinery involved in the generation of gaze strategies and actions.

The present chapter has provided an account of the reasons for studying gaze control in natural tasks and a brief history of the subject. Chapter 2 deals with reasons why eye movements are made and gives a brief account of the types of eye movements (saccades, reflex stabilizing movements, smooth pursuit, and vergence) that make up the repertoire of components of the strategies used in natural tasks. Chapter 3 raises the fundamental question of what drives eye movements. The evidence for bottom-up (i.e. image-driven) and top-down (e.g., task-driven) control is discussed here in some detail.

In Part II, Chapter 4 describes gaze strategies in relatively sedentary activities, from reading (text and music) to drawing pictures. Readers may feel that reading, a subject with a huge literature and much controversy, is somewhat underrepresented here, but this is deliberate. It is only one of a great many equally interesting tasks. In Chapter 5 we consider 'domestic' activities, in particular food preparation. These typically consist of a series of different actions carried out one after the other. Of particular interest here are the relative timings of gaze changes and the actions they enable, and the functions of individual fixations, in terms of the kinds of information they provide. Chapter 6 deals with locomotion on foot, and with questions such as how far ahead do we look when placing our feet on uncertain terrain and what sources of information are used to guide locomotion. It also examines the roles of eye, head, and body movements during turns, and of the reflexes that coordinate them. Chapter 7 is devoted to driving, and the main questions here are how, when, and from where do we obtain the information needed to negotiate curves, turn corners, avoid obstacles, and brake effectively. Also discussed are the ways that learner drivers on the one hand and racing drivers on the other differ from ordinary competent drivers. Chapter 8 examines the use of visual information in a variety of ball sports. The timing required in some of these can be extraordinary: in cricket, for example, an effective shot must be timed to within 5 ms, probably even less in baseball. Changing gaze position at the right time can be crucial in these sports, and eye movement studies have thrown some light on how this is achieved. Chapter 9 is slightly different in that it discusses the eyes both as receivers and providers of information. In social contexts, it is often important to know who is looking at whom, and eye contact is an essential part of many kinds of interaction. People also pick up on the direction that others are looking and follow suit, a phenomenon often used by magicians to distract the gaze of the audience.

The final three chapters (Part III) are concerned with the cognitive and neural machinery involved in gaze control. Chapter 10 deals with the representation of the visual world in the mind and returns to some of the issues raised in Chapter 3. Evidence from 'change blindness' studies in the 1990s showed that each time the eyes are moved most of the direct pictorial information in the image is lost. However, it is equally clear that selective information is retained over successive fixations although not in its original form. Indeed, life would be very difficult if we could not remember the locations and appearances of objects that we make use of in a task, or could not recall the landmarks on the way home. The chapter discusses the possible nature of the various representations that originate in the retinal image. Chapter 11 outlines what we know of the neural machinery involved in the initiation and coordination of actions and their associated gaze patterns. Much of this knowledge comes either from macaque electrophysiology or from brain-scan studies, and there are obvious limitations: macaques cannot do most of the tasks discussed here, and real action in scanners is limited. Nevertheless, it seems that it is possible to locate the major pathways corresponding to the components in Fig. 1.1a, even if the details are far from clear. Chapter 12 discusses the roles of attention and various types of memory in the control of action and then addresses the function of frontal lobe structures in the generation of goals and action schemas. We discuss the possible relevance of new ideas from control engineering, such as predictors and inverse controllers, particularly in relation to fast-skilled behaviour. The book ends with suggestions for the future.

Chapter 2

The human eye movement repertoire

Why we need to move our eyes

Before we can discuss the eye movement strategies employed in different tasks, we need to review briefly the individual types of eye movements that people are capable of making. Surprisingly, perhaps given the fluidity of our motor behaviour in general, this repertoire is small, well defined, and very similar from one individual to another. It is also well understood not only in terms of the movements themselves but also in terms of the neurophysiological mechanisms that generate them. We will begin with a discussion of why we have the eye movements that we do and not others (e.g. we do not let our eyes wander smoothly across a scene: they always jump from one point to another). This will be followed by an account of the eye muscles and the neural machinery that controls them and subsequently, brief descriptions of the different types of eye movement. One of the first accurate and admirably succinct descriptions of the human eye movement repertoire comes from the surgeon John Hunter:

> From all of which we find these three modes of action produced; first, the eye moving from one fixed point to another; then the eye moving along with an object in motion; and last, the eye keeping its axis to an object, although the whole eye, and the head, of which it makes a part, are in motion.
>
> (John Hunter, 1786, pp. 209–210)

Today we would recognize Hunter's three categories as saccades, smooth pursuit, and stabilized fixation, and would probably add vergence as a separate category. Good accounts to augment the brief framework given here can be found in the works of Carpenter (1988, 1991).

Throughout the animal kingdom, in animals with as diverse evolutionary backgrounds as men, fish, crabs, flies, and cuttlefish, one finds a consistent pattern of eye movements that can be referred to as a 'saccade and fixate' strategy (Land, 1999). Saccades are the fast movements that redirect the eye to a new part of the surroundings, and fixations are the intervals between saccades in which gaze is held almost stationary. As Dodge showed in 1900, it is during fixations that information is taken in; during saccades we are effectively blind.

In humans there are two reasons for this strategy. First, the fovea, the region of acute vision, is astonishingly small. Depending on exactly how it is defined, its angular diameter is between 0.3° and 2°, and the foveal depression (fovea means pit) covers only about one in four-thousandth of the retinal surface (Steinman, 2003). Away from the fovea, resolution falls rapidly – to a tenth of its maximum value at an eccentricity of 20° (Fig. 2.1). To see detail in what we are looking at, we need to move the eye so that the object of interest is centred on the fovea. Because a combination of blur and active suppression causes us to be almost blind during these relocations, we have to move the eyes as fast as possible, and saccades are indeed very fast, reaching speeds of 700° s^{-1} for large saccades (Carpenter, 1988). Second, gaze must be kept still between saccades, during the fixations when we take in visual information. The reason for this is that the process of photoreception is slow: it takes about 20 ms for a cone to respond fully to a step change in the light reaching it (Friedburg et al., 2004). The practical effect of this is that at image speeds of greater than about 2 to 3° s^{-1} we are no longer able to use the finest (highest spatial frequency) information in the image (Westheimer and McKee, 1975; Carpenter, 1991); in short, the image starts to blur, just as in a camera with a slow shutter speed. As we discuss in the following text, vertebrates have two powerful mechanisms – the vestibulo-ocular reflex (VOR) and the optokinetic reflex (OKR) – for stabilizing gaze even when the head and body are in motion. An interesting

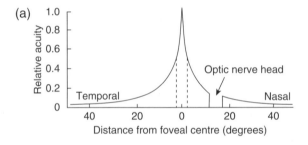

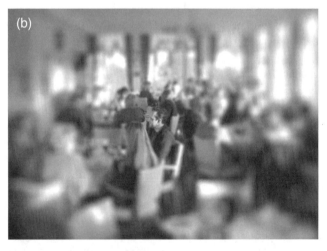

Fig. 2.1 (a) The decrease in acuity with eccentricity from the centre of the fovea. By 20° acuity is reduced by a factor of 10. (b) A reconstruction of the image of a scene on the retina blurred by the function shown in (a). The sharply resolved figure at the centre is one of the authors (BWT). Figure supplied courtesy of Ben Vincent, from Snowden et al. (2006).

finding is that animals such as goldfish without well-defined foveae still employ the saccade and fixate strategy (Land, 1999). Keeping gaze rotationally stable is the primary requirement whatever the retinal configuration, but in addition mobile animals necessarily require saccadic gaze-shifting mechanisms to prevent the eyes from becoming trapped at the ends of their movement range (Walls, 1962). Thus fish need the same machinery as primates, even though most do not use their eyes in the same inquisitive fashion.

The eye movement machinery

Eye muscles

In humans the eyeball is supported and moved by six muscles (Fig. 2.2). The same six muscles are present in lampreys, relatives of the earliest jawless fish from the Ordovician (450 M years ago), so the design has a history as old as vertebrate vision.

To a reasonable approximation, the four *rectus* muscles (lateral, medial, superior, and inferior) rotate the eyeball in the horizontal and vertical planes, thereby shifting the line of sight of the fovea relative to the surroundings. The two *oblique* muscles (superior and inferior) rotate the eyeball around the visual axis (torsion), providing partial compensation for head roll. The superior oblique is unusual in that its tendon runs through a pulley, a loop of cartilage that changes the muscle's line of action. The other five muscles connect the eyeball to the skull directly. In reality, the muscles do not work entirely independently. For example, the superior and inferior recti produce a small amount of lateral movement and torsion as well as predominant motion in the vertical plane. Thus any eye movement requires the action of all the eye muscles to varying degrees and a correspondingly complex pattern of activation from the oculomotor nuclei.

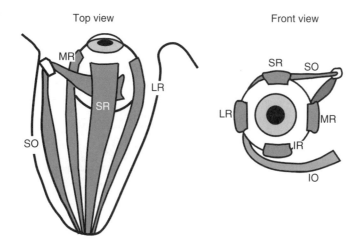

Fig. 2.2 Muscles of the right human eye. SR, IR, LR, MR, Superior, inferior, lateral, and oblique rectus muscles; SO, IO, superior and inferior oblique muscles.

The oculomotor system of the brain

We give here only the briefest of descriptions of the regions of the brain that control the movements of the eyes. A more detailed discussion is postponed until Chapter 11. Extensive accounts can be found in Carpenter (1988), various chapters in Carpenter (1991) and in Chalupa and Werner (2003). The control can be thought of as operating at three levels: the cerebral cortex, responsible for 'voluntary' eye movement control; midbrain structures, particularly the superior colliculi that have an important role in saccade generation; and the nuclei of the brain stem that put together the motor output that directly controls the eye muscles.

Working backwards from the eye, the eye muscles receive their motor innervation from three nuclei in the brain stem. The *oculomotor* nucleus supplies the superior, inferior, and medial recti and the inferior oblique via cranial nerve III; the *trochlear* nucleus supplies the lateral rectus via nerve VI; and the *abducens* nucleus supplies the superior oblique via nerve VI. Upstream of these motor nuclei is a complex series of pre-motor nuclei (PMN, Fig. 2.3) in which the specific patterns of neural activity required for different types of eye movement are constructed. Of these the *paramedian pontine reticular formation* is particularly associated with the generation of saccades. This region contains neurons that provide a burst of impulses to move the eye to a new position (*burst units*) and others that produce a continuous output to hold the eye in its new position (*tonic units*). The *nucleus reticularis tegmenti pontis* is involved in smooth pursuit movements. Other important inputs to the pre-motor brainstem complex come from the *vestibular nuclei* that provide a signal that compensates for head movements (via the vestibulo-ocular reflex, see *The stabilizing mechanisms*),

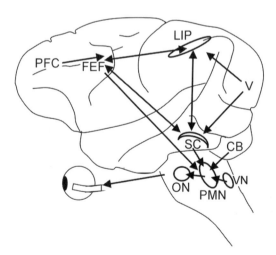

Fig. 2.3 The major regions of the brain concerned with eye movement control in the macaque. CB, cerebellum; FEF, frontal eye field; LIP, lateral intraparietal region; ON, oculomotor nuclei (oculomotor, abducens, and trochlear); PFC, pre-fontal cortex; PMN, pre-motor nuclei; SC, superior colliculus; V, visual cortex; VN, vestibular nuclei.

from the *cerebellum*, from the *superior colliculus*, and from the cortical *frontal eye fields*.

The two superior colliculi in the roof of the midbrain are homologous with the optic tecta of other vertebrates, where they have a major role in visual orientation, not just of the eyes but of the head and trunk as well. In primates their role was thought to be confined to the organization of eye saccades, but it now seems that they can also control the head movements associated with eye saccades (Gandhi and Sparks, 2003). The collicular surface contains maps of cells responsive to sensory stimuli. These are exclusively visual in the superficial layers, but in the deeper layers auditory and somatosensory modalities are also represented. These deeper layers also contain motor cells involved in generating commands for saccades. These are organized as a map whose coordinates represent the size and direction of saccades. The output from these deep layers goes predominantly to the ocular PMN of the brain stem, mentioned above. The colliculi receive direct input from the cortex (the frontal eye fields (FEF), the lateral intraparietal area (LIP), and from V1, the primary visual cortex). They are reciprocally connected to FEF and LIP via the thalamus.

The regions of the cortex most concerned with eye movements are the FEFs and the nearby supplementary eye fields, and parietal area LIP. The FEFs and LIP are strongly reciprocally connected, and both receive input from various parts of the visual cortex. It appears that saccades can be initiated either from the FEFs or the superior colliculi: lesions of either region on its own have relatively little observable effect, but destruction of both virtually abolishes saccadic activity. It seems that the FEFs can control the oculomotor systems of the brain stem either directly or via the superior colliculi. The FEFs are also involved in the initiation and maintenance of smooth pursuit eye movements. The role of LIP is less well understood, but a primary function seems to be to translate visual information from retinal coordinates into coordinate frames representing different motor effectors, such as the eye, head, trunk, and hand (Colby and Goldberg, 1999). The cortical eye fields receive an important input from the dorsolateral prefrontal cortex, a region associated with behavioural goals and the planning of actions, that is, with the schema system of Fig. 1.1.

Types of eye movement

Saccades

The term saccade comes from the French for 'jerk' or 'twitch', and was first used by Javal in 1879 to mean a rapid eye movement. It was introduced to the English eye movement literature by Dodge in 1916 (see Wade and Tatler, 2005). The maximum frequency with which saccades can be made is about 4 s^{-1}, although it is usually lower. This frequency is reached, for example, during reading or when quickly scanning a scene. If a typical saccade lasts 30 ms, and the fixation that follows it lasts 300 ms, then one-tenth of the waking day is spent making saccades. This means that for about one-and-a-half hours each day we are effectively blind. Saccades made by the two eyes are conjugate, that is, they are simultaneous and are of the same size and in the same direction, although the sizes may be slightly different if there is a change in fixation distance and vergence is involved.

Saccades make up a family of fast eye movements, whose velocities and durations vary with their size, but, with some pathological exceptions, are very similar from one individual to another (Fig. 2.4). The velocity and duration of saccades vary somewhat with their direction, but not greatly. Saccade duration is an almost linear function of saccade amplitude, at least up to about 40°, and can be described by the equation,

$$D = D_0 + d.A$$

where D is the duration, A the amplitude in degrees, D_0 is a minimum duration of 20 to 30 ms, and d is the duration increase per degree of amplitude. This is in the range 2 to 3 ms per degree. The velocity profile of a saccade has an inverted-U shape, increasing to about half-way through and then decreasing. The way the peak velocity (PV) increases with saccade amplitude is approximately exponential, rising to a maximum (saturation) value (PV_m) that is typically around 500° s^{-1}. The appropriate equation is as follows:

$$PV = PV_m \left(1 - \exp(-A/A_{63})\right)$$

where A_{63} is the amplitude for which the peak velocity reaches 63% of its saturation value. A typical value for A_{63} is 11 to 12°. The average velocity of a saccade is its amplitude divided by duration (A/D).

Saccades can be triggered by external stimuli, for example, by a movement or the appearance of a novel object, but as we have seen already (Fig. 1.2), they are also triggered by internally generated instructions. For externally triggered saccades reaction times (latencies) are typically in the range 150 to 200 ms. There appears to be a second smaller population of shorter latency saccades (90–130 ms) known as express saccades that can be evoked in particular attentional situations. Saccade latency increases with increasing target eccentricity (angular distance from the fovea) by up to 100 ms and also increases as light level decreases. When several saccades are made in rapid succession, as in reading or simply looking round a room (e.g. Fig. 2.7), there is a minimum interval between saccades of about 130 ms, although average intervals are longer: 225 ms is typical of silent reading.

Saccades are pre-programmed, and changes to the target position during a saccade cannot modify its end-point, except in very unusual circumstances. Saccades are sometimes referred to as 'ballistic', but this is slightly misleading as there is internal control of the trajectory even though external feedback from vision is ineffective. The generation of a saccade, in terms of the activation of the eye muscles, is a two-stage process. To get the eye to its new position requires a high frequency *pulse* of action potentials, followed by a sustained lower frequency *step* to hold the new eye position against the tension of the other eye muscles. Because the eye muscles operate in antagonistic pairs, the opposing muscle must have an inverted pulse-step activation pattern.

Larger saccades (>20°) do not always land exactly on target. In laboratory conditions they usually undershoot by about 10%. The error is made up by a secondary or 'correction' saccade of a few degrees, which follows the initial saccade after an interval of 100 to 150 ms. It interesting to note that this interval is usually shorter when the initial saccade is larger, but the latency of the correction saccade from the onset of the initial saccade is relatively constant (about 200 ms; Fig. 2.4). The implication of this is that the secondary saccade is not the result of a visual correction but is actually

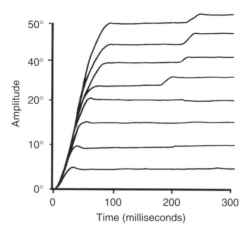

Fig. 2.4 Series of human eye saccades of increasing amplitude. The larger saccades have greater maximum velocities and longer durations. Under laboratory conditions saccades greater than 20° are typically followed by a 'correction' saccade after an interval of about 150 ms. From Robinson (1964).

programmed at the same time as the first saccade. Thus the secondary saccade is apparently a built-in component of the whole gaze shift. Whether this result applies to subjects with freely moving heads in a visually complex scene is not yet clear.

In normal life saccadic gaze changes are made by moving both eyes and head. Head and eyes can of course be moved independently, but for ordinary saccades there is a 'default' condition in which the head contributes about one-third of the total for gaze changes of up to about 30°. For larger shifts the contribution of the head becomes larger as the eyes approach their maximum excursion. The physical limit to eye movement is about 50° from the primary (straight ahead) position, but in practice the eyes rarely rotate beyond ±30°. For gaze movements of less than about 20° the saccade is made almost entirely by the eyes, with the much heavier head catching up slowly, and the eyes counter-rotating so that gaze remains stationary (Fig. 2.5a). This counter-rotation is mediated by the VOR (see below). For larger gaze changes the situation is more complicated, with the eyes being carried passively by the head and with VOR switched off until the final destination of gaze is reached (Fig. 2.5b). The trunk and feet may also be involved in the gaze shift: these large gaze shifts are discussed in Chapter 6. The rules governing eye and head movements are different. The amplitudes of eye saccades are determined by a combination of velocity and duration (Fig. 2.4), but head saccades have an almost fixed duration of about 0.5 s (when not made deliberately slowly or fast) and their velocity is a function of their amplitude (Zangemeister et al., 1981).

Starting about 50 ms before a saccade, and continuing for 100 ms or more after the saccade has begun, the visibility of a test flash is reduced. The biggest reduction, to less than 10% of normal visibility, occurs about 20 ms into the saccade. This is the phenomenon of saccadic suppression and accounts for at least some of the insensitivity to external changes that is characteristic of saccades. According to Burr et al. (1994) the

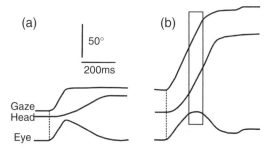

Fig. 2.5 Combined eye and head saccades. For the smaller saccade in (a) the head has hardly begun to move before eye saccade is complete. When the head starts turning the eye counter-rotates, resulting in stationary gaze. In the much larger saccade (b) eye and head move together to begin with, then the eye remains almost stationary in the head (rectangle) and gaze is carried entirely by the head. After this the eye starts to counter-rotate and gaze stabilizes. (Redrawn after Guitton, 1992).

imposed suppression acts specifically on the magnocellular pathway from the retina, which normally responds to rapid movement. Without suppression it would become undesirably activated by the image motion caused by the saccade. The parvocellular pathway, which is slower and responsible for detailed vision rather than motion, will suffer so much blur at the image speeds typical of saccades that it will not be responding anyway and so suppression is not required. Interesting changes in the structure of perceptual space occur at the same time as saccadic suppression (Burr and Morrone, 2003). These are not detectable in normal viewing, but when spots of light are flashed during saccades their positions are consistently mislocalized in a direction that indicates a compression of visual space. This may be related to the problem of why the world does not appear to move when we make a saccade, even though the retinal image does, but this is not yet clear.

The stabilizing mechanisms

During ordinary activity the body and head rotate in space at velocities as high as several hundred degrees a second, so that for fixation to be maintained during such motion powerful compensatory mechanisms are required to move the eyes in the opposite direction to the rotation of the head. There are two such mechanisms: the VOR and the OKR (Fig. 2.6). In the VOR the semicircular canals of the inner ear measure head rotation velocity, and the signal they provide is fed to the eye muscles via the vestibular and oculomotor nuclei. Over a wide range of velocities the gain of this reflex is close to 1, so that a rotation of the head evokes an eye movement that almost exactly counteracts it. The latency of the reflex – the delay between head and eye movements – is extremely short, about 15 ms, compared with 150 ms for the visually mediated optokinetic reflex (see below). If rotation is maintained, for example, by using a revolving chair, the eyes would rapidly reach the limit of their range. This does not happen because fast saccade-like movements (quick phases) are made in the

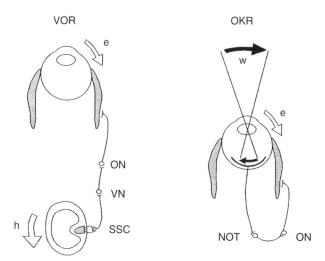

Fig. 2.6. The two mechanisms that stabilize gaze. In the vestibulo-ocular reflex (VOR) head rotation (**h**) is sensed by the semicircular canals (SSC) of the inner ear, and this information is passed via the vestibular nucleus (VN) to the oculomotor nuclei (ON) that activate the eye muscles, resulting in an eye movement (**e**) equal and opposite to **h**. In the optokinetic response (OKR), motion of the world relative to the eye (**w**) is sensed by the retina, and this information goes via the nucleus of the optic tract (NOT) to the oculomotor nuclei, causing an eye movement (**e**) in the same direction as **w**. This is a closed velocity feedback loop which tends to make **e** equal to **w**.

opposite (anti-compensatory) direction, resulting in a saw-tooth-like *nystagmus*. With prolonged rotation the compensatory rotation declines because the fluid in the semicircular canals catches up with the tube walls and the hair cells in the ampullae are no longer deflected. If the rotation suddenly stops, the fluid carries on moving resulting in a post-rotatory nystagmus in the opposite direction as well as dizziness. With natural head movements these effects are not important.

At slower velocities a second reflex, the OKR, augments VOR, and at velocities close to zero takes over from it. It operates by measuring the actual velocity of the image on the retina and causing the eye muscles to rotate the eye in the same direction as the retinal motion, thus nulling it out. The OKR is a feedback system, working on the error between the desired image speed ($0°\ s^{-1}$) and actual image speed. The VOR on the other hand is not a feedback mechanism, as the movements of the eyes have no effect on the sensor – the semicircular canals. The OKR is evoked when large regions of the image move together; this distinguishes it from smooth pursuit (see below) that is used for tracking small targets by the fovea. As with VOR, prolonged rotation of the visual environment – produced, for example, by putting the subject's head in a striped drum – produces optokinetic nystagmus in which quick phases repeatedly bring the eye back closer to the straight ahead position. Of course the real world does not rotate, except perhaps in earthquakes, so the real function of OKR is not to follow a moving scene but to glue the retinal image to the stationary world.

The difference in speed between OKR and VOR can be appreciated by holding a hand in front of the face and gently moving it to and fro while keeping the head still. This evokes OKR, and the hand does not have to move very fast (about 1 Hz) before it becomes difficult to count the fingers. Now keep the hand still and shake the head (inducing VOR). Even with the fastest head shakes, perhaps 5 Hz, the view of the fingers remains unblurred. Between them the two reflexes keep eye rotation in space within acceptable limits. Residual image motion, under conditions of realistic natural head rotation, is in the range 0.5 to 5° s^{-1} (Collewijn et al., 1981; Kowler, 1991), that is, just below the limit at which blur starts to set in.

The combined operation of saccades and stabilizing reflexes is illustrated in Fig. 2.7, which shows a record of eye, head and gaze movements made while a subject was turning to look from one side of a kitchen to the other. This was not a deliberate search pattern, and most of the saccades landed on nondescript regions of the room's walls and surfaces. Nevertheless, the eyes are not wandering smoothly across the scene, and the successive snapshot pattern of stationary gaze fixations is very clear. (The slight downward slope of some of the later fixations is because of the subject's body movements during the turn, causing relative motion of the points of fixation). Although the eye makes a total of 10 saccades in 3 s, it is not these saccades but the head movement that carries gaze across the room. The function of the saccades is to minimize the time that gaze is in motion (when vision would be blurred). Between saccades the eyes move in the opposite direction to the head, presumably mainly as a result of VOR, and

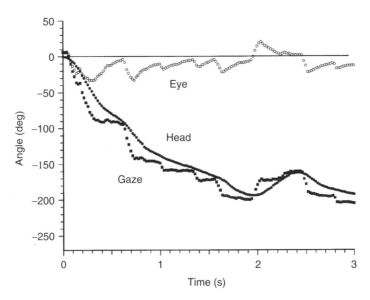

Fig. 2.7 Eye, head, and gaze movements while looking around a room. The overall gaze movements are made by the head, with the eyes making saccades and counter-rotations that result in near-stationary gaze fixations. Taken from an eye-camera video of tea making.

the sum of the head and eye movements results in the series of well stabilized gaze fixations.

Pursuit

In ordinary active life saccades and stabilizing movements dominate. A third kind of movement, smooth pursuit, augments these movements when the target of fixation is a small moving object. Here the target is kept on the fovea by smooth movements not unlike those of OKR. However, OKR operates on large areas of the image, whereas pursuit requires a small target, and when a target is being tracked the pursuit system is actually pitted against the wide-field OKR system, whose function is to keep the over-all image still. Smooth pursuit eye movements on their own work only up to target velocities of about $15° \text{s}^{-1}$. Above this speed the smooth movements are supplemented by saccades (Fig. 2.8b), and above about $100° \text{s}^{-1}$ pursuit becomes entirely saccadic. In practice these ranges are extended because the head also moves, and so the velocity contribution of the eyes to overall gaze motion is lower.

The pursuit system, in its simplest form, can be thought of as a feedback loop with image velocity as its input and eye velocity its output (similar to OKR, Fig. 2.6). When a stationary fixated object begins to move, the eye starts to follow it after a latency of 100 to 150 ms. For slow image movements, less than about $2° \text{s}^{-1}$, pursuit occurs on its

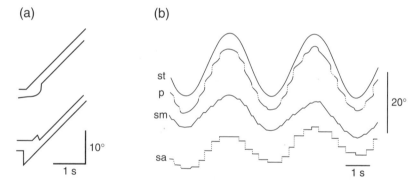

Fig. 2.8. Smooth pursuit. (a) The beginning of smooth pursuit in a monkey. In the upper record a target starts to move at constant speed of $10° \text{s}^{-1}$. The eye starts to move in the same direction after a short latency, and there is a 'catch-up' saccade that brings gaze direction closer to the target. The lower record shows the response to a 'step-ramp' stimulus in which the target jumps in one direction but moves off in the opposite direction. In spite of the initial position jump, the smooth pursuit system follows the target velocity, but the saccade is made in the direction of the position change. (From Fuchs, 1967). (b) Human subject tracking a stimulus (st) that moves from side to side with a sinusoidal trajectory. At this speed the pursuit response (p) has both smooth (sm) and saccadic (sa) components, and these have been separated here by artificially taking out the saccades from the pursuit record and accumulating them separately. In this case the contributions of smooth pursuit and saccades are roughly equal. (From Collewijn and Tamminga, 1984).

own, but for faster speeds there is usually a 'catch-up' saccade that makes up the position error caused by the pursuit delay and brings the fovea back close to the target (Fig. 2.8a). Typically this occurs about 75 ms after pursuit has begun. For targets moving at constant velocity, the pursuit system operates with a closed loop gain of about 0.9, meaning that a target moving at $10° s^{-1}$ is tracked at $9° s^{-1}$, leaving a retinal image velocity of $1° s^{-1}$. This also means that at the maximum pursuit speed of $100° s^{-1}$, there will be a position error of $10°$ after 1 s. In practice the position error never reaches this value as it is corrected by small saccades made several times a second (Fig. 2.8b).

There is considerable evidence that the pursuit system has anticipatory powers and that its ability to track predictable stimuli, such as targets moving with a sine-wave trajectory, is much better than a simple feedback model would permit. In particular, the lag between target velocity and eye velocity can be reduced dramatically after only one movement cycle. Whether the predictor simply supplements the basic mechanism or is an inextricable part of it is not clear (Pola and Wyatt, 1991). Related to this predictive ability is the observation that the eyes may continue to track a constant speed target if it disappears briefly, and under some circumstances a sine-wave target may be tracked for a cycle or more after it disappears. Presumably this is because the predictor continues to operate for a while in the absence of a target.

Vergence

Vergence movements are responsible for adjusting the angle between the eyes to different distances, and they are unique in that the eyes move in opposite directions relative to the head (i.e. they are non-conjugate). Vergence movements are smooth, relatively slow (at least in the laboratory) and typically have a latency of about 160 ms. They can be driven by disparity (the difference in position, relative to each fovea, of the image of a target in the two eyes), or they may accompany accommodation, driven by defocus in the image. The role of vergence in real tasks is unclear. In principle the eyes should converge so that the two foveal directions intersect at the target, but during a task where the subjects had to use vision to guide tapping, Steinman (2003) recorded 'Vergence tends to be set 25% to 45% *beyond* the attended plane; in other words, subjects do *not* adjust gaze to intersect the attended target.' (p. 1350). It may well be that, out of the laboratory situation, vergence control is quite imprecise.

Vergence control is a fascinating subject, but in this book we are mainly concerned with the direction in which the eyes are looking, and the adjustments of the eye to distance are rather taken for granted. We will go into no more detail here but refer interested readers to Carpenter (1988) and Mays (2003).

Eye movements and gaze control

These, then, are the components from which eye movements strategies in real life tasks are constructed. They are essentially the same as those studied under various kinds of restraint in laboratories over the past century. There are other issues that have been less well studied in laboratory conditions, for example, the co-operative actions of eye, head, and body, which become important in the behaviour of freely moving individuals. We may not necessarily expect the same constraints on eye movements outside the laboratory as we find when subjects are asked to do their best at some artificial task. To quote Steinman (2003) again,

> Under natural conditions gaze control is lax, perhaps even lazy. One could just as easily call it *efficient*. Why should the oculomotor system set its parameters so as to make it do more work than is needed to get the job done?
>
> (Steinman, 2003, p. 1350)

Summary

1. Balancing the need to keep the retinal image stable to avoid blur with the need to direct the high-resolution fovea where required has resulted in a particular limited repertoire of eye movements. These are effected by six eye muscles and controlled by a hierarchy of cortical and subcortical brain regions.

2. Saccades are a family of fast eye movements that redirect gaze in as short a time as possible. Vision is suspended during saccades.

3. Two mechanisms (the vestibulo-ocular reflex and the optokinetic reflex) keep the retinal image stable during fixations despite movements of the head and the body in space.

4. Small targets can be tracked smoothly providing the velocities are relatively low ($<100°\ s^{-1}$). Faster moving targets are tracked saccadically.

5. Vergence movements are non-conjugate movements that align the eye axes to objects at different distances.

Chapter 3

How our eyes question the world

The previous chapter provided a brief account of the repertoire of individual eye movements available to humans. Of course these eye movements are not isolated events: to understand eye movements in natural behaviour we must consider sequences of eye movements or, more properly, sequences of fixations because it is where people look that is now our primary concern rather than the mechanics of the saccades that get them there. Take, for example, the sequence of fixations shown in Fig. 3.1 as an observer looks at Georges de la Tour's famous painting *Le tricheur à l'as de carreau* (more prosaically, 'The card sharp'). What drives these fixation sequences? For example, did the observer in Fig. 3.1 look at people's eyes because they are highly visible (dark irises against white scleras) or because the observer was interested in trying to guess the intentions of and relationships between the players? A fundamental question, therefore, is whether the eyes are driven primarily by the visual features of the external world or by the viewer's internal agenda. This is a complex problem because it depends on what the viewer is thinking about at that time. Looking at a scene with

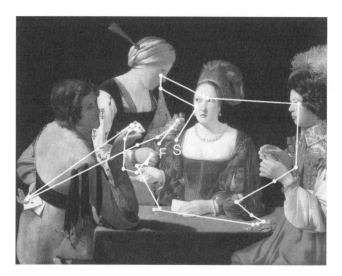

Fig. 3.1 The sequence of fixations made by an observer looking for the first time at Georges de la Tour's painting *Le tricheur à l'as de carreau*. The dots denote locations where the eyes paused for fixations. The lines represent saccadic shifts of gaze. The first fixation is indicated by the S. The record was made and kindly supplied by Iain Gilchrist.

nothing particular in mind is quite different from looking at the same scene while trying to identify the objects in the scene. This is again different if one is physically interacting with the scene, driving through it perhaps, or changing the positions of the
objects it contains. We would not expect there to be a one-size-fits-all way of predicting what pattern of fixations viewers will adopt.

We begin the chapter by asking whether it is actually meaningful to talk about fixation sequences. How repeatable is the pattern of fixations that an individual uses to
view a scene, and how similar is this pattern between individuals? If there were nothing in common between one viewing and the next, there would be very little to study.
Fortunately, this is not the case: there are important, if somewhat elusive, constraints
on how we view the world. We will go on to discuss some of the ideas that have been
put forward to account for the extent of similarities between fixation sequences and
for the structure of these sequences. We consider the different issues involved when
subjects are simply viewing a scene compared with when they have some behavioural
task to complete while inspecting it.

Characterizing sequences of fixations

Questions about the sequences or patterns of eye movements were a prominent
feature of the earliest investigations of saccades and fixations. It was the sequence of eye
movements during reading that first revealed the saccade and fixate strategy
(e.g. Hering, 1879; Lamare, 1892; see Tatler and Wade, 2003) and subsequently inspired
the development of objective devices for recording eye movements (see Wade and
Tatler, 2005). Early investigations of eye movements when viewing simple forms, patterns, and illusions also emphasized the role of sequences rather than individual eye
movements: Judd and Stratton both set out to consider whether the pattern of
eye movements when viewing simple illusions such as Müller–Lyer explained the experience of the illusion but reached opposing conclusions (Judd, 1905; Stratton, 1906).
Stratton (1902) was also interested in the path taken by the eye when viewing simple
shapes and whether our aesthetic appreciation of symmetry in simple shapes was
reflected by symmetry of eye movement paths when viewing such shapes (Stratton,
1906). Stratton was surprised to observe the discontinuity of eye movements and the
lack of symmetrical movement paths when viewing symmetrical forms. It is interesting,
however, that after this early interest in sequences of eye movements, for much of the
twentieth century research effort focussed more strongly on the mechanics of individual eye movements or the placement and stability of individual fixations than it did on
these sequences (Wade and Tatler, 2005). There were, however, two notable exceptions
to this shift in research emphasis, and their work would later reignite interest in understanding how sequences of fixations are generated: Buswell (1935) and Yarbus (1967)
each conducted extensive studies of the similarities between sequences of fixations
made by subjects when viewing pictures and came to similar conclusions about how the
eyes are used to inspect the scene. These pioneering works highlighted many of the
issues of eye movement behaviour that remain the subject of contemporary research.

The question of how similar sequences of eye movements are to each other can be
asked at three levels. Do the two eyes of the same individual follow identical paths?

How similar are the eye movement sequences of the same individual viewing the same picture on different occasions? Finally, how similar are the sequences of fixations of different individuals viewing the same picture? In his book *Eye Movements and Vision*, Yarbus (1967) provided comprehensive answers to all three questions, and in this section we will draw heavily on his account.

Yarbus recorded eye movements using a variety of suction cups attached to the eye on which a small mirror was mounted (Fig. 3.2). A collimated light beam was reflected from the mirror onto a photographic plate, and as the eye rotated this produced a trace on the plate corresponding to the subject's eye movements while looking at the picture. To make such recordings, the subject's head had to be restrained. In these records saccades come out as thin lines and fixations as thickenings or knots on the lines as gaze dwells for a few hundred milliseconds near particular points.

Fixation sequences of the two eyes

Figure 3.3 shows simultaneous records of a subject's two eyes while looking for 30 s at the happy scene in the painting. Only one eye was actually viewing the picture, but both eyes were being monitored. Two features of the records stand out. First, they are both very clearly related to the main features of the composition. The fixations mainly cluster around the three heads, the accordion, and the child's feet. These are joined for the most part by long saccades. This is clearly nothing like a random walk. Second, the paths of the two eyes are almost identical. Sometimes one seems slightly displaced relative to the other. This is roughly what one would expect when viewing a real scene with both eyes open as objects at different distances result in different degrees of vergence. However, the same saccades are made between the same fixation points, and the fixations are all identifiable from one trace to the other. This similarity was by no means a novel finding. The realization that the two eyes normally move together is enshrined in Hering's Law of Equal Innervation, first published in 1868. This yoking

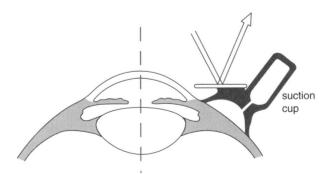

Fig. 3.2 Device used by Yarbus to record eye movements (the 'P1 cup'). A plane mirror is mounted on a suction cup attached to the sclera. A beam of light reflected from the mirror writes directly onto a photographic plate. Modified from Yarbus (1967).

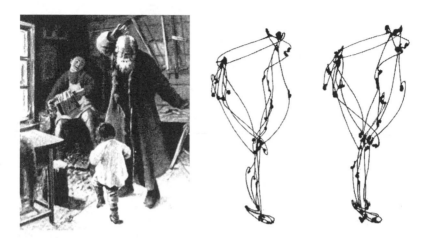

Fig. 3.3 Record of the movements of both eyes while the subject looks at a picture (A Happy Moment) for 1 minute. The records are nearly identical. From Yarbus (1967).

of the eyes is found in most but not all vertebrates: chameleons, sea-horses, and some other fish have eyes that move independently (Land and Nilsson, 2002).

Sequences of fixations made by the same subject

In Figure 3.4a to 3.4d a single subject is looking at the same picture (An Unexpected Visitor by I.P. Repin) on four different occasions. The viewing lasts 3 minutes, and the subject was given no specific instruction about what to look for. As in Fig. 3.3, the movements of the subject's gaze trace out the main features of the more interesting regions of the picture. The four scan patterns (there were seven in Yarbus' original figure) are clearly similar, but they are certainly not identical. Similar clusters of fixations occur around the same features (mainly faces and clothes), but none of the saccades follows exactly the same path in the different records, as they do in Fig. 3.3, and outside the clusters the fixations are all to different locations.

Scan patterns of different viewers

Figure 3.4e to 3.4h shows four records of different subjects viewing the same picture. Again they show the same overall pattern of fixations, in particular, picking up the heads of the figures, but clearly the records are more different from each other than those of the individual in Fig. 3.4a to 3.4d. Some of these differences are quite marked. The subject in Fig.3.4e looks all round the outline of the picture; subject g seems to be interested only in the faces; and none of them is as interested in clothes as the subject in Fig. 3.4a to 3.4d. Buswell (1935) reached similar conclusions, namely that there were certain elements in pictures that most individuals fixated during viewing, but that there were also clear individual differences evident in the eye movement records.

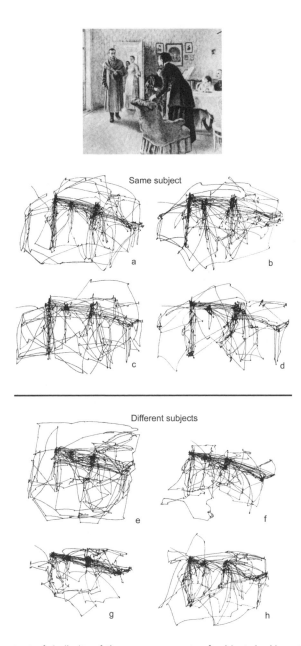

Fig 3.4 The extent of similarity of the eye movements of subjects looking at a picture (An Unexpected Visitor) for 3 minutes. a–d: the same subject on four separate occasions. e–h: four different subjects. From Yarbus (1967).

It would be an interesting task to try to quantify the extent of the differences illustrated in Fig. 3.4, but even without such a numerical estimate, it is evident that the trajectories of the two eyes on one occasion are more similar than those of the same individual on different occasions, which are again more similar than those of different individuals looking at the same scene.

Three questions arise from these studies. First, what is it in a scene that induces a viewer to fixate certain features of the scene, but not others? Second, what processes lead to a particular sequence of fixations? Third, what processes, within an individual and between individuals, introduce variation into the scan patterns, even under what appear to be identical viewing conditions? Note that in the examples given above the subjects were all simply examining pictures freely, with no imposed agenda. We will see later that this may not be the best conditions under which to understand eye movement behaviour.

What drives the eye around a scene?

The first thing to be said is that saccadic movements of the eyes are spontaneous. In awake humans the natural state is for the eyes to move to a new viewpoint several times a second. So we are not concerned so much with the fact that the eyes move – that happens anyway – but what constrains the places they move to and the sequence in which they move.

There are two very different schools of thought that attempt to explain the patterns of fixations seen in everyday life. The first are 'bottom-up' explanations that assume that eye movements are driven principally by the properties of the image on the retina. The sum of the image properties that result in eye movements are usually referred to as their *image salience* (or often simply as their *salience*). Explanations of this kind provide an essentially reflex account of eye movement behaviour and ignore possible influences from higher cognitive processes. 'Top-down' accounts emphasize that movements of the eyes are largely directed by the goals of the current behaviour rather than simply by image properties. These goals may involve the need to find particular information from the scene, or they may be concerned with the execution of an ongoing physical task. They derive from the agenda currently being pursued by the brain as a whole. It is worth noting that the 'property' that both Buswell and Yarbus believed defined the locations selected for fixation was 'interestingness' to the viewer, a view that combines both bottom-up and top-down elements. Indeed many contemporary authors would argue that it is most likely that saccade target selection involves a combination of bottom-up and top-down factors, but the relative weightings of these remains a matter of much debate. In the rest of this chapter, we will first examine salience-based accounts of fixation patterns, then discuss objections to them, and finally consider other types of explanation based on cognitive control strategies.

Salience-based accounts of eye movement control

Something is 'salient' if it sticks out. Salience is a much-used word in visual psychology, usually meaning 'intrinsic conspicuousness', but its origins are not related to vision.

The noun 'salient' meant a jutting out or prominent part of a fortification and comes from the same Latin root (*salire*, to leap) as 'sally', meaning a sudden charge or outburst. Somehow, leaping changed into bursting forth, then into jutting out, and finally into being conspicuous. In ordinary conversation 'salient' often just means important. In visual terms objects may be considered salient if they are bright, colourful, contrasty, detail-containing, flashing, moving, and so on. Salience and saliency are synonyms.

Salience and attention

If something 'sticks out' then it can also be said to draw attention to itself. Salience is thus about the features of an object or part of a scene that result in attentional capture. Most accounts of visual attention distinguish between 'overt attention', in which the shift in attention from one object to the next is accompanied by an eye movement, and 'covert' attention, where no eye movement occurs, but the target object is nevertheless the subject of increased visual awareness (e.g. Posner, 1980). William James (1890, p. 437, original italics) phrased it as follows:

> Usually, as is well known, no object lying in the marginal portions of the field of vision can catch our attention without at the same time 'catching our eye' – that is, fatally provoking such movements of rotation and accommodation as will focus its image on the fovea, or point of greatest sensibility. Practice, however, enables us, *with effort*, to attend to a marginal object whilst keeping the eyes immovable. The object under these circumstances never becomes perfectly distinct – the place of its image on the retina makes distinctness impossible – but (as anyone can satisfy himself by trying) we become more vividly conscious of it than we were before the effort was made.
>
> (William James, 1890, p. 437, original italics)

The analogy of a spotlight is often used to describe the way that covert attention is directed around the visual field (Posner, 1980; Posner et al., 1978). However, although the notion of a spotlight implies a fixed spatial extent of attentional allocation, an alternative to the spotlight is that attention may have a variable spatial extent. This is known as the zoom lens model of attention (Erikson and St James, 1986).

In contrast to James' effortful process, which we can all recognize, a current idea suggests that covert attention is a much more common process. The link between covert and overt attention remains unclear. One possibility is that these two processes are independent (Klein, 1980): although a target may attract both covert and overt attention, this coincidence need not imply any causal link between these processes, and different mechanisms are involved in guiding these two types of attention (Remington, 1980). Alternatively, covert attention may serve to lead overt attention to targets of potential interest: when orienting to a peripheral target, covert attention is first oriented to the target location and used to process the target, after which a saccade may be initiated to orient overt attention to this location (e.g. Deubel and Schneider, 1996; Henderson, 1992; Shepherd et al., 1986). In this account it is possible that covert attention is directed to a location but overt attention does not follow; however, the inverse is not possible. Finally, it has been suggested that covert attention serves only to plan saccades to target locations and as such can be thought of more as a by-product of overt attention than a form of attention in its own right (e.g. Rizzolatti et al., 1987).

In this chapter, we are concerned with the question, 'What is it that determines where we direct the next saccade?' A reasonable answer might be that the saccade target had just been visited by the spotlight (if we wish to use this analogy) of covert attention and found to be of interest, so whether covert attention is independent of overt attention, leads overt attention, or is a by-product of preparing to move overt attention is not of particular concern. However, there is now much evidence, both psychophysical and neurophysiological, for a linkage between covert and overt attention (e.g. Hoffman and Subramaniam, 1995; Kustov and Robinson, 1996, reviewed in Itti and Koch, 2001). If we accept this relationship between eye movements and attention, then salience refers to the properties of an object that first cause the deployment of covert attention. Because attention has yet to be activated, such features are often referred to as 'pre-attentive'.

Parallel and serial search

Evidence for the pre-attentive selection of certain attributes comes from visual search studies, in which subjects are asked to detect objects with particular properties in a field of 'distractors' with somewhat different properties (see Wolfe, 1998). It was found that objects of a different colour from the distractors, or with simple differences of geometric form (e.g. O vs X), are detected very rapidly (the search rate of <10 ms per item is far too fast for eye movements to be involved), and, crucially, the number of distractors present has no effect on the ease of detection (Treisman, 1988; Treisman & Gelade, 1980). The targets 'pop out' from the distractor field. Detecting more complex differences between targets and distractors, such as conjunctions of features, is slower (25–50 ms per item, which is still faster than eye movements can be made), and the greater the number of distractors the longer the task takes, suggesting that each object has to be scrutinized separately after it has been attended to (Fig. 3.5). The implication of this difference is that the first pop-out kind of search is carried out

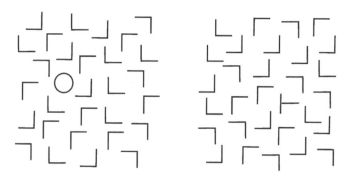

Fig. 3.5 Examples of an element that shows 'pop-out' in an array of distractors (left), and one that does not (right).

in parallel across the retina by low-level detectors of the kind involved in pre-attentive selection, whereas the slower kind of search is post-attentive and serial, with the properties of each object being checked out after it has been targeted by covert or overt attention. (For constructive critiques of this account see Wolfe, 1994, 2003). Although search is a task, and so is different from simply looking at a picture or scene, Occam's Razor suggests that the low-level mechanisms that lead to pop-out in parallel search are also likely to be those that contribute to salience in uncommitted viewing, and indeed this has often been assumed. However, whether this assumption is valid will be considered in more detail later.

Salience-driven schemes of eye movement control

A number of attempts have been made to quantify and model the pre-attentive features of a scene region that contribute to its salience. Probably the most influential was developed by Koch and Ullman (1985) and elaborated by Itti (Itti and Koch, 2000). It begins by identifying a series of low-level image features that are known to be extracted by the early stages of the visual pathway, including the primary visual cortex (V1). These are generally features that are extracted in parallel across the whole retina, and include colour, brightness, and orientation at several different spatial scales (Fig. 3.6). Each of these parallel arrays produces a feature map, and after a stage in

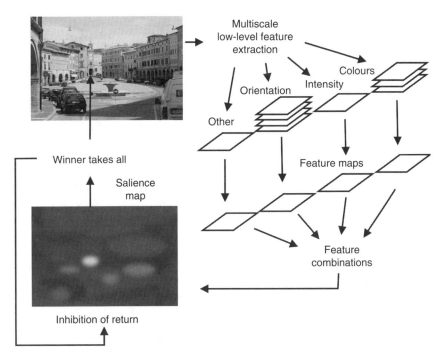

Fig. 3.6 Organization of a salience map that controls attentional orienting. See text for details. Based on Itti and Koch (2001).

which competitive processes such as centre-surround inhibition occur, these maps are combined additively (although individual maps may have different weightings) to produce a single salience map. Different regions of the scene excite the salience map to different extents, depending on how strongly the various pre-attentive features are stimulated, and so the map will have 'hot spots' corresponding to regions where a lot of visually conspicuous things are going on. Before a saccade can be made a choice process must occur – a 'winner-takes-all' mechanism – so that only one locus is left to become the target of covert attention and then a saccade. In this model, and other similar models, the choice of saccade targets relies on the image-based low-level features of the scene and is independent of the nature of the task. Several authors accept that this is only part of the story (Einhäuser, Rutishauser et al., 2008; Findlay and Walker, 1999; Itti and Koch, 2001), but so far salience, in the sense of conspicuity, is the only component of saccade initiation that it has been possible to model in a computationally satisfying way.

A potential problem with the salience scheme is the question of how the visual system moves on from its current attentional state, given that the salience map has already found the most interesting structure in the field of view. There has to be a mechanism for inhibiting the just-attended location on the map, once an eye movement has been made (in retinotopic space this location will now, after the saccade, be at the centre of the map). Transient inhibition of recently visited locations has been reported in simple search experiments, and this phenomenon has been termed 'inhibition of return' (Klein, 2000). This mechanism offers a convenient way of avoiding the salience model becoming stuck on a single location: with the main source of salience removed, gaze would be free to visit targets lower down the salience hierarchy. However, this solution does come with two important caveats. First, a transient inhibition of salient locations means that once the inhibition is removed, the viewer will look at the most salient location again. In other words, fixation patterns will form a repeating cycle with the cycle length depending on the transience of the inhibition. Some cyclical looking behaviour is seen in human observers (Fig. 3.3), but often no clear cycles are apparent (Figs 3.4, 3.9, and 3.10). Second, whether inhibition of return is evident when viewing complex scenes such as photographs is unclear. Reports suggest that there is no avoidance of refixating the previous fixation location, and indeed observers show an increased tendency to refixate, suggesting a form of facilitation of return rather than inhibition (Hooge et al., 2005; Smith and Henderson, 2009; Tatler and Vincent, 2008).

Problems with salience models

In this section we will consider some of the recent objections that have been raised about the original salience map model. For a more extensive discussion of the factors that underlie saccade target selection and of the support for and challenges to salience-based models of eye guidance, we refer the reader to Tatler (2009).

Does salience account for fixation selection?

Although the salience map framework of Itti and Koch (2000) is appealing, and apparently based upon biologically plausible principles of feature extraction, the acid test of any such theoretical framework is of course whether it can account for behavioural data. The natural consequence of a winner-takes-all salience-driven scheme is that the salience at locations selected for fixation should be higher than that at other non-selected locations. Consequently, the most common method for evaluating whether salience might indeed underlie fixation selection is to examine computationally the salience at locations that were fixated by human observers and compare this with the salience at randomly selected locations in the same scene. The logic is that if selection involves salient features, then there should be higher levels of salience in the fixated locations than in the control locations. In essence we are presented with a signal detection problem: we can collect a distribution of salience at fixations and a distribution of salience at control locations (Fig. 3.7). The question then becomes, can we reliably discriminate fixated and control locations on the basis of salience? If we can then we can say that selection of salient features was different from that expected by random sampling by the eye. Any such correlations between salience and fixation have been taken to imply that salience is involved in the decision about where to fixate (but see below for why this conclusion may be unwise).

Across a range of studies, robust differences have been found between the low-level feature content of fixated locations and control locations (e.g. Parkhurst et al., 2002; Parkhurst and Niebur, 2003; Reinagel and Zador, 1999; Renninger et al., 2005).

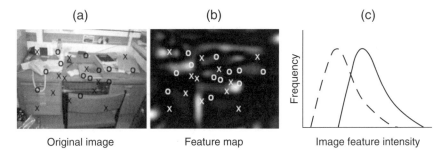

(a)   (b)   (c)

Original image   Feature map   Image feature intensity

Fig. 3.7 A standard technique for evaluating low-level features or salience at fixation. The example illustrates the principle for a single participant looking at a single scene. Human fixations (Os) on a scene (a) are used to look up low-level feature content (or salience) at fixated locations, using a feature (or salience) map of the scene (b). Across a number of participants and scenes, a distribution of image feature intensities at fixation can be constructed (solid curve in c). An equal number of control locations (Xs) are selected in the scene (a) and used to look up feature content at these control locations (b) to construct a distribution of feature (or salience) intensities at control locations (dashed curve in c). To evaluate whether fixation selection is correlated with low-level feature content of scenes, the two distributions are compared, using a technique such as signal detection theory (Tatler, Baddeley et al., 2005). If the two distributions differ then we can conclude that there is some correlation between fixation selection and the feature being evaluated. The control locations must be selected appropriately, incorporating behavioural biases of humans when viewing scenes, to obtain meaningful results (Tatler, Baddeley et al., 2005; Tatler and Vincent, 2009).

The particular features that appear to correlate most strongly with fixation selection vary between studies. Tatler, Baddeley et al. (2005) found stronger correlations with fixations for contrast and edge information than for luminance or chromaticity information. However, Jost et al. (2005) found a stronger association between colour and fixation. From all of these results, we could argue that salient or conspicuous scene regions are targeted for fixation by the eye.

One issue with creating a salience map that combines multiple feature channels in an essentially arbitrary manner, or trying to assess the relative importance of different features for fixation selection, is that there will be strong correlations between the different features. For example, a border between two coloured surfaces will involve not only local chromaticity differences but also an edge, and most likely a local luminance contrast. For this reason, Baddeley and Tatler (2006) used a Bayesian approach to take these correlations into account and thus more accurately considered the relative predictive power of different image features for fixation selection. They found that of contrast, luminance, and edge information, it was high frequency edge information that was the most predictive feature of where observers fixated in complex photographic scenes. Low spatial-frequency edge information was actually inhibitory of fixation, and neither contrast nor luminance made significant contributions to fixation selection. Another conclusion was that the area over which edge information is integrated has a diameter of 1.5 to 2°. This is about the size of the fovea, and because saccades need to bring the fovea to the next point of interest with roughly this degree of accuracy, this result seems to correspond to what would be expected for a targeting system. However, these results seem to be at variance with the idea that saccades are driven, ultimately, from a salience map in which the contributions of many low-level features are summed (Fig. 3.6). If Baddeley and Tatler are right then there is essentially only one key feature.

Interpreting correlations between fixation and salience

The above-mentioned results would seem to suggest that salient locations are in some way selected for fixation. This appears to support the premise of salience-based models of eye movement behaviour that where we look is determined by the visual conspicuity of those regions rather than by any internal agendas. However, we will now argue that caution must be exercised in making such conclusions from these findings.

Importantly, the correlation between fixation selection and salient locations need not imply a causal link (see Henderson et al., 2007 for a similar position). It may be for instance that selection is not driven by raw image properties but instead involves a higher-level strategy of, for instance, looking at particular objects. Objects will be likely to stand out from their background, having features that are unlike their surroundings – a teapot is likely to be visually quite unlike the worktop on which it is placed – and so looking at objects will inevitably result in different image feature properties at fixation than at control locations. Indeed, when the predictive power of low-level image features is compared with that for objects in photographic scenes, fixation locations could be predicted better using object-level information than image features (Einhäuser, Spain et al., 2008). This result suggests that the weak associations between image features and fixations may be artefacts of object-level selection criteria.

The apparent selection of salient locations may also be confounded by other behavioural biases, such as the well-known tendency for human observers to have a bias towards looking at and near the centre of screens and monitors rather than at their margins (Tatler, 2007). This behavioural bias could inflate the apparent selection of salient locations if there is a central tendency in the distribution of salience in the scenes displayed on the monitor. Indeed this is often the case, because photographers tend to place objects of interest at the centre of the viewfinder, and thus salience will tend to be higher in the centre of the scenes used in many eye movement experiments (Tatler, 2007; Tatler, Baddeley et al., 2005). By selecting natural scene images in which the distributions of visual features was biased towards particular parts of the scene, Tatler (2007) showed that human observers continued to display a strong central tendency in fixation behaviour that was independent of the distribution of features in the scenes (Fig. 3.8). This result highlights two important factors for the current discussion. First, the link between salience and fixation is clearly weak at best because varying the distribution of salience across scenes did not influence the distribution of fixations. Second, if much of the eye movement behaviour we record when people are looking at computer monitors is a product of looking at a screen, then extracting and modelling the image feature information at these locations will give a misleading account of the factors responsible for target selection.

Although evaluations of salience models do show statistically significant differences between fixated and control locations, the magnitude of these differences, and thus the predictive power of low-level image features, is small. For example, Tatler,

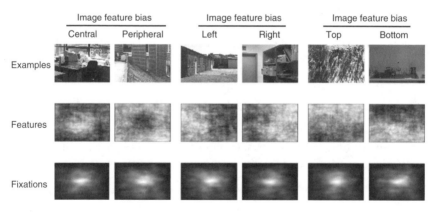

Fig. 3.8 There is a strong tendency to fixate the centre of the screen. The distributions of human fixations (bottom row) show that this bias prevails irrespective of the bias of the low-level feature content of scenes (middle row). If features were causal, the fixation distributions should be influenced by the feature distributions; this was not the case. In the distributions plotted, brighter pixels reflect higher frequencies of fixations (bottom row) or of image features (middle row). Adapted from Tatler (2007).

Baddeley et al. (2005) used a signal detection measure (the receiver operating characteristic area) to estimate how well a salience model would discriminate between the most predictive regions of the image compared with control areas. They found that the model gave a 65% correct performance compared with 50% for chance. Parkurst et al. (2002) found similarly unspectacular effects: the correlation between salience and fixation when viewing photographs was 0.45. Low performances and correlations are common in evaluations of salience-based models (e.g. Einhäuser, Spain et al., 2008; Nyström and Holmqvist, 2008). As such, even if we were to interpret the correlation between fixation and salience as causal, the amount of data it would explain is quite limited.

Eccentricity and salience

The idea of a salience map of 'pre-attentive' features being constructed in parallel across the entire visual field (see above) may be plausible. However, the implementation of this in computational models has tended to neglect a fundamental characteristic of the visual system: the variable resolution across the retina. In general, salience models assume that features of all spatial frequencies are extracted across the visual scene, but in reality peripheral sampling limits mean that the higher spatial scales are not available from peripheral locations (Vincent et al., 2007). For example, Tatler, Baddeley et al. (2005) found that the most predictive spatial scale that they tested was around 10.8 cycles per degree, but this scale of information is not available at eccentricities of more than about 14 degrees (see also Fig. 2.1). Thus, larger amplitude saccades could not be targeted based on the information that is not detectable. Few empirical studies have considered this question. However, Tatler et al. (2006) approached this by splitting their dataset of fixations according to the amplitudes of the saccades that brought the eye to each location. They found that there were greater differences between image features at fixated and control locations for small amplitude saccades than for large amplitude saccades, which tended to show no difference between fixated and control locations. This result demonstrates that any ability for salience models to account for saccade target selection may be limited only to saccades of small amplitude. Larger amplitude saccades could not be predicted based on salience.

Oculomotor tendencies and fixation selection

When we look at scenes, there are systematic tendencies to select certain eye movements rather than others. For example, although we have the musculature to make saccades over a wide range of amplitudes (Chapter 2), we are far more likely to make smaller amplitude saccades than larger ones. Similarly, at least when looking at images on a screen, we make more horizontal eye movements than vertical ones, and oblique saccades are the least frequent. Tatler and Vincent (2009) showed that these systematic tendencies in how we move our eyes are an important source of information for predicting saccade target selection. In fact, saccade targeting could be better predicted based on these tendencies alone (and therefore with no direct information about the visual stimulus) than it could based on salience. This result offers a strong challenge to the utility of the salience model and also demonstrates that understanding how we move our eyes, and why we exhibit particular oculomotor tendencies during viewing, will be an important avenue to explore in future research.

In conclusion, correlations between the distribution of salience and the distribution of actual fixations are not impressive, and their interpretation is fraught with problems. It is indisputable that objects of high salience sometimes 'catch the eye', but whether this effect is an important determinant of where we look in our everyday dealings with the world seems very questionable.

Evidence for high-level control: the effect of task

Looking at scenes with particular questions in mind

It is important to remember that for much of the data we have described so far, the task of the viewer was simply to look at the scenes. This 'free viewing' of scenes has often been used as it is thought to result in a state in which the observer is free from any high-level goals, and thus it is possible to study how salience influences eye movement behaviour, free from any cognitive 'contaminants'. Of course, in reality it is unlikely that subjects' minds are simply blank when asked to view scenes: in fact it may be that this condition simply gives the observer free reign to select their own high-level approaches to looking at scenes. So rather than improving consistency between the cognitive states of the observers this instruction may have the opposite effect. Whether or not free viewing does result in participants viewing images with effectively no high-level control, this is unlike most, indeed perhaps all, natural behaviour. The function of vision is rarely to contemplate the scene before us, but to assist in shaping our actions to our needs.

In fact, the cognitive activity of the subject turns out to be very important in how people look at scenes. This was first described by Buswell (1935). In one experiment he showed a subject a photograph of the Tribune tower in Chicago. In one trial,

> [The eye movement record] was obtained in the normal manner without any special directions being given. After that record was secured, the subject was told to look at the picture again to see if he could find a person looking out of one of the windows of the tower.
>
> (Buswell, 1935, p. 136)

The scan paths are reproduced in Fig. 3.9. The pattern of eye movements in the first case was a rather open scan with only a few fixations on the tower itself, but the second case was quite different. There was a much greater concentration of fixations on the tower and particularly around the regions with windows. It seems obvious now, and perhaps it did then, that one should look at the places from which information is requested, but Buswell was, to our knowledge, the first person to show that this was so.

Yarbus (1967) greatly extended Buswell's result, and it is Yarbus' demonstration that is in most recent textbooks. He asked his subject to inspect a picture (the same 'Unexpected Visitor' as in Fig. 3.4) with several different questions in mind (Fig. 3.10). These included 'remember the clothes worn by the people' and 'estimate how long the visitor had been away from the family'. He found that each question evoked a different pattern of eye movements, clearly related to the information required by the question.

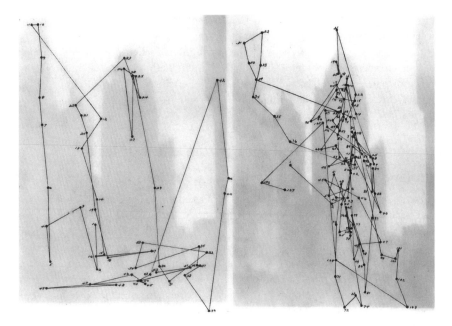

Fig. 3.9 Two of Buswell's eye movement recordings of a subject looking at a photograph of the Tribune tower in Chicago. Left: free viewing. Right: viewing when asked to see whether anyone is looking out of a window. From Buswell (1935).

Thus the question about clothes evoked mainly vertical eye movements, as the clothes were scrutinized. The length of absence question, on the other hand, caused a great many horizontal saccades from one face to the other, as the subject sought clues to the nature of the relationships between the main actors. An interesting finding was that the maid who opened the door was not fixated, presumably because her face could not help to answer the question. In another question the subject was asked 'to remember the positions of the people and objects', a task so daunting as to produce something like oculomotor panic. The message from this famous study is clear: eye movements are not simply related to the structure of the picture itself but also to top-down instructions from executive regions of the brain.

Given the striking effect of the cognitive goals of the observer on how people look at scenes, a challenge for any salience-based account of eye guidance is to what extent it can generalize beyond the artificial situation of free viewing. From a theoretical viewpoint of course a purely salience-driven system could never result in different patterns of eye movements for different tasks when viewing the same image. However, it may be that a salience model can still explain a certain amount of this behaviour. When comparing free viewing of scenes to searching for objects within a scene, it has been found that although salience has some ability to predict free viewing behaviour, it falls well short of explaining eye movements during search tasks (Einhaüser, Rutishauser et al., 2008; Henderson et al., 2007; Underwood and Foulsham, 2006; Underwood et al., 2006).

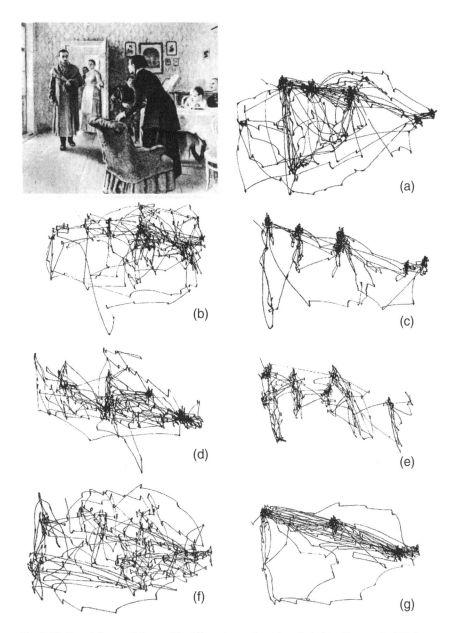

Fig. 3.10 Examining a picture with different questions in mind. (An Unexpected Visitor, as in Fig. 3.4). Each record lasts 3 minutes. (a) Free examination. (b) Estimate the material circumstances of the family in the picture. (c) Give the ages of the people. (d) Surmise what the family had been doing before the arrival of the 'unexpected visitor'. (e) Remember the clothes worn by the people. (f) Remember the position of the people and objects in the room. (g) Estimate how long the 'unexpected visitor' had been away from the family. From Yarbus (1967, Fig. 109).

Can a salience basic framework accommodate top-down attention?

We have argued that the original notion of visual conspicuity driving fixation selection is limited in its ability to account for where people look, especially when high-level goals influence behaviour. William James (1890, p. 416) distinguished between attention that is 'passive, reflex, non-voluntary, effortless' from attention that is 'active and voluntary'. The first of these categories roughly corresponds to salience-driven attention and the second to the kind of cognitively directed (or script-driven) attention seen during the execution of a task. The question is whether the salience map model of the generation of covert and overt attention can be modified to embrace script-driven attention or whether something else entirely is needed.

One problem is the use of the word salience itself. If the useful idea of a single map whose landscape leads to shifts of covert attention and ultimately to eye movements is to be retained, then it has to be accessible to influences other than salience (in the original sense of conspicuousness). Task relevance, in particular, needs to be represented. The objects that populate the script of a task are rarely the most conspicuous, but they nevertheless have to win the battle over more conspicuous objects. One way round this is to redefine salience as 'that which is fixated' (many have adopted this usage), but then 'salience' loses its etymological roots, and its definition becomes circular. A better solution, advocated by Serences and Yantis (2006) and Fecteau and Munoz (2006), would be to retain the original meaning of salience and to use 'priority' to refer to the map upon which the saccade target battle is fought.

A key problem in real-world target selection is the process by which particular objects with complex geometries are recognized. In a script-driven task, each object has to be located and recognized. In a situation (say, a kitchen; see Chapter 5) that is only partly familiar, this will involve summoning what information is available about the location of the next object in the sequence, which may even be out of sight at the time, orienting to it, and recognizing it. In our experience it is remarkable how little actual search behaviour occurs in such settings: locations are recalled remarkably well even after what seem to be quite cursory inspections of the scene. The question of when and how objects are recognized is also important. Are they recognized, partially at least, in the periphery, before a saccade is made to them, or is it only when they are close to the fovea that their identity is verified? The former would imply a greater degree of peripheral analysis than is generally accepted (e.g. Nelson and Loftus, 1980), but the latter would mean that the targeting saccade is driven entirely by remembered location information, with no input from peripheral vision, or indeed by covert attention. Whether in the periphery or the fovea, recognition must occur at some stage. There seem to be two possible classes of mechanism.

In one, loosely following the salience/attention model, it might be that an object is recognized from its particular combination of low-level attributes and that by tweaking the parameters of the various low-level feature maps, by top-down intervention, the salience map can be engineered to favour a particular class of object. A successful computational model of this kind, based on the kind of low-level filters used by Itti and Koch (2000), has been produced by Navalpakkam and Itti (2005). Here, the weightings of the different features and spatial scales of information that are used to create the master salience map can be differentially weighted according to the behavioural task of the viewer: essentially each task could be represented by a profile of channel weightings that contribute to the master map. Whether this approach will provide an adequate account of the complexities of eye guidance during natural behaviour remains to be determined, but theoretical concerns about the power of such a scheme have been raised (Vincent et al., 2007). Another model (Rao et al., 2002), based on a hierarchy of multiple-scale oriented filters, has been found to be able to mimic human eye movement strategies in certain object-finding tasks.

Alternatively, as the script of a task progresses, the executive system might set up a series of high-level images – schematic pictures of what the eyes are supposed to find. These could, for example, be akin to the '2.5D sketches' of Marr (1982) or assembled from the 'geon' primitives of Biederman (1987). This idea is appealing because when you are looking for something it does feel as though you are trying to effect some kind of match with what ethologists call a 'search image'. However, it is very difficult to imagine how such 'holistic' images could be accommodated in the framework of a purely salience-based model of the kind outlined earlier. One approach to reconciling this possibility in salience-based models has been to suggest that some kind of object detector operates alongside the salience map and is used to modify the map's output. Ehinger et al. (2009) included a face detector in their model of eye guidance while looking for people in photographic scenes. The salience map was subsequently constrained to locations in which the face detector signalled that there might be a face present, such that only salience peaks within these regions were represented in the final decision map. A similar approach of including a probabilistic object detector as a modifier of the salience map has been employed by Kanan et al. (2009). In both cases, including a notion of object detection in the models drastically improved their ability to account for human fixation behaviour while searching the images. What is not clear in these models is whether there remains a need to include the salience map if there is an effective system for detecting objects anyway. In the Findlay and Walker (1999) saccade generation model the final salience map (better, priority map) is fed by separate topographically mapped channels for intrinsic salience (as in the Itti and Koch, 2000, model), search selection, peripheral visual events (sudden unexpected intrusions), and spatial selection (the kind of input that a script-driven task would produce). Such an outline model has the flexibility to deal with processes that are probably very different from each other, at least until the decision to move the eyes is finally made.

In our example of the script-driven task of making tea (Chapter 5) we argue that we summon what information we have about where the next object will be found. Although direct visual input from the scene is a valuable source of information in this respect, when we search for an object in a real scene, we can use our past experience of this or similar scenes to narrow down the search. For example, if looking for a cup in a kitchen we are more likely to find it on work surfaces than the floor, walls, or ceiling. Torralba and colleagues (Torralba and Oliva, 2003; Torralba et al., 2006) developed an account of eye guidance that integrated low-level feature information and high-level context based on previous knowledge of similar scenes. Global low-level features in scenes (Oliva and Torralba, 2006) can be used to discern the gist of a scene, and this

gist can be used to look up a spatial prior probability distribution for the likely location of the target object (Fig. 3.11). A model that included this component far outper-
formed the ability of a feature-only model to account for human search behaviour
(Fig. 3.11) suggesting that these spatial expectations about where objects are likely to
be found are used by humans when searching for objects.

These new developments in modelling eye guidance are providing far better insights
into eye movement behaviour when viewing images than was previously possible, but
we remain some way from understanding the complexities of eye guidance during
natural behaviour. It is interesting to note that all of the emerging models discussed
above still place the salience map at their heart. High-level factors exert their influence
by modulating the output of the salience map. The decision to retain the salience map
in new models is worth considering critically. The assumption is that there exists some
'default' mode of looking that we revert to in the absence of high-level factors. We
have seen in this chapter that salience is at best a poor predictor of fixation behaviour,
even in free-viewing conditions where no task is explicit. It remains to be seen whether
treating high-level factors merely as modulators of a salience map is a useful approach.
Thus, one challenge for the future will be to decide whether it is still worth including
a salience-driven component in models of eye movement behaviour, or whether alternative approaches that centre upon targeting higher-level 'features' such as the
informativeness of objects or other scene regions might provide better understanding
of how we select where to fixate.

Interest, meaning, and informativeness

It seems self-evident that the objects that our visual system singles out for closer
inspection are in some sense more interesting than others. As Mackworth and Morandi
(1967) put it, 'gaze selects informative detail'. The scan path records of Yarbus (Figs
3.3, 3.4, and 3.10) exemplify this perfectly. The question here is the extent to which
terms such as 'informativeness' imply something more than 'salience' in the strict
bottom-up sense of Itti and Koch (2000). Are there features more complex than colour, brightness, orientation, and spatial scale to which we nevertheless respond 'automatically'?

It is interesting at this point to return to what the pioneers of the subject, Buswell
and Yarbus, thought about fixation selection. Although their evidence regarding the
consistency between observers when viewing scenes has been used to argue for low-
level features driving fixation selection, this was not how these authors described their
findings. Buswell framed his conclusions about where the eyes dwell in terms of
'centres of interest': 'The density plots do give a rather clear indication as to what
parts of a given picture are likely to prove most interesting to a random selection of
subjects' (Buswell, 1935, p. 24). From Buswell's records of fixations on pictures it is
not possible to be sure whether his more top-down interpretation was the correct one.
However, one other observation of Buswell can certainly be interpreted as weakening
the simple salience explanation: 'The perceptual pattern for various types of repetitive
designs showed clearly that the pattern of eye movements does not resemble even
remotely the general pattern of the design' (p. 143).

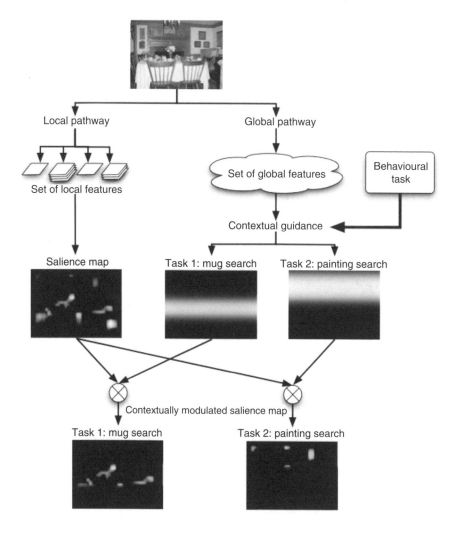

Fig. 3.11 Schematic of Torralba's contextual guidance model (Torralba et al., 2006). Images are analysed via two parallel pathways. A local feature pathway, in which a salience map is constructed much as in Itti and Koch's (2000) model (see Fig. 3.6). A global pathway is used to extract global features across the entire scene to rapidly derive the gist of the scene. This gist is used in combination with the observer's behavioural task to look up a learnt spatial probability map of where target objects are likely to occur in scenes of the current type. The spatial probability map (or contextual map) is then combined with the salience map to effectively inhibit any salience peaks that occur outside the region in which the target is likely to be found. The resultant contextually modulated salience map constrains eye movements to the region in which the target is expected. (Adapted from Torralba et al., 2006.).

On a salience scheme one might have expected that attention, released from the confines of one design element by an eye movement and inhibition of return, might become similarly entrapped by the next element. But it seems that this is not so.

Like Buswell, Yarbus (1967) was very clear that it was the informativeness of different components of the scene that attracts attention:

> Records of eye movements show that the observer's attention is usually held only by certain elements of the picture. As already noted, the study of these elements shows that they give information allowing the meaning of the picture to be obtained.
>
> (Yarbus, 1967, p.190)

In relation to the attributes that might contribute to salience, in the sense of conspicuity as discussed above, Yarbus (1967) was dismissive:

> First we will note that special attention or indifference to the elements of a picture is in no way due to the number of details composing the elements.

> Similarly, the brightest or darkest elements of a picture are not necessarily those that which attract the eye (if the brightness of these elements is considered alone).

> Sometimes both colored and black-and-white reproductions of the same size taken from the same picture were used. However, in no case did the corresponding records reveal any appreciable influence of color on the distribution of points of fixation.
>
> (Yarbus, 1967, pp. 175, 182, 183)

These comments appear to rule out spatial frequency, brightness, and colour as attractors of the eye. Yarbus was more equivocal about outlines, which do receive attention, but he commented as follows:

> Borders and outlines are only elements from which, together with other no less important elements, our perception is composed and the object recognized. Clearly the outlines of an object will attract an observer's attention if the actual shape of the outline includes important and essential information.
>
> (Yarbus, 1967, p.190)

Unlike the studies of the painting of 'The Unexpected Visitor', where different eye movement patterns were evoked when different questions were asked (Fig. 3.10), the comments just quoted relate to pictures being inspected freely, without prior instruction. Under these circumstances one might have expected straightforward salience cues to dominate the fixation pattern. In Yarbus' view this is not the case, and even free viewing is governed largely by top-down, meaning-driven, instructions.

> Eye movements reflect the human thought processes; so the observer's thought may be followed to some extent from records of eye movements. ... It is easy to determine from these records which elements attract the observer's eye (and, consequently, his thought), in what order, and how often.
>
> (Yarbus, 1967, p.190)

Of course, one possible resolution of the apparent differences between salience and informativeness would be to suggest that informative locations in a scene coincide with peaks in the master salience map. Elazary and Itti (2008) have argued just this: they found that the most salient regions in scenes tended to fall within the boundaries of objects labelled as interesting by observers. Indeed it would be very surprising if this were not so, as interesting objects are often prominent. Thus visual conspicuity may offer a rough approximation of interestingness in scenes, but again we cannot draw any causal links between salience and selection on this basis. Indeed, just because interesting objects may show some degree of salience, this should not imply that salient locations will necessarily be interesting to the observer. Evidence that this coincidence between salience and informativeness or interestingness may be nothing more than a correlation comes from the work by Nyström and Holmqvist (2008). These authors showed that removing the salience of semantically informative locations such as faces, by blurring them, did not reduce the likelihood that these locations would be fixated.

When we come later to consider fixation sequences made during the performance of domestic tasks, such as those discussed in Chapter 5, it will become clear that the objects fixated are those needed for the task, and all other are ignored, irrespective of their conspicuity.

Although quantifying informativeness or interestingness in natural scenes can be very difficult, faces may provide a useful set of stimuli in this respect. Faces contain collections of features that appear to draw attention effortlessly. There is now general agreement that faces are more readily detected in scenes than other objects with similar low-level characteristics (i.e. they show 'pop-out', see Fig. 3.5). Hershler and Hochstein (2005) found that human faces were easily detectable in composite pictures with a variety of distractors, that the speed of detection (<10 ms per item) was consistent with pop-out, and that the number of distractors did not influence search times. In contrast animal faces and other objects did not produce pop-out, neither did 'scrambled' faces with the same features but in randomized positions. They conclude that face search is mediated by 'holistic face characteristics rather than face parts'. It seems from this that objects with a high-order structure can, under some circumstances at least, access the low-level machinery responsible for pre-attentive processing; whether this machinery is the same as that involved in saccade targeting is still not yet clear.

The temporal sequence of fixations

Changes in fixation behaviour during prolonged viewing

At the head of this chapter we stated that we are interested in understanding sequences of eye movements when viewing scenes. However, much of the work described above is aimed at understanding *where* people fixate but with no notion of *when* in the sequence this might be. For example, in typical evaluations of salience at fixation, whether the location was selected early or late in the viewing period is not considered. However, it has long been recognized that inspection behaviour changes as we view a scene for a prolonged period of time. Buswell (1935) found that fixation patterns changed during the viewing period. If we consider the first few fixations on a scene by a number of different observers, we see a high degree of consistency in where they fixate. In contrast, consistency between observers is much less for the last few fixations on a scene (Fig. 3.12). One possible explanation for this result is that following the onset of a new scene, the first few fixations are driven more strongly by salience than later fixations (which may be under more strategic control). If so, we should see that the amount of salience at fixation would be higher for the first few fixations than for later fixations. Indeed, the winner-takes-all salience model requires that locations will be selected in rank order of salience, meaning that the salience at early fixations should be highest. Parkhurst et al. (2002) found that salience at fixation was highest for the first fixation on any scene and decreased over the next few fixations. From this result, they concluded that salience was driving early fixations more strongly than later fixations.

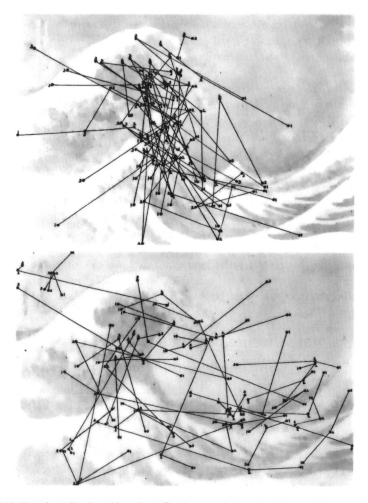

Fig. 3.12 First three (top) and last three fixations made by 40 subjects while viewing the Hokusai print 'The Wave'. From Buswell (1935).

This result, however, has since been challenged. Tatler, Baddeley et al. (2005) asked the same question but came to a very different conclusion: these authors found that there was no evidence for any change in the salience at fixation over viewing time. Tatler and colleagues argued that the Parkhurst result was an artefact of the sampling method used for selecting the control locations: because early fixations are more strongly biased towards the centre of the monitor – especially if a central pre-trial fixation marker is used – and images tend to have higher salience at the centre. If these biases are not accounted for in selecting the control locations, salience will appear inflated for early fixations. When they did not account for these biases, Tatler and colleagues were able to replicate the Parkhurst result, but when they did take these biases into account, they found no change in salience at fixation over the course of viewing a scene. Thus the relative role of salience early and later in viewing remains controversial. Carmi and Itti (2006) argued that an early prominence of salience in fixation selection was still observed, using movie sequences as stimuli. Nyström and Holmqvist (2008), on the other hand, showed that if contrast and edge density were locally reduced at a location in a scene that attracted early fixation, this region continued to attract fixation early in viewing in much the same way. This is not what would be predicted if early fixations were targeted on the basis of low-level image features.

Not only does consistency in where people look change with viewing time, but so do other aspects of oculomotor behaviour. Buswell (1935) found that later fixations were of longer duration than earlier ones (273 ms for the first five fixations, increasing to 367 ms for the last five). Using this evidence, together with the changes he observed in where people fixate over time, Buswell suggested that the viewer changed from an initial quick survey to a more detailed study of limited regions. This finding was repeated by Antes (1974) who found an increase in fixation duration from 215 ms initially to 310 ms after a few seconds. On the matter of these two modes of viewing, Buswell (1935) commented, somewhat wryly: 'It is probable that most of the visitors to an art gallery look at the pictures with this [*quick survey*] type of perception and that they see only the main centers of interest' (p. 142).

Apart from the general trends in fixation, duration, and location over the course of several seconds of viewing, it has also been found that the characteristics of each saccade and fixation can be quite intricately linked to the characteristics of the saccades and fixations that immediately precede or follow it (for a review see Tatler and Vincent, 2008). For example, Motter and Belky (1998) found that small saccades tend to be followed by large saccades and vice versa. In contrast, in photographic scenes Tatler and Vincent (2008) found evidence for sequences of small amplitude saccades. Fixation duration also appears to be influenced by the amplitude of the saccade that is about to be launched (Tatler and Vincent, 2008; Unema et al., 2005). Evidence from a range of studies of sequential dependencies in eye movement behaviour appear to support Buswell's notion of different modes of viewing: it would appear that there are periods of localized scanning of the scene interspersed with global relocations to new parts of the scene (Frost and Pöppel, 1976; Tatler and Vincent, 2008; Unema et al., 2005). Interestingly, we will later see that when performing real tasks such as preparing food, the same distinction is found between local scanning (of the object being manipulated) and more global relocation (to the next target of action; see Chapter 5).

Scanpaths and scan paths?

Describing the general trends in oculomotor behaviour over time or dependencies between successive saccades and fixations is still some way short of fully capturing the unfolding behaviour of the eyes as they inspect a scene. The sequence of eye movements we make when viewing a scene is often called a scan path or scan pattern, and the importance of the full sequence of fixation locations in scene inspection has been the subject of a number of studies. Perhaps most prominent among these was the work of Noton and Stark (1971), who referred to the sequence of eye movements with the single word *scanpath*, a term that has attracted much controversy. Noton and Stark proposed that the trajectory of gaze across a scene had a more important role in the perception of that scene than previously supposed. They pointed out that when a subject is asked to recognize a drawing out of a series of drawings that they have previously viewed, the scanpath they used in identifying the drawing is again similar to the one they used to examine it in the first place (Fig. 3.13). They suggested that on initial viewing a memory trace of the sequence of eye movements from feature to feature is laid down and that when subsequently recognizing the drawing: 'the subject is matching the internal representation with the pattern, by reproducing the successive eye movement memories and verifying the successive feature memories, a successful completion of the scanpath indicating recognition of the pattern' (p. 310).

It is interesting to note that the suggestion of a pivotal role of the course taken by the eye in perception (rather than simply emphasizing the fixation points) is in some ways a return to ideas that were found in the literature around the turn of the twentieth century. Prior to Erdmann and Dodge's (1898) chance discovery that they could not see their own eye movements in a mirror, it was not realized that vision was suppressed during eye movements; rather it was thought that it was during eye movements that information was gathered (Cattell, 1900).

Since Noton and Stark proposed their scanpath ideas, some limited support has been offered for their findings. Using simple chessboard-like stimuli, Brandt and Stark (1997) found similar scanpaths during viewing and later imagining the patterns. Similar findings were reported by Holsanova et al. (1999). Laeng and Teodorescu (2002) found decreased memory performance when central fixation was maintained during the recall phase (where no scene was present) than if they were allowed to move their eyes. They interpreted this as support for a necessary link between reproducing eye movement sequences made while encoding, during the recall phase and being able to form a mental image of the scene. Noton and Stark's ingenious idea, however, has not found much favour in recent years, partly because pattern recognition can occur without eye movements, and because there are many other explanations for scanpath-like eye movement patterns. The other problem with the scanpath idea is that sequential viewings of the same scene are really not very similar. Even the published records from Noton and Stark (1971) require a certain generosity to be seen as really alike (Fig. 3.13).

Although unpopular for some time, the notion of scanpaths is now being revisited in the context of salience- and task-driven schemes of eye movement control (see Foulsham and Underwood, 2008; Humphrey and Underwood, 2008). Using photographic scenes,

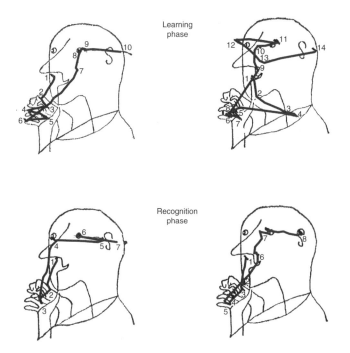

Fig. 3.13 Scanpaths, redrawn from Noton and Stark (1971). Sequences of fixations made while subjects viewed one of five patterns they had not previously seen. In the 'learning phase' the pattern was viewed for 20s, and two extracts from these sequences made by one subject are shown. In the subsequent recognition stage subjects were asked to identify the pattern from a set of 10, and two examples from the same subject's performance are shown. In these examples there is a repeated pattern (mouth, hands, eye, ear), but there are many differences in detail.

similarities between successive viewings of a scene have been found but to a far lesser extent than in previous work (Foulsham and Underwood, 2008). These authors also found that on average only one of the first five fixations on a scene landed in one of the five most salient locations. This work highlights that not only the replicability of scan-paths, while above chance, is low but also that when sequential information is taken into account the winner-takes-all salience framework is ineffective at explaining much about the order in which locations are fixated.

To distinguish the rather special meaning of scanpath used by Noton and Stark from the more general sense of a particular sequence of fixations, we will revert to the two-word *scan path* or more neutral phrases such as scan pattern or sequence of fixations, for the latter.

From lab to life

Most if not all of the work reviewed in this chapter was conducted in laboratory settings as subjects viewed images on screens or computer monitors. We were not really equipped by evolution to do experiments on screens in darkened rooms, although it is a tribute to the versatility of the human visual system that it can become quite at home in this strange situation. In natural behaviour, our eyes help us to steer a course, on foot or in a vehicle; they make it possible to play sports; they find the things we need and then guide our hands in the manipulations of these objects; they enable us to read, write, type, and play music; and they act as social signals. Given the contrast between the medium in which we have developed much of our understanding of vision and the medium in which it normally operates, we are certainly entitled to wonder whether conclusions drawn from laboratory settings transfer to natural behaviour? This simple question is not easy to answer, but it is the topic of Part II of this book and also of an increasing amount of research.

In a pioneering series of experiments, Epelboim and her colleagues (1995, 1997) compared tapping a series of coloured pegs, to looking at the same pegs and imagining tapping them (reviewed in Steinman, 2003). Despite the fact that the two conditions were identical apart from whether they involved the act of tapping, there were striking differences in the oculomotor strategies employed by the subjects. For example, the involvement of the head in achieving gaze shifts was very different: when only looking at the pegs, little head movement was observed, with gaze shifts being achieved by the eye alone. However, when tapping the pegs, the head made a strong contribution to shifting gaze. These studies demonstrate that the way in which we employ our oculomotor system to sample the world may be rather different when involved in an active task than when simply looking at scenes.

With regard to the issue of eye guidance by salience, little or no supporting evidence has been found for it during natural activity (Jovancevic et al., 2006; Turano et al., 2003). High-level task information appears to dominate fixation behaviour even more in natural behaviour than in laboratory settings, with fixations highly constrained to task-relevant objects even in the presence of many salient distractors (Chen and Zelinsky, 2006; Hayhoe et al., 2003; Rothkopf et al., 2007). Similarly, the temporal patterns of fixations are largely determined by the action sequences required as a task progresses. We will now turn our attention to more natural settings and consider how the eyes are deployed to sample the information we require to complete our behavioural goals.

Summary

1. Simple psychophysical search tasks suggest a role for basic image features in capturing attention and guiding eye movements.

2. Models emphasizing low-level image features (salience) have been prominent in recent research. However, many lines of evidence indicate that they fail to capture many aspects of human viewing behaviour.

3. Classic studies by Buswell and Yarbus showed that cognitive factors profoundly influence how people look at pictures.

4. Attempts to reconcile the influence of task in eye guidance with image-based salience favour the idea that high-level factors modulate the salience map. However,

this assumes a default stimulus-driven mode of viewing that may prove unnecessary if selection operates on higher-order features such as objects.

5. Most studies of eye guidance have involved viewing static images, employing a limited set of cognitive tasks. We argue this is fundamentally different from the way vision is used in active tasks during real behaviour.

Part 2

Observations

Chapter 4

Sedentary tasks

In the chapters that make up Part II we shall be dealing with the roles of vision, and in particular fixation sequences, in the activities of everyday life. In all of these, the eyes have two basic roles: finding and identifying the objects needed for the various tasks and guiding the actions that make use of these objects. As head-mounted eye movement cameras were not available until the 1950s, all studies before that period involved tasks that could be performed in constrained laboratory situations, in which the head had to be normally kept still. This effectively limited work to reading, playing the piano, typing, and drawing. It is with these sedentary activities that this chapter is principally concerned.

Reading

Silent reading

Although silent reading involves no overt action, it nevertheless requires a particular eye movement strategy to make possible the uptake of information in a way that allows meaning to be acquired. Thus visual sampling and comprehension are parallel processes and need to be matched in speed. Reading is one of best studied (as well as the most atypical) examples of a clearly defined eye movement pattern. Eye movements in reading are highly constrained to a linear progression of fixations to the right (in English) across the page, which allows the words to be read in an interpretable order. In this, reading differs from many other activities (such as viewing pictures; see below) where order is much less important. Reading is a learned skill, but the eye movements that go with it are not taught. Nevertheless they are remarkably similar between normal readers. There is a huge literature on eye movements in reading, including many excellent reviews; only the principal facts need to be included here. Much of what follows is derived from an extensive review by Rayner (1998) and chapter 5 in Findlay and Gilchrist (2003). The reader is referred to Radach et al. (2004), or parts 4 and 5 of Van Gompel et al. (2007) for accounts of recent issues in reading research.

During normal reading, gaze (foveal direction) moves across the line of print in a series of saccades, whose size is typically 7 to 9 letters (Fig. 4.1). Within limits this number is not affected by the print size, implying that the oculomotor system is able to make scaling adjustments to its performance. For normal print the saccade size is about 2°, and the durations of the fixations between saccades have a mean of 225 ms. It is interesting to note that this varies with the apparent difficulty of the text, from 202 ms for light fiction to 264 ms for biology textbooks (Rayner and Pollatsek, 1989).

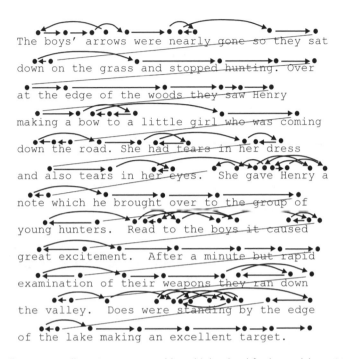

The boys' arrows were nearly gone so they sat
down on the grass and stopped hunting. Over
at the edge of the woods they saw Henry
making a bow to a little girl who was coming
down the road. She had tears in her dress
and also tears in her eyes. She gave Henry a
note which he brought over to the group of
young hunters. Read to the boys it caused
great excitement. After a minute but rapid
examination of their weapons they ran down
the valley. Does were standing by the edge
of the lake making an excellent target.

Fig. 4.1 Silent text reading. A passage read by a high school freshman (about 14 years old) with good reading skills for his age. Dots above the text show fixations and arrows indicate the progression of saccades across the text. Most saccades are to the right, but 28 (31%) are regressions, of which 8 result from starting new lines too far to the right. There are a number of grammatical or lexical surprises in the text, some of which appear to cause a flurry of regressions (e.g. 'bow' in line 4, 'Read' in line 8 and 'Does' in line 11). Data from Buswell (1920) plate 35.

The frequency of right-to-left regressions also increases with difficulty, and saccade length decreases slightly from 9.2 to 6.8 characters. Most saccades (in English) are to the right, but 10% to 15% are regressions (to the left) and are associated in a poorly understood way with problems in processing the currently or previously fixated word (e.g. Fig. 4.1 especially lines 8 and 11). Words can be identified up to 7 to 8 letter spaces to the right of the fixation point, but some information about the shape of words is available up to 14 to 15 letter spaces away. From studies in which words were masked during fixations it appears that the visual information needed for reading is taken in during the first 50 to 70 ms of each fixation. Adult readers typically read at 250 to 300 words per minute – or 0.2 s per word.

A key tool for studying information uptake during reading is the 'moving window' technique, introduced by McConkie and Rayner (1975). This allows changes to be made to the text, either in the regions on either side of the word being fixated or, in the 'foveal mask' technique, around the fixation point itself (Fig. 4.2). These methods involve monitoring the eye movements and introducing changes while saccades are

Window

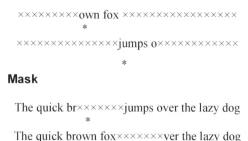

Mask

Fig. 4.2 Foveal window and foveal mask techniques. Two successive fixations with asterisks indicate the current fixation point.

being made ('gaze contingent' modifications). Because of blur and saccadic suppression this means that the changes are effectively invisible to the subjects who are usually unaware of them. These gaze contingent techniques have provided a number of important insights into how we read. First, interfering with the letters around the fixation point severely compromises reading: a 7-letter mask centred on the fovea reduces reading to 12 words per minute (from 250) and even then many mistakes are made. Second, with a window in which only a 7-letter foveal region is intact, reading accuracy is relatively unaffected, although reading rates are lower, implying that the region outside the fovea does contribute something to normal reading. In fact some loss of speed is detectable when letters are interfered with up to 15 characters to the right of the current fixation point, although this effect only extends to about 4 characters to the left. This range of letter spaces for which manipulations can be shown to influence the fluency of reading is known as the *perceptual span* for reading.

The moving window technique also allows an exploration of how more peripheral regions of text might influence reading behaviour. By varying the nature of the extra-foveal mask, it is possible to consider whether properties such as the size of words or the overall word structure (in terms of ascenders and descenders in letters such as d and p) influence reading. The influence of word size on reading can be considered by comparing extra-foveal masks of Xs in which spaces between words were preserved to extra-foveal masks in which the spaces were also filled with Xs. This comparison showed that for windows of up to 25 characters (symmetrical about the fixation point), reading speed was slower when the spaces were filled. However, when the visible central window was larger than this, reading fluency was unaffected by whether the spaces were filled or not. This result suggests that extra-foveal word spacing information does influence reading but only up to a certain range ahead of the current point of fixation. The influence of word structure can be considered by using extra-foveal masks where the letters are replaced by other letters rather than Xs. Here, the letters used as the mask can either preserve or not the word structure of ascending and descending letters. This manipulation showed that word structure did influence reading speed but only for central windows of fewer than 21-letter spaces. Word structure therefore appears not to be encoded as far ahead of fixation as does word spacing information. These findings by Rayner and colleagues seem to suggest that the primary influence of extra-foveal information in reading is to control the landing points of upcoming saccades. However, as we shall see below, this may not be its only function.

The way gaze progresses along the line of print raises two separate questions: where do the eyes move to next, and when do they move there? The 'where' question is the less controversial and can largely be explained by non-linguistic, 'low-level' factors such as word length. Generally saccades land near the middle of the first half of the next word. The size of the saccade that achieves this is influenced by two factors: the length of the next word, and the launch point on the current word (McConkie et al., 1988). If the next word is long the saccade reaching it is lengthened accordingly, so that it lands 1 or 2 characters deeper into the word than it would with a short word. This implies that an estimate of upcoming word length has been made in extra-foveal preview. If the saccade is launched from a long way back in the current word then it will 'fall short' on the next word. If, for example, it is launched from 7 characters back in the current word it will typically land 1 to 2 characters into the next word, whereas if launched from only 1 character back it will land around characters 4 or 5. Word length and launch point also affect two other features of gaze progression: whether a word is skipped altogether and whether it requires a second fixation. Words of one, two, or three letters are often skipped, especially if the saccade launch site is towards the end of the preceding word: a 2-letter word is likely to be skipped 90% of the time when the launch site is one character to the left and 50% when it is launched 8 or more characters away. When a saccade lands near the beginning of long word there is likely to be a refixation within the word, so that for 8-letter words the rate of refixation is 31%, falling to 13% for 4-letter words. Saccades that land near the end of a word can lead to regressive saccades that refixate close to the beginning of the same word. Thus the mechanisms that control the spatial sequence of fixations are flexible within broad limits and are tuned to a considerable degree by information from the parafoveal region to the right of the currently fixated word.

The explanations given above focus on the dominance of non-linguistic factors on the decision about where to fixate. However, some linguistic effects on landing position and the probability of skipping a word altogether have been reported. The landing position in a word can be altered by misspelling a word (orthography), with fixation landing closer to the beginning of a word when misspelled (White and Liversedge, 2004). However, Pynte et al. (2004) ran a similar study of misspelled words, but in their study the misspelling was present only before the word was fixated and thus visible only in the parafovea. These authors found no effect of misspellings on landing positions, although they did find reliable effects on the duration of the fixation before the misspelled word was targeted. Word predictability and morphology may also influence landing position in words. Whether a word is skipped or not depends partly on non-linguistic factors such as saccade launch site and word length but also on linguistic factors such as word frequency (how common it is) and how predictable the word is from its preceding context (see Drieghe et al., 2007 for a thorough review of word skipping).

The question of when the eyes move on during reading has proved more controversial than the question of where they are targeted. One school of thought (O'Regan, 1990) argues that fixation duration is indeed mainly controlled by the same kind of low-level factors that influence saccade landing. The prevailing view, however, is that it is the rate at which words are processed that makes fixations longer or shorter. Individual fixations vary in length between about 0.1 and 0.4 s (Fig. 4.3). Fixations on more difficult words – those that have a low frequency in the language – elicit longer fixation durations than high frequency words of the same length (Inhoff and Rayner, 1986). The average difference is about 20 ms, or 10% of the average duration. This is consistent with the idea that low-frequency words take longer to activate their corresponding unit in the mental dictionary ('lexical access'). Other linguistic features such as ambiguity and syntactic complexity can also affect the duration of a fixation within its lifetime. A challenge to the evidence for linguistic effects on fixation duration was mounted by Yang and McConkie (2001) who suggested that most of these apparent linguistic effects could in fact be accounted for non-linguistically using a model of saccade initiation based on Findlay and Walker's (1999) scene viewing model (see Chapter 3). However, despite these challenges, most researchers favour linguistic processing effects on fixation duration in current accounts of reading.

Of those who favour linguistic influence on fixation duration, two distinct theoretical accounts of reading have emerged, which differ fundamentally in their position on the processing that underlies reading. The key question that distinguishes these theoretical positions is whether reading is a serial or a parallel process? Given that we know that eye movements must themselves be serial (we can only look in one place at a time), this question might seem redundant. Yet the serial nature of fixations does not itself impose a serial *processing* strategy. Perhaps the most prominent current model of reading behaviour is the EZ Reader model (Reichle et al., 1998, 2006), now on its tenth iteration. Like Morrison's (1984) original model of reading, EZ Reader assumes that processing is strictly serial: attention moves on to the next word (word $n+1$) *only* when processing of the currently attended word (word n) is complete. Note that where attention is directed in this model is not always the same as where the eye is fixating. It is possible for attention to move on to word $n+1$, and begin processing, before the eye has moved to it. This decoupling of fixation and attention also allows word skipping to be explained: if word $n+1$ is short the processing of that word may also be completed before the eyes are moved from word n. As a result, the saccade will be made directly to word $n+2$, skipping word $n+1$. The latest version of the EZ Reader model is able to account for many such empirical phenomena of reading, including regressions to previously fixated words (a phenomenon that the first versions of EZ Reader could not explain).

But why should we assume that processing of words in text is subject to such strict serial ordering? In other visual domains, such as scene viewing, it is widely accepted that extra-foveal processing is undertaken during a fixation. Rayner and colleagues argue that reading is a special case of vision in which processing is strictly serial, but other authors have considered the possibility of parallel processing in reading, just as with scene viewing. The leading competitor to EZ Reader is the SWIFT model (Engbert et al., 2005). Here lexical processing occurs in parallel across a region of the central

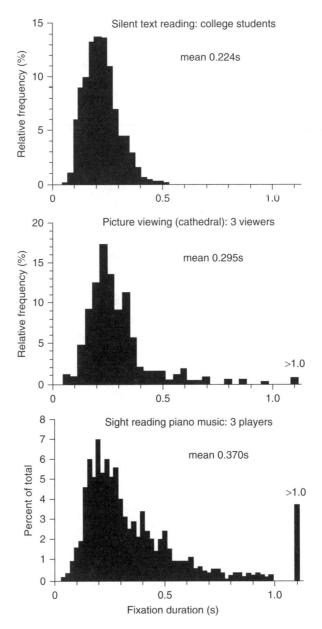

Fig. 4.3 Fixation durations during text reading (data from Rayner and Pollatsek, 1989), picture viewing (three individuals viewing a photograph of a cathedral interior; data from Buswell, 1935), and piano playing (three individuals of different skill levels reading double-stave music; data from Furneaux, 1996). The ordinate scales are not numerically comparable because the time bin widths are different.

visual field encompassing several words within a processing gradient or 'field of acti-vation', and the decision about when and where to move the eyes does not depend on completing visual processing at the current word. Rather the decision about where to fixate next depends on competition between lexical activation at each of the possible target words, with the most active becoming the target of the next saccade. This expla-nation is very similar to the Findlay and Walker (1999) activation model for saccade targeting in scene viewing. The decision about when to saccade is based on a random timer that can be locally inhibited according to processing requirements. SWIFT has proved successful at accounting for such empirical phenomena as the effects of para-foveal words on the current fixation duration (so-called parafoveal on foveal effects). These effects cannot be explained in the strictly serial EZ Reader account, and they strongly suggest parallel lexical processing (Kennedy et al., 2002).

One problem for both models is how to explain fluent reading despite disordered input. 'Disorder' can arise in the serial framework of EZ Reader, partly owing to skip-ping, but primarily because of regressions back to skipped or other words. 'Disorder' is certainly a feature of parallel models where processing may not reflect the serial ordering of words in the text, and proponents of EZ Reader have challenged the SWIFT model on these grounds: if read in parallel according to competing activations, how can the fluent and serial understanding of text emerge (Pollatsek et al., 2006)? Kennedy and Pynte (2008) considered disordered reading and found that not only is disordered reading rather common, but it does not adversely affect comprehension. These findings present a considerable challenge to the strictly serial EZ Reader model

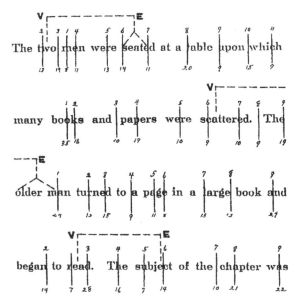

Fig. 4.4 Eye–voice span (V-E) when reading aloud by a high school student (freshman, about 14 years) recorded by Guy Buswell. Vertical bars are fixations. Upper numbers give the sequence along the line, and lower numbers their durations in multiples of 0.02 s. From Buswell (1920) plate 4.

and favour parallel models such as SWIFT. However, how the disordered input is integrated into a coherent understanding of the sentence has yet to be explained in the SWIFT framework.

Reading aloud

How long it takes to process words all the way from vision to meaning is hard to assess. However, the delay between reading and speech during reading aloud (the eye–voice span) can be measured (Fig. 4.4). In a classic study Buswell (1920) managed to integrate signals from a microphone and eye camera. He found that for high school students (ages 13–17) the time from fixating a word to uttering it (the eye–voice span) was about 13 letters, or 0.79 s (average word length of 4.7 letters and a reading speed of 3.5 words per second). On a simpler reading piece elementary school students (5th grade, age 10–11) had an eye–voice span of 11 letters, or 0.91 s. The eye–voice span of 'good' and 'poor' readers differed by 4 to 5 letters. These delay times are very similar to those later found in music reading (see below), stepping (Chapter 6) and driving (Chapter 7).

Typing

Copy-typing, like reading aloud, has a motor output, and according to Butsch (1932) typists of all skill levels attempt to keep the eyes about 1s ahead of the currently typed letter – much the same as in both reading aloud and music reading. This represents about 5 characters (Fig. 4.5). Inhoff and his colleagues (Inhoff and Wang, 1992) found more variability in the eye–hand span and also showed that it was affected by the nature of the text. Using a moving window technique they showed that typing starts to

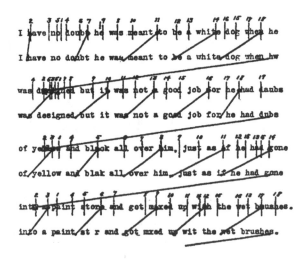

Fig. 4.5 Record of typing from Butsch (1932) showing the fixation sequence (upper vertical lines, numbers give fixation order) and the line actually typed (including errors). Oblique lines show eye positions at the instants the keys were pressed.

become slower when there are fewer than three letter spaces to the right of fixation, indicating a perceptual span about half the size of that used in normal reading. The potential word buffer is much bigger than this, however. Fleischer (1986) found that when typists use a read/check cycle of approximately 1 s each, while typing continuously, they would typically take in 11 characters during the read part of the cycle, and exceptionally, strings of up to 30 characters could be stored.

Reading music

Musical sight-reading shares with text reading the constraint that gaze must move progressively to the right. It is, however, more complicated in that – for keyboard players – there are two staves from which notes must be acquired. Weaver (1943) recorded eye movements of trained pianists and found that their gaze alternated fixation between the upper and lower staves (Fig. 4.6a):

> Notes on the treble and bass parts of the great staff are usually so far apart that both vertical and horizontal movements of the eyes must be used in preparing two parallel lines of material for a unified performance.
>
> (Weaver, 1943, p. 27)

This alternation means that notes that have to be played together are viewed at different times, adding a task of temporal assembly to the other cognitive tasks of interpreting the pitch and length of the notes. For the Bach minuet illustrated in Fig. 4.6a, Weaver's pianists acquired notes from the score at between 1.3 and 2.0 notes per fixation (making a note roughly equivalent to a word in text reading). Interestingly, the fixations on the upper stave were much longer (average 0.44 s) than those on the lower stave (0.28 s), presumably because more notes were acquired during each upper stave fixation. The time from reading a note to playing it (the eye–hand span) was similar to what Buswell (1920) had found for reading aloud: for the minuet the average for 10 performances was 3.1 notes, or 0.78 s. Fixation durations in sight-reading are longer than in text reading (mean 370 ms compared with 224 ms), and, in common with most activities other than reading, the distribution has a tail extending to beyond a second (Fig. 4.3).

Furneaux and Land (1999) and Furneaux (1996) looked at the eye–hand spans of pianists of differing abilities (Fig. 4.6b and c, Fig. 4.7). They found that the mean eye–hand span did not vary with skill level when measured as a time interval (typically close to 1 s), but that when measured in terms of the number of notes contained within the eye–hand span professionals averaged 4 to 5 compared with 2 for novices. Thus the processing time is the same for everyone, but the throughput rate of the processor is skill dependent, as is the preview distance when measured in notes rather than time (a 'note' was defined here as all individual note heads that are played simultaneously, and thus could be a single note or a chord). The variation in eye–hand span, measured on a fixation-by-fixation basis, was much greater for novices than professionals (Fig. 4.7), which fits with the subjective impression one has of barely being in control during the early stages of learning the piano. A final difference between professional performers and novices was in the number of note heads actually fixated: professionals viewed only about 40% of the printed notes (Fig. 4.6a and b), whereas novices tended to fixate almost every note or chord (Fig. 4.6c). Novices also made more regressions than advanced players.

The only factor that had a major effect on the eye–hand span for all players was tempo, with fast pieces having an eye–hand span of 0.7 s, increasing to 1.3 s for slow pieces. Interestingly this difference was not reflected in the number of notes contained in the eye–hand span, which was almost independent of tempo. Faster tempos produced shorter duration fixations rather than fewer fixations, which would have been the alternative. What seems to emerge from this is that the eye–hand buffer can contain a more or less fixed number of notes independent of tempo, and this number depends mainly on skill level. The time a note spends passing through the buffer lengthens or shortens to fit the speed of the performance.

A feature of the performances of players of all skill levels was the presence of glances down to the keyboard to check finger position. Although piano teachers tell you to avoid looking at the keys, even the professional accompanists made these glances (Fig. 4.6b). The impressive feature of these glances was the accuracy of the return saccade which, at least for the more skilled players, usually landed within a degree of where one would expect the next fixation to be located, had the fixation on the hands not been made (Fig. 4.6b). 'Corrective' saccades, such as are often seen in laboratory

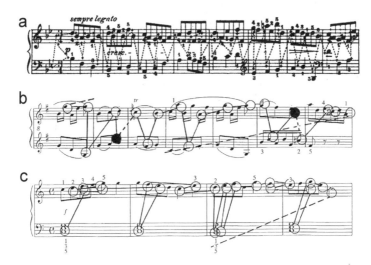

Fig. 4.6 Fixations while sight-reading piano music. (a) Record by Weaver (1942) of the eye movements made by an expert pianist playing a Bach minuet. Dotted lines join successive fixations and show how gaze alternates between the staves. (b) A professional accompanist playing line from a sonata by Scarlatti (presto). Circles (diameter ~ 1°) show fixation positions. The filled circles are fixations followed by brief glances down to the keyboard, about 30° below. The return saccade is not made to the same point but to the next fixation in the sequence, apparently without interrupting the progression. (c) A novice playing 'The five fingers', an exercise by Czerny. In contrast to (a) and (b), where fewer than half the note heads are fixated, the novice fixates almost all the notes, sometimes more than once. (b) and (c) from Furneaux and Land (1999).

orienting tasks to correct an undershoot of a primary saccade (e.g. Becker, 1991), were not seen when playing, even though the keyboard was located 30° below the score. Interestingly both the fixations on the fingers and the fixations immediately preceding them were unusually short (means 214 and 256 ms, compared with 370 ms for other fixations on the stave). This implies that the fixation on the fingers and the one preceding it are planned as a pair whose total duration (470 ms) is by no means unusual (Fig. 4.3). The fixation following the return to the stave is of normal duration.

What happens to the pattern of gaze as a piece of music is learned from initial sight-reading to fluency? Furneaux (1996) examined the eye movements of one intermediate player as she learned to play a sonata by Dušek (Royal Schools of Music Grade IV).

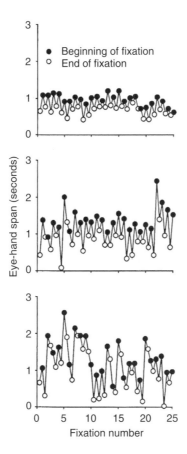

Fig. 4.7 The eye–hand span (time between fixating a note and playing it) for three 25-fixation sequences played by a professional (top) intermediate grade 6 to 7 (middle) and novice grade 3 to 4 (bottom). The mean eye–hand span is similar for all three – about 1 s – but the standard deviation for the professional is less than half that of the novice. Pieces and speeds were appropriate to the ability levels of the performers. From Furneaux and Land (1999).

This was a difficult piece to sight-read but not hard to learn to play fluently after a learning period totalling 5 hours. The player did not learn the piece 'by heart' and still needed the score to play from. Differences between initial and final performances included an increase in tempo and note accuracy, with fewer refixations and regressions. There was also a halving of the number of fixations made to the notes. Initially the subject fixated almost all the notes, but by the final performance major chunks of the score were not viewed at all. This was particularly true of the lower (left-hand) stave, in which only 17 of the 50 notes were fixated, compared to 48 fixations made during sight-reading. It seems likely that the strategy of this player was to learn many of the chords and phrases of the left hand, retaining more direct visual prompting for the melodic line of the right hand. Other players may have different learning strategies.

The three activities discussed so far – reading, typing, and musical sight-reading – are all similar in that they involve the continuous processing of a stream of visual information. Although this information is taken in as a series of stationary fixations, this probably has more to do with the visual system's need for an unblurred image (see Chapter 2) rather than with any cognitive requirement. The auditory system, for example, takes in and processes speech as an unbroken continuum. The visual information is translated and processed into a stream of muscular activity of various kinds (or into 'meaning' in the case of silent reading). In each case the time within the

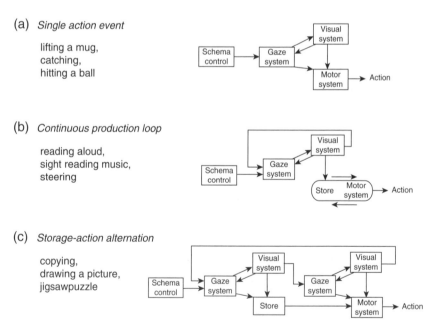

Fig. 4.8 Three versions of the gaze-action scheme (Fig. 1.1) applicable to (a) single actions, (b) continuous processing in which visual information is entered into a store which continuously translates it into action, and (c) storage-action alternation in which the first set of fixations provides information that is stored temporarily. The stored information is then used to guide actions during the second set of fixations. Further details in the text. From Land (2009).

processor is about a second. Once the appropriate action has been performed the original visual information is overwritten, so the operation is more like a production line than a conventional memory system. In these respects the pattern of information flow in the gaze, visual, and motor systems is different from that in a simple operation such as lifting a mug (Chapter 1, Fig. 1.1, and Fig. 4.8a). The gaze system has a self-generated pattern of movement, and the visual system does not monitor the motor system directly (as in Fig. 4.8a) but deposits information onto the conveyor that processes it into movements of the muscles of throat and mouth, or of the fingers, over the course of the next second (Fig. 4.8b).

Copying tasks

The block copying task of Ballard and Hayhoe

A pioneering study of the relationship between eye movements and actions was undertaken by Dana Ballard and his colleagues in 1992. They devised a task in which a model consisting of coloured blocks had to be copied using blocks from a separate pool. Thus the task involved a repeated sequence of looking at the model, selecting a block, moving it to the copy, and setting it down in the right place (Fig. 4.9). The most

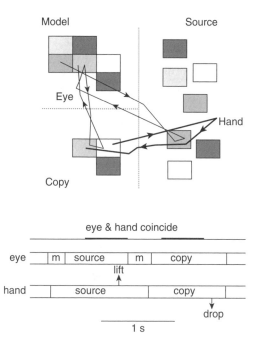

Fig. 4.9 Block copying task devised by Ballard and colleagues. The Model is recreated in the Copy space by picking up blocks from the Source pool on the right. Movements of the eyes and hand are shown during one of the moves, and the average timings in a cycle are shown below. Details in the text. Based on Ballard et al. (1992).

important finding was that the operation proceeded in a series of elementary acts involving eye and hand, with minimal use of memory. Thus a typical repeat unit would be as follows: fixate (block in model area), remember (its colour), fixate (a block in source area of the same colour), pick up (fixated block), fixate (same block in model area), remember (its relative location), fixate (corresponding location in model area); move block, drop block. The eyes have two quite different functions in this sequence: to supply the information needed to guide the hand in lifting and dropping the block and to gather the information about the attributes of particular blocks (Fig. 4.8c). The only times that gaze and hand coincide are during the periods of about half a second before picking up and setting down the block. Memory use is minimal, as shown by the fact that separate glances are used to determine the colour and location of the model block. This, incidentally, was the first study to examine in detail the temporal and spatial relationships between eye movements and actions.

The main conclusion from this study was that the eyes look directly at the objects they are engaged with, which in a task of this complexity means that a great many eye movements are required. Given the relatively small angular size of the task arena, why do the eyes need to move so much? Could they not direct activity from a single central location? Ballard et al. (1995) found that subjects could complete the task successfully when holding their gaze on a central fixation spot, but it took three times as long as when normal eye movements were permitted. Because the 1° blocks were within 5° of the fixation point it is unlikely that this was caused by difficulty in seeing them. For whatever reasons, this strategy of 'do it where I'm looking' is crucial for the fast and economical execution of the task. As we shall see, this strategy seems to apply almost universally. With respect to the relative timing of fixations and actions Ballard et al. (1995) came up with a second maxim: the 'just in time' strategy. In other words the fixation that provides the information for a particular action immediately precedes that action; in many cases the act itself may occur, or certainly be initiated, within the lifetime of a single fixation. This re-emphasizes that memory is used as little as possible. These conclusions appear to be borne out by nearly all the studies detailed in Chapters 4 to 8 of this book and can be regarded as basic rules for the interaction of the eye movement and action systems. However, they are not quite universally applicable, and some caution is needed.

An implication of the 'do it where I'm looking' strategy is that vision can only be engaged with one task at a time, and that is not always true. When driving, for example, looking at a road sign does not necessarily mean that the driver is out of visual contact with the road. The English language has expressions such as 'seeing out of the corner of one's eye' or 'keeping one eye on at the traffic and another on the road'. In practice these statements may mean that gaze alternates rapidly between rival attractions (e.g. when sight-reading both staves of a piano, see Fig. 4.6), but they may also mean that two tasks are monitored simultaneously by different regions of the retina: on winding roads, for example, the distant part of the road is observed by the fovea, but the near lane edges are monitored at the same time by regions about 5° obliquely below the fovea (Chapter 7). In the context of normal activity, the extent to which attention can be divided between sub-tasks remains to be explored, as does the related problem of the relative roles of fovea and periphery. It would be an over-simplification to think that only one vision-requiring process is active at any one time.

This leads to the question of whether looking at something is evidence that that is the object or location you are attending to or dealing with at the time. Conversely, if you are manipulating something does that also mean you are fixating it? It is clear that the answer to both questions is generally 'yes', as Ballard's dictum would imply, but it is also easy to find exceptions (see the section on magic in Chapter 9).

Jigsaw puzzles

Jigsaw puzzles resemble Ballard's block copying task (Fig. 4.9) in that the objective is to copy a model – the picture on the box – by assembling pieces drawn from a random source. They are, however, much more demanding because they require pattern fitting at three levels. The pieces have to be recognized by pattern and colour as belonging to a part of the overall source pattern; they must be chosen so that their pattern fits in with some part of the puzzle already completed; and the outlines of suitable new pieces have to be examined and oriented so as to produce a mechanical fit with other existing pieces in the puzzle. Together with two students at Sussex (see Acknowledgments) we recently examined the fixation patterns of two subjects as they completed a puzzle. The overall cycle loosely followed a model-source-copy pattern, with the pick-up and place movements of pieces occurring near the end of the fixations of the source and the beginning of those on the copy. However, the timings were very different from the task of Ballard et al. because of the need to search the source for suitable pieces and to manipulate each new piece in the area around the copy to get a suitable fit. Here the average times spent fixating the model, source, and copy were 1.3 ± 0.9 (s.d.), 2.8 ± 1.7, and 3.2 ± 2.6 s. The 'cycle time' between the fetching of new pieces from the source was 15.5 ± 7.2 s, which contrasts with the cycle time in the block copying task of just over 2 s.

Figure 4.10 illustrates an interesting 30 s episode during which the player has two loose pieces (*a* & *b*) that he eventually joins and fits to the completed part of the puzzle. The pattern of fixations allows us to reconstruct his thought patterns with some confidence. In the first few seconds, between 1 and 2 piece *a* is rotated anti-clockwise in three stages (i). While this is happening, the glances to the completed part of the puzzle are all to region *x*, indicating that the player is trying to fit *a* to this region. However by 2 it is clear that this will not work. He consults the picture on the lid and thereafter directs gaze on the puzzle itself to region *y*. About a second later (ii) he moves piece *a* to the right of piece *b*, probably having also noticed that the right-hand side is a straight edge. Interestingly, this move is completed while the eyes are looking at the picture about 20° above, so presumably its trajectory was set up during the previous fixation. Between 3 and 4 the player concentrates on piece *b*. He moves *a* and *b* to the left (iii, iv) and just before 4 he rotates *b* (v) so that its new right-hand profile matches the left profile of *a*. Just after 4 piece *b* is lifted and joined to *a* (vi). After 5 there is quite long period when both pieces, now joined, and the profile of the completed section are fixated and presumably appraised for goodness of fit. The two pieces are lifted together and finally joined to the rest of the puzzle (vii).

This episode illustrates a number of general points. First, the eyes only fixate the parts of the field that are important – the two pieces, the relevant regions of the part-completed puzzle, and on two occasions the relevant region of the picture. When looking at the individual pieces *a* and *b* fixation is accurate: the mean fixation distance from the centre of each piece (approximately 2° by 3°) was 1.4°. Second, during the various movements of the pieces they are either fixated during the move or during the half second before the move. This seems to bear out both the 'do it where I'm looking' and the 'just in time' rules (see above). Third, comparisons between patterns and outlines are mostly made by looking from one element to the next and back again, rather than sizing up the situation from a single gaze location. This is particularly clear between 1 and 2 where gaze moves repeatedly from *a* to the completed part of the puzzle and back again as *a* is rotated. This leads to the rejection of the hypothesis that *a* can fit to *x*, and the development of the new idea that it might fit near *y*, which is then checked by consulting the picture. Similar 'aha' moments precede the move at (vi), again accompanied by much to-and-fro checking, and also before move (vii), although here the relevant profiles are now within 2° of each other, and there is a lull in the overt cross-checking seen elsewhere. Overall, this sequence and many others like it demonstrate the information-gathering function of eye movements and their close moment-by-moment relationship with the thought processes involved.

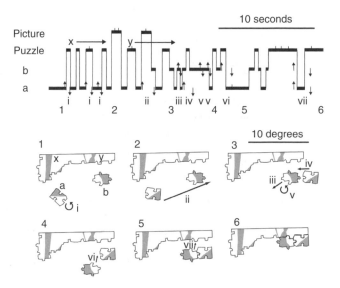

Fig. 4.10 Gaze movements during a 30 s excerpt from a jigsaw puzzle. Upper part shows the gaze shifts between two pieces (a and b), the part-completed puzzle, and the picture on the box. Numbers refer to the sketches below, and roman numerals to the seven movements of the pieces. All the gaze shifts are made with single saccades, and other saccades within each area are shown by short vertical lines. Hand contacts resulting in movement of the pieces are shown by upward (contact) and downward (release) arrows. The lower part of the figure shows details of the movements of the pieces. The movements shown refer to movements made between the current illustration and the next. More details in the text.

Drawing and sketching

The task of producing a picture is very different from simply looking at one, as described in Chapter 3. In drawing a portrait the artist has to acquire information from a sitter, formulate a line to be drawn and execute this on the drawing itself. There is thus a repeating sitter – drawing gaze cycle, with vision employed in different ways in each half cycle: a limited amount of information is collected from the sitter, which is then converted to a mark on the paper, checked by the eyes (Fig. 4.8c). In the first study of its kind Miall and Tchalenko (2001) recorded the eye and hand movements of the portrait artist Humphrey Ocean as he made first a pencil sketch of a model (12 minutes) and then a finished drawing (100 hours over 5 days). In both cases there was a very regular alternation between sitter and drawing, with 0.6 to 1.1 s spent on the sitter and rather longer (2–4 s) on the drawing. Miall and Tchalenko estimated that while drawing a line Ocean was capturing about 1.5 cm of detail per fixation on the model and that his visual information was being refreshed roughly every 2 s (Tchalenko et al., 2003).

Portrait sketching

A problem in trying to probe deeper into the way vision is used in the production of each line during a long drawing session is that the functions of each sitter-drawing cycle are not all the same. Sometimes a line is drawn, sometimes it is just checked, sometimes a line is altered or added to, and often, particularly in Henry Ocean's portrait, a line is simply rehearsed without the pencil contacting the paper. One way to remove this ambiguity is to make a fast sketch in which there is no checking, and a line is drawn every cycle. In our laboratory we asked a painter and art teacher, Nick Bodimeade, to make some portrait sketches for us as well as a longer more measured drawing, while wearing an eye tracker with a head-mounted scene camera that showed both the sitter and the drawings (Fig. 4.11). Figure 4.12 shows the whole sequence for one sketch, together with the 'average cycle' in which the various timings are indexed to the beginning of each drawn line. The principal findings were that a typical cycle lasted 1.7 s (35 cycles per minute), with 0.8 s on the sitter and 0.9 s on the sketch (Fig. 4.12b). On average the pen made contact with the paper about 0.1 s after gaze transferred to the sketch, and lasted for the time gaze remained on the sketch. However there was much variation, as Fig. 4.12a shows, and standard deviations for all these measures (relative to the beginning of the drawn line) were in the range 0.3 to 0.5 s, so the cycles were far from metronomic, and no event was absolutely synchronized to any other. It is worth noting here that sketching is essentially a copying task and can be compared with the block copying task of Ballard et al. (1992), described above (Fig. 4.9). The timings of the repetitive cycles, and the components within them, are remarkably similar (Figs 4.9 and 4.12).

It was possible to work out something of what was happening as the artist formulated his next line. Between one and four fixations were made on the sitter's face (mean 2.3), and by the last fixation the point to be addressed on the sketch had been selected. When gaze left the sitter, it was transferred accurately (<2° error) to the corresponding point on the sketch. However, this was not the point that the next line was to be drawn

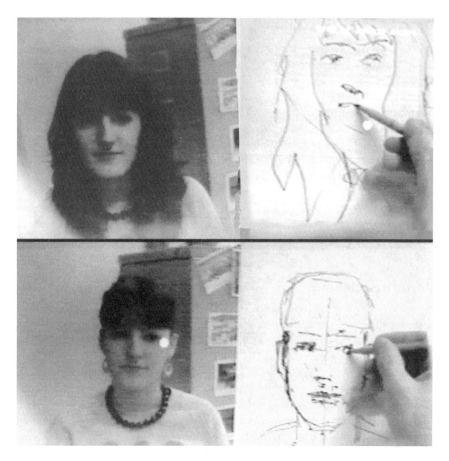

Fig. 4.11 Eye tracker views of sitter and sketch (top) with fixation on the sketch just below the pen, and sitter and measured drawing (below) with fixation on the sitter. Diameter of fixation spot is 1°. From a study by G. Baker and M.F. Land, in Land (2006).

from, but the point drawn *to*, that is, the end of the line (Fig. 4.13). This surprised us as well as the artist. It does, however, make some sense. In a sketch each line is a new entity, almost unrelated to the last. Thus the start of the next line must be determined by some process of internal selection by the artist. (This contrasts with the detailed drawings made by both Nick Bodimeade and Humphrey Ocean, where one line usually continued on from its predecessor, or was closely related to it spatially.) The course of the line and its end-point, however, have to be derived from features on the sitter, once the start of the line has been established.

The selection of the target point (i.e. the first fixation on the sketch and the end-point of the next line) occurred during the first fixation on the sitter, which was unusually short (~0.15 s). Subsequent fixations were longer (~0.28 s) but did not bring gaze closer to the target. Interestingly, when only one fixation was made on the sitter it was of long duration (~0.43 s), equal to the sum of the first and second fixations when two were made. We speculate that in this case it takes 0.15 s to make the decision that the gaze is already on target and that the function of the rest of that fixation and of subsequent fixations when more than one is made, is to obtain and store information about the form of the line to be drawn. The timing of the selection of the position of the start of the line is more problematic because the first sign of hand movement to the start point does not occur until about half a second after the end-point is established

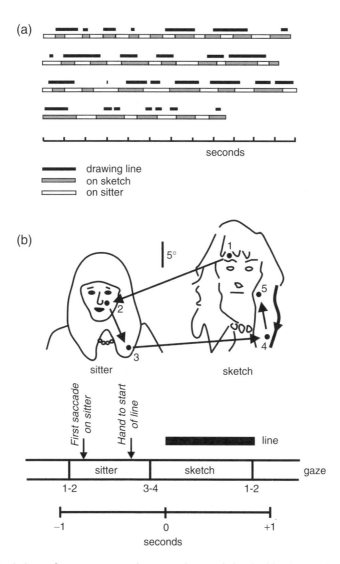

Fig. 4.12 Timings of eye movements between sitter and sketch. (a) All gaze alternations during the production of one sketch, and their relation to the periods of line drawing. (b) Average cycle, using data from (a); all events are indexed to the start of each drawn line (0 s). From Land (2006).

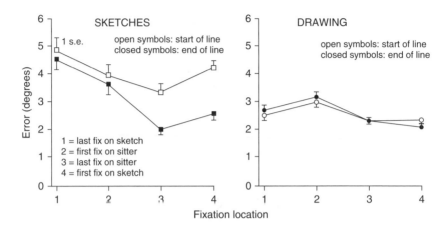

Fig. 4.13 Selection of the start and end of the next line to be drawn. The ordinates show the angular distance (error) between the current point of regard (fixation location, see Fig. 4.12b) and the start and end of the next line to be drawn. For the sketches (left) the angle to the end-point is halved between the first and last fixations on the sitter (2 and 3), but there is no corresponding decrease in the angle to the start point. For the measured drawing (right), where one line typically follows on from the next, there is a much smaller decrease in error angle, and no difference between the angles to the start and end-points of the line.

(Fig. 4.12b). However, it seems logical that the beginning and end of the line would be determined at about the same time. The last fixation on the sketch itself was a very poor predictor of either the start or end-point of the next line, so it seems that all decisions about the position and shape of the line to be drawn are made while gaze is on the sitter. This contrasts with the situation in the more measured drawing, where one line often followed directly from the last, and so fixations on the sitter were necessarily related to previous fixations on the drawing. In the case of the sketches there was no evidence from the eye movements of strategic planning beyond the next line.

When gaze returns from the sitter to the picture, the predominant behaviour is for gaze to follow the pen tip as it proceeds across the paper. This tracking is always saccadic and is not particularly precise. As Fig. 4.14 shows, gaze is usually maintained within a roughly elliptical area centred about $1°$ to the right of the pen tip, and about $2°$ below it in the case of the sketch, but level with it on the drawing. The reason for this difference is that in the sketch there are many long lines all drawn downwards, and because gaze tends to go first to the end (bottom) of the line to be drawn this means that the distribution of gaze positions is biased to a region below the pen. In the drawing there is a preponderance of short lines of different orientations, so this bias is not evident. In the drawing the area containing 90% of fixations is about $6°$ high and $4.5°$ wide, meaning that gaze is rarely more than $3°$ from the pen tip. For the sketch this area is slightly larger ($8.5°$ by $6.5°$) and displaced $2°$ downwards as just mentioned,

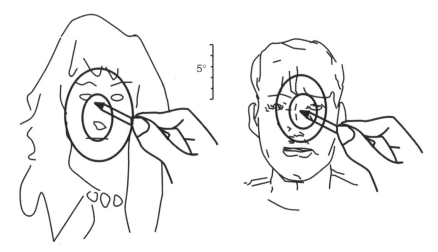

Fig. 4.14 Location of gaze, relative to the pen tip, when the artist is drawing lines on the sketches (left) and measured drawing (right). Generally, gaze follows the pen tip saccadically around the paper as each line is drawn: the particular positions of the pen shown here are only examples to indicate scale. Ellipses enclose areas containing 50% and 90% of all fixations, measured every 0.1 s during the execution of two 40 s sketches and one 4 minute drawing.

meaning that gaze may be as much as 6° from the pen tip, particularly at the start of long downward lines.

The fixations outside the 90% ellipses are scattered widely, up to 10° from the pen tip and appear to be different in nature from the more usual pen-following fixations. They seem to be excursions to other parts of the sketch or drawing, to check on some other feature. Occasionally the pen will follow gaze to this new position and begin a new line, indicating that some composition does take place on the drawing, without reference to the sitter. However, this is rare, and usually gaze returns to the vicinity of the pen tip.

Drawing lines

In a study of simple point-to-point line drawing, Tchalenko (2007) distinguished between two modes of eye–hand behaviour that he referred to as Close Pursuit and Target Locking. In Close Pursuit, gaze followed the pen saccadically as the line was drawn, but in Target Locking, gaze went directly to the end-point of the line, and the line was drawn to this new gaze location. In our study (above) most of the gaze movements on the sketch can be classified as Close Pursuit, and their function seems to be to check that the pen is properly executing the instructions devised while gaze was on the sitter. However, the first movement from sitter to sketch, especially where a long line is to be drawn, is of the Target Locking type, with gaze moving to, and in a sense marking, the new line's end-point. A similar distinction was made by Sailer et al.

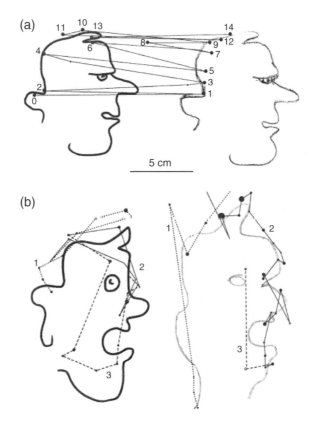

Fig. 4.15 (a) Direct copying, in which the location of each fixation on the original (left) is transferred to the corresponding point on the copy and information from the original is used to guide the next line segment. Only the fixations on the back of the head are shown. (b) Memory copying in which the original is scanned in a somewhat haphazard sequence of three ill-defined sections (1–3). When the original is removed the copy is made in three similar segments, with the eye following the pencil (Close Pursuit mode). Size of dots indicate fixation durations. From Tchalenko and Miall (2009).

(2005), discussed in Chapter 12. They studied the acquisition of a skill in which a novel mouse-like device was used to move a cursor from one target to another on a screen. In the early stages of learning how to use the device gaze followed the cursor, providing feedback about the accuracy of the hand movements. Later, however, when the motor skill had become proficient, gaze went straight to the next target with the cursor following behind. It seems that these two forms of visuo-motor control involving following and feedback provision on the one hand, and anticipatory targeting on the other, are likely to be common features of skilled eye–hand tasks.

In a subsequent study Tchalenko and Miall (2008) examined the strategies of beginner art students when copying more complex lines – outlines of caricature heads – in four different copying conditions. These were as follows: direct copying in which both original and copy were visible and side by side; direct blind copying in which the subject could not see the drawing hand and the copy; memory copying in which the original was memorized and then removed before drawing began; and non-specific memory copying in which the subject was told that this was a recognition rather than a copying task, before being asked to make a copy without the original. Direct copying produces the most accurate results, with the eye alternating rhythmically between the pencil and corresponding section of the original (Fig. 4.15a). This is a similar strategy to the portrait sketch in Fig. 4.12. In direct blind copying the hand draws the line in a continuous movement while the eye moves along the line on the original in Target Locking mode, leading the hand. The drawing is accurate in details of shape, but the overall scale changes across the copy. In memory copying the eye covers the original in one or more rapid passes with fixations linked only approximately to the line. The copy, in the absence of the original, is drawn in a series of consecutive segments (1–3 on Fig. 4.15b) with the hand leading the eye in Close Pursuit mode. Shape reproduction and spatial positioning are fair but not as good as in direct copying. In non-specific memory copying the initial view of the original is made looking at the central region rather than the outline. When making the copy the hand draws the components of the head separately, with the eye only very loosely linked to hand position. The accuracy of both shape and spatial positioning is poor.

From these observations Tchalenko and Miall (2008) concluded that the drawing of shape is the result of a visuo-motor mapping developed while perceiving the original, before looking back to the drawing surface. Accurate spatial positioning, however, requires vision of the drawing surface while drawing the line. Conventional accounts of drawing assume that what is stored when looking at the original is a mental image of the picture element and that this image is only converted to a motor action at the time of drawing the line. In Tchalenko and Miall's scheme, which they refer to as the *Drawing Hypothesis*, no mental image is stored, and each element of the drawing is achieved by a direct translation of visual information to motor command. When some kind of evocation of an image is required, as in memory copying, the results are much worse than when copying is direct. Drawing in this direct mode requires very little memory, and this conclusion is entirely in line with other results, particularly those of Ballard et al. (1992, 1995) described above.

In a companion study to that just described Miall et al. (2009) performed a functional imaging study of drawing cartoon faces. Normal participants were scanned while they viewed simple line-drawings and then after a brief retention period drew them either blind from memory or when the cartoon was again visible but not the drawing hand. They found that face-sensitive areas of the lateral occipital cortex and fusiform gyrus were strongly activated while viewing the cartoon. During the retention interval there was no activation of these areas – arguing against the maintenance of a visual image. However, during drawing itself these areas became again active, even during blind copying, implying a continued role for the cortical visual system in guiding motor action. 'Dorsal stream' regions were also active – the posterior parietal and premotor areas as well as parts of the cerebellum. In memory copying the left inferior parietal area and the anterior cingulate were more active than when the original was visible, suggesting that they have a planning and monitoring function not required during direct copying.

Summary

1. Silent reading involves a stereotypical pattern of saccades that move the eyes about 7 characters at a time. How long we spend in each fixation depends on linguistic factors such as processing difficulty.

2. In tasks such as reading aloud, typing, and sight-reading music information is taken in by the eyes in a systematic series of fixations but is processed continuously and emitted as motor output about 1 s later.

3. In tasks involving copying there is an alternation between gathering information in one fixation and translating it into motor output at a subsequent fixation, often in a different location. Copying tasks involve a minimal use of memory, with information gathered just before its use is required.

Chapter 5

Domestic tasks

Throughout their history humans have manipulated objects. Early tools and weapons were fashioned from bone, horn, and stone. Shelters required the bending and shaping of wood. Animal skins were dressed for clothing, and eventually plant and animal fibres were woven into cloth. When fire was tamed the skills of cooking began to be developed. Humans, more than other primates, have specialized in allying vision to action in the development of skills for making life more secure and comfortable. Modern activities such as food preparation, carpentry, or gardening typically involve a series of different visually guided actions, rather loosely strung together by a 'script'. In this chapter we examine the way in which vision is used to make such activities possible. We are particularly interested in what information the eyes supply to the hands, when they provide it, and how they acquire it.

In the kitchen: making tea and sandwiches

Scan paths and actions

Land et al. (1999) studied the eye movements of subjects while they made cups of tea. When made with a teapot, this simple task takes 3 to 5 minutes and involves about 45 separate acts, where an 'act' is defined as 'the movement of an object from one place to another or a change in the state of an object' (Schwartz et al., 1991, p. 384). Land et al. (1999) used a head-mounted eye camera that recorded foveal direction onto a video of the scene taken from eye position and a separate synchronized scene camera recording the movements of the subject's hands and body. Fig. 5.1 shows the same scene (putting a sweetener into the mug) from the scene camera (a) and the eye camera (b).

Figure 5.2 shows three examples of the fixations made during the first 15 s of the task. The subjects first examine the kettle, then pick it up and move towards the sink while removing the lid from the kettle, place the kettle in the sink and turn on the tap, then watch the water as it fills the kettle. There are impressive similarities both in the form of the scan path and in the numbers of fixations required for each component of the action. In each case there is only one fixation that is not directly relevant to the task (the sink tidy and the trays to the left of the kettle and to the left of the sink). The two fixations to the right of the sink in JB's record correspond to the place where he put down the lid. Other minor differences concern the timing of the lid removal and details of the way the taps are viewed, but overall the similarities of the two records suggest that the eye movement strategies of different individuals performing similar tasks are highly convergent.

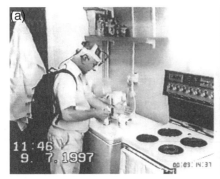 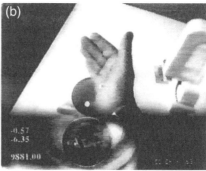

Fig. 5.1 (a) MFL in the kitchen wearing the eye camera and about to put a sweetener into a mug. (b) The same scene viewed from the eye camera, showing the sweetener on the hand and gaze directed into the mug. Note that the eye camera reverses the scene left to right. From Land et al. (1999).

Two principal conclusions can be drawn from these scan paths. First, saccades are made almost exclusively to objects involved in the task, even though there are plenty of other objects around to grab the eye. Second, the eyes usually deal with one object at a time. The time spent on each object corresponds roughly to the duration of the manipulation of that object and may involve a number of fixations on different parts of the object.

In a parallel study Mary Hayhoe examined the eye movements of students making peanut butter and jelly (jam for readers in the United Kingdom) sandwiches (Hayhoe, 2000; Hayhoe et al., 2003), a task that takes about 2 minutes. They found the same attachment of gaze to task-related objects and the same near absence of saccades to irrelevant objects. Two versions of the table top layout were presented to the students, one with just the objects and materials needed for the task – knife, peanut butter, bread, and so on – and another with a more cluttered layout containing other food items, forks, and irrelevant tools such as pliers. In the first (simple) layout there were irrele-vant items in the background, but these only attracted about 2% of the fixations, although in the cluttered layout the irrelevant objects attracted 20% of fixations. Of particular interest was an observation on the cluttered table before and after the task had started. Before starting, relevant and irrelevant objects were fixated roughly equally, but after the task had begun the proportion of fixations on the irrelevant objects fell from 48% to 16%. Clearly the execution of the task had made gaze direc-tion much more selective. Furthermore, Hayhoe (2000) commented that 'the sequence of fixations and reaches were almost identical for four subjects despite the unspecific nature of the instructions' (p. 45). As in Fig. 5.2, it seems that different individuals evolve convergent eye–hand strategies, at least in straightforward tasks.

Timing of movements and actions

In the tea-making study it was initially difficult to work out how the records of body movements, eye movements, and manipulations fitted together in time. We had to

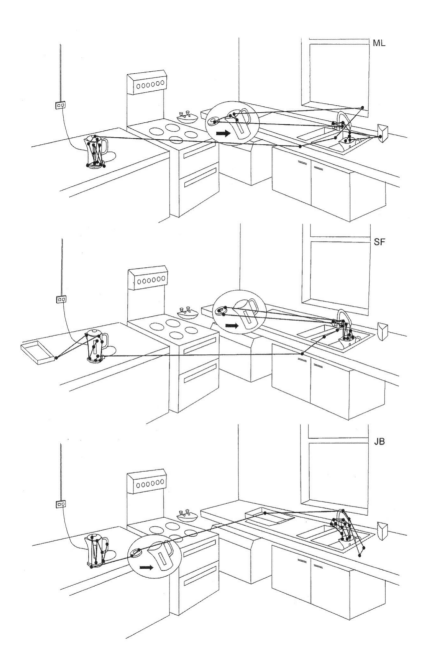

Fig. 5.2 Fixations made by three subjects while filling a kettle prior to making a cup of tea. The records last approximately 15 s. The subjects first examine the kettle, pick it up, and walk to the sink while removing the lid. They then turn on one tap, place the kettle in the sink, and watch the water stream as it fills the kettle. From Land et al. (1999).

resort to drawing out each 4-minute sequence on a roll of paper as a time-line, recording the beginnings and ends of all acts and all the visual fixations that accompanied them. This is shown in Fig. 5.3a for a 10 s sequence; the record of the entire 4-minute sequence was 12 m (40 ft) long. These cartoons were subsequently tidied up to give a more concise account of the sequences (Fig. 5.3b). What emerged from this exercise was that for most component acts, there was a definite temporal pattern. This involved first, a movement of the whole body towards the next object in the overall sequence; second, a gaze movement to that object; and finally the initiation of manipulation of the object by the hands. To work out the timings of these elements we needed to establish appropriate time markers. Even though trunk movements usually began each sequence, their start was often hard to define precisely, and in many cases they were not made because no shift in body position was required. We found that the best temporal marker to use to define the beginning of each act was the saccade that was made when the eyes left one object and moved on to the next, typically with a combined head-and-eye movement. This provided a 'defining moment' against which the timing of the other components of the action could be measured. Thus these 'next object' saccades could be used to 'chunk' the task as a whole into separate 'object-related actions' (which might consist of more than one act on the same object). They acted as time markers to relate the eye movements to movements of the body and manipulations by the hands. In this way the different acts in the task could be pooled, to get an idea of the sequence of events in a 'typical' act. The results of this are shown in Fig. 5.4. Not all acts could be included in these histograms because they involved waiting for something to happen – the kettle to fill, for example – which meant that the eyes tended to explore other parts of the room not relevant to the current action. On a few occasions the two hands were engaged in different acts at the same time, and these too were excluded.

At first it seemed surprising that it was the body as a whole that made the first movement in an object related action: that the trunk should receive the 'new instructions' first, rather than the eyes. In fact the reason for this was often obvious: when the next object in the overall sequence was on a different work surface, a turn or a few steps were required before it could be reached with an eye movement. As Fig. 5.4 shows the first saccade was made about half a second after the start of the trunk movement, and half a second after that the first movements of the hands towards the object occurred. Thus the eyes nearly always led the hands, presumably because manipulation required information from vision before it could begin. An interesting finding was that at the end of each object-related action, the eyes moved on to the next object about half a second before manipulation was complete. This means that the information that the eyes had supplied was still available in a store until the motor system required it.

Part of the reason why it had been so difficult to see the temporal pattern of the trunk, eye, and hand movements in the first place was that these movements were not simultaneous but staggered over a second or more. Equally important, however, was that these lags were quite variable. For the three subjects the standard deviations of the lags were in the range 0.6 to 1.6 s, rather larger than the mean lag times, which only ranged between 0.4 and 0.7 s. Evidently the brain is tolerant of asynchronies of up to

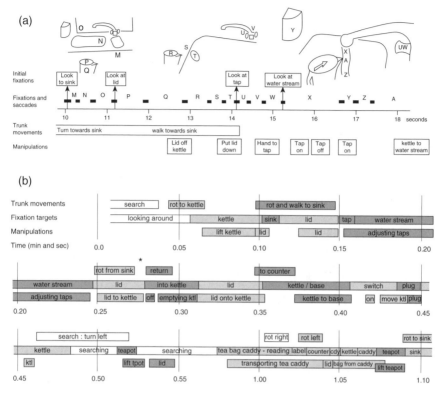

Fig. 5.3 (a) Copy of the original 'cartoon' record of the latter part of the first sequence shown in Fig. 5.2. The locations of the different fixations are shown on the sketches and their timings above the time scale. Trunk movements and manipulations are shown below the scale. Arrows indicate the transitions from one object to the next and mark the beginnings of new object-related actions. Note sketches come from the raw video images and are left–right reversed compared with Fig. 5.2. (b) Cleaned up version of the first 70 s of the first record in Fig. 5.2, showing the beginnings and ends of periods of body movement, gaze on single objects, and manipulations. Note the stepped body-gaze-manipulation sequences, especially at 0.05 and 0.35 s. The asterisk marks a verbal intervention ('You're not making tea for the army'), which seemed to synchronize actions. The shading is used only to distinguish successive actions. Sequences not linked to actions are unshaded.

at least 2 s in the timing of the components of an action. Similarly large variations in eye–hand lead times are seen during portrait drawing (Chapter 4), so this apparent temporal sloppiness may be a feature of all self-paced activities.

In Hayhoe's study of sandwich making gaze also led manipulation, although by a rather shorter interval (Hayhoe et al., 2003). This difference is possibly attributable to the fact that the sandwich making was a sit-down task involving only movements of the arms. Two other differences that may have the same cause are the existence of

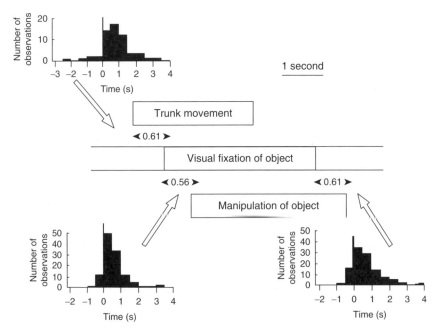

Fig. 5.4 Average relative timings of trunk movements, fixation on particular objects (usually involving several individual fixations), and manipulation of those objects. Fixations with long waiting periods (e.g. for the kettle to fill) have been excluded, and the data represent 94 object-related actions from three subjects. The typical duration of the visual fixation component was 3.04 s. Trunk movements precede visual fixation, and fixations precede the beginning of arm or hand movement each by about 0.6 s. Gaze leaves objects about 0.6 s before manipulation is complete. From Land et al. (1999).

more short duration (<120 ms) fixations than in the tea-making study and the presence of more 'unguided' reaching movements (13%) mostly concerned with the setting down of objects.

Another study that is relevant here is that of Johansson et al. (2001) who studied with great precision the relationships of eye and hand movements in a simple repeated task of lifting a bar to touch a target switch while avoiding a projecting obstacle (Fig. 5.5). As in the tea and sandwich making, subjects almost exclusively fixated the landmarks that were crucial for the control of the task. These included the grasp site on the bar, the target, and the support surface onto which the bar was returned. The obstacle was also fixated, although this was not obligatory. Gaze reached each landmark (to within a 3° radius zone) well before contact was made or, in the case of the obstacle, before gaze passed the closest point. These lead times were surprisingly long, gaze reaching the grasp site almost 2 s before finger contact, although this was more like 0.5 s when passing the obstacle. Interestingly, the time that gaze left a landmark coincided closely with the time that contact was made suggesting that gaze waited just long enough to monitor completion of the sub-task.

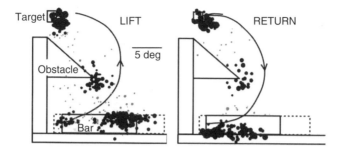

Fig. 5.5 Accuracy of fixation in a task in which a bar is lifted past an obstacle to make contact with a target, and then set down again. All fixations are shown for nine subjects. Black dots are fixations within 3° of one of the landmarks (bar, obstacle, target, set-down point), grey dots are fixations outside these regions. Area of each dot indicates fixation duration. From Johansson et al. (2001).

Saccade amplitude and timing statistics

A striking difference between the eye movements made during active tasks such as food preparation and sedentary tasks such as reading was the size of saccades. Typical saccades when reading a book have amplitudes of about 1.3°, whereas during tea making the average amplitude was 19° (Fig. 5.6). Presumably this difference is related to the scale of the objects under scrutiny. On the retina the dimensions of objects contacted during tea making ranged from 1° (taps, switch, sweetener box) to 20° (kettle, teapot). This compares with 0.2° or less for letters on a page at reading distance. Saccade size is known to scale with letter size in reading and with object size in scene viewing (Wartburg et al., 2007), so this result simply shows that this scaling ability of the saccadic system extends to ordinary objects as well. In both tea making and sandwich making, there was a clear distinction between 'within-object' saccades made during single object-related actions, and 'between-object' saccades when gaze moved on to the next sub-task. The former had mean amplitudes of about 8° in both studies (Fig. 5.6a and b), but the latter were much larger: up to 30° during sandwich making on a restricted table top and 90° in tea making in the less restricted kitchen (Fig. 5.6c and d; Land and Hayhoe, 2001).

The distribution of inter-saccade intervals (the time from the start of one saccade to the start of the next) in the tea making task was unremarkable, with a mean value of 497 ms and a mode at 300 ms (3 subjects) for the tea making. The mean fixation duration in sandwich making was 398 ms (Hayhoe et al., 2003), but allowing 40 ms for saccade duration this gives a mean inter-saccade interval of 438 ms, only slightly shorter than in tea making. However the modal value for fixation durations was very much shorter, about 120 ms. This resulted from considerable numbers of very short (<100 ms) fixations, seen in all subjects. Hayhoe et al. attributed them to saccades that are part of pre-programmed sequences, but quite why they were not seen to anything like the same extent in the tea making study remains a mystery. In both studies the tails of the fixation distributions were long, with many fixations lasting more than 1 s.

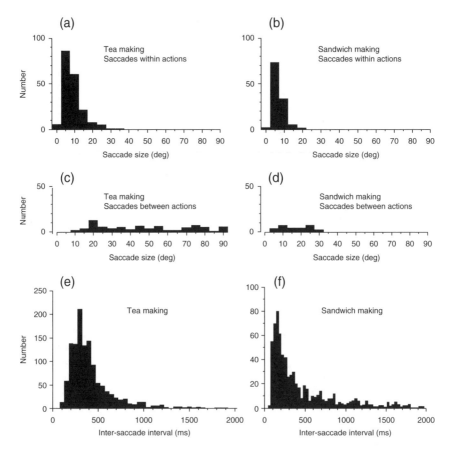

Fig. 5.6 (a) to (d) Sizes of saccades made within actions and between actions in tea making (total for three subjects) and sandwich making (total for seven subjects). From Land and Hayhoe (2001) (e) and (f) Distribution of inter-saccade intervals during tea making (data from Land et al., 1999) and for sandwich making (data from Hayhoe et al., 2003). The original sandwich data were for fixation durations, and these have been converted to inter-saccade intervals by adding 40 ms to each x-value.

This can be explained by the long times spent monitoring such extended processes as spreading peanut butter, filling a kettle, pouring tea, and so on.

Saccade targeting accuracy

Can we use data from natural behaviour to estimate the accuracy with which we target objects with the fovea? From what we have learnt about the precision with which the eye can target specific portions of a word during reading, or return to specific notes in a piece of music after looking down to the keyboard (Chapter 4), it would seem logical to suppose that targeting by the foveae is very precise. Furthermore, when isolated targets are presented in laboratory-based paradigms, saccades that bring the eye close to but not onto the target are typically corrected (Becker, 1991). For targets presented some way into the periphery, the initial saccade tends to be hypometric, undershooting by about 10%. When this occurs a small corrective saccade will usually follow so that the foveae end up brought to bear rather precisely on the isolated target. The existence of corrective saccades suggests precise targeting: why else would there be a need to correct a saccade that had already brought gaze close to the target? Is the same degree of precision seen in saccade targeting within a complex natural environment?

The accuracy of saccade targeting is hard to estimate during natural behaviour, or indeed when viewing any complex scene, because it is usually not clear exactly which part of an object was being targeted. The question of accuracy when viewing complex photographic scenes has been approached by looking for evidence of corrective saccades. If these are present in the data then this might imply that some degree of precise targeting is necessary. Tatler and Vincent (2008) did find evidence for a distinct population of saccades that fit the normal characteristics of corrective saccades: they were of very small amplitude, continued in the same direction as the previous saccade, and were preceded by a very brief fixation pause. However, the role of these saccades is unclear, and the evidence is not sufficient to allow estimates of saccade targeting precision.

When viewing a complex scene without an active motor task, it is very hard to determine what was the 'target' of any saccade. However, in a natural task such as making tea, the field of possible targets can be narrowed down given the intimate link between action and vision. During object-related actions when making both tea and sandwiches saccades had average amplitudes of 8°. This implies that no viewed target was likely to be more than 4° from a fixation point. This is about six times larger than the equivalent accuracy in reading. Other estimates of accuracy are between these values. Johansson et al. (2001), in a bar raising task where targets locations were well defined, estimated the sizes of circles that enclosed 90% of fixation points for nine subjects (Fig. 5.5). For the target object and the bar tip this circle was 3 to 4° in diameter, implying a maximum target eccentricity of 1.5 to 2°. They regarded 3° as the diameter of the 'functional fovea' for this particular task.

These estimates of how accurately we place our foveae are perhaps much sloppier than might be expected. Of course, it is likely that the accuracy with which we target relevant entities in the environment is a function of the size of the target. Nevertheless, if there are situations during natural scene viewing in which targeting is so loose, this raises serious concerns over the way saccade target selection in natural scenes is evaluated (Chapter 3). We described in Chapter 3 the standard technique for assessing what factors may underlie fixation selection. Almost all these are based on characterizing what is at the centre of fixation, usually within a maximum of 0.5 to 1° from the centre. If the relevant features or objects only need to be within 2 to 4° of fixation, then we are not only failing to capture the true nature of target selection, but we are probably overestimating the importance of features lying closest to the fixation point. This raises the obvious question of whether we can really learn about how we decide where to sample in the visual environment by studying only what is on the fovea.

The functions of single fixations

During tea making Land et al. (1999) found that about one-third of all fixations could be clearly linked to subsequent actions. These were mainly the first fixations to new objects. The remaining two-thirds were made after an action had been initiated so that although they may well have had similar functions in guiding action, it was less clear how they were specifically related to the ongoing motor behaviour.

Of particular interest in this context was a subject, AI, who had almost no eye movements because of fibrosis of the eye muscles, and who made head saccades instead (Findlay and Gilchrist, 2003; Land et al., 2001). These gave her an almost bird-like appearance when looking around. Head saccades are both slow and energetically expensive, and in executing the same tea-making task as normal subjects, AI made only a third as many of these head saccades as normal subjects made eye saccades. As AI made tea with normal speed and competence, the implication is that the rest of us make more saccadic eye movements than we really need. An example of this apparent profligacy is shown in Fig. 5.7, when the subject was waiting for the kettle to boil. Perhaps when there is little else to do, the oculomotor system reverts to some more primitive function, such as keeping the image refreshed.

Land et al. (1999) found that the functions of fixations could be classified into four categories, which were designated as locating, directing, guiding, and checking (Fig. 5.8). Locating fixations are concerned with establishing the locations of objects, even though there was no associated motor activity at the time of the fixation. In a hand-washing task Pelz and Canoza (2001) also found a number of 'look-ahead' fixations that anticipated future actions, and these are consistent with this category. They will

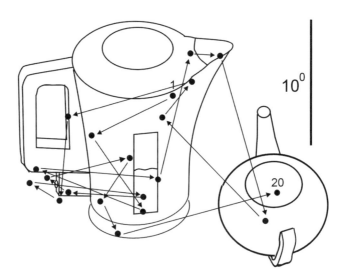

Fig. 5.7 Sequence of 20 fixations made over a 14 s period while waiting for the kettle to boil. Fixations cluster very loosely around the switch at the left, the gauge in the centre, and the spout. The average saccade amplitude is 7.2°. It is not clear in this case what is gained by changing fixation so many times.

be considered later in the chapter. *Directing* fixations accompany either a movement of the hand to contact an object (in which case the object is fixated) or the movement of hand and object to a particular position (when the set-down position is fixated). Typically only a single fixation is involved, and the eye usually moves away from the object or set-down point just before the hand reaches it. Thus visual feedback is not involved in the last stage of the act. It seems that the main function of the directing fixation is to provide fovea-centred goal-position information to guide the arm (the transformations involved here are discussed in Chapter 10). *Guiding* fixations are concerned with manipulations involving more than one object, for example, a kettle and its lid. Here the objects have to be guided relative to each other so that they dock in an appropriate way. Most tool use is of this nature (e.g. spanner and nut, hammer and nail). It is more complicated than simple directing and usually involves a number of fixations that alternate between the objects, and the action is normally completed under visual control. Some guided actions may involve more than two objects, for example, knife, bread, butter. *Checking* fixations determine when some condition is met, for example, the kettle is full, the water boils, the top is off the bottle. These checking operations may require the eye to dwell on some appropriate region of an object, either in one long fixation or in a series of repeated fixations. When the specified condition is met, a new action is triggered. For example, when the kettle is full the tap is turned off. It is interesting to note that there are some things that are rarely if ever fixated during sequences of this kind. The hands themselves are never fixated, and once objects have been acquired by the hands they are not fixated either. In their study, Johansson et al. (2001) also noted that subjects never fixated either their hands or the moving bar. The implication of these surprising findings is that vision is a scarce and valuable resource

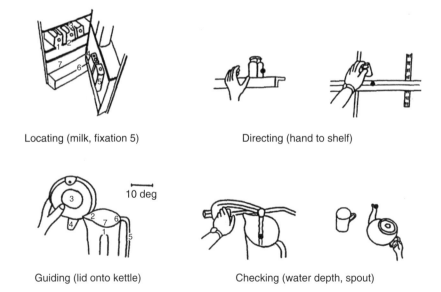

Locating (milk, fixation 5)   Directing (hand to shelf)

Guiding (lid onto kettle)   Checking (water depth, spout)

Fig. 5.8 General functions of fixations during tea making. Most of the initial fixations on each new object fell into one of these four categories. From Land et al. (1999).

and is disengaged from action as soon as the task can be delegated to the haptic or proprioceptive senses.

It is clear that this classification, although appropriate here, does not fit all types of information gathering for which the eyes are employed. In particular a fixation may simply establish a particular attribute of an object. Thus in the block-copying study of Ballard et al. (1992), shown in Fig. 4.9, the logic of the task dictates that the first fixation on the model establishes the colour of a block, which is then used to locate a similar block for use in the copy. The next fixation on the model is used for another purpose, to check the block's location. In sketching and other copying tasks one or more fixations acquire the form of a feature so that it can be reproduced (Fig. 4.12). Continuous tasks such as reading text or music are also rather different, as each fixation acquires a small part of an information stream that is then compounded internally with those preceding and succeeding it to produce a sequence that has meaning.

Look-ahead (locating) fixations

As mentioned above, some of the fixations on objects in natural tasks are not followed immediately by manipulation of the object, but may anticipate the use of that object at some future time (Hayhoe et al., 2003; Mennie et al., 2007; Pelz and Canoza, 2001). The significance of these 'look-ahead' or locating fixations is twofold. First, they imply that action plans sometimes start to be formed well in advance of the act itself rather than simply being 'taken off the shelf' at the time of execution, as the 'just-in-time' strategy might suggest (see Chapter 4). Second, they indicate that not all information is lost when a saccade is made and that there is some degree of trans-saccadic memory for the location of objects (Chapter 10). In the Mennie et al. study, look-ahead fixations preceded reach-and-grasp actions during a model-assembly task in about 20% of occasions, and they occurred an average of 3 s before the act itself. Mennie et al. found some evidence that look-ahead fixations do affect subsequent operations when the target object is refixated. Interestingly a look-ahead fixation actually increased subsequent eye–hand latency from 230 ms to 353 ms. They interpret this as a facilitation effect on refixation, with the eyes making saccades earlier in the eye–hand movement sequence but with no effect of the look-ahead fixation on the timing of the hand movement itself. There was also an improvement in the accuracy of refixation saccades. It thus seems that look-ahead fixations do improve both the timing and accuracy of subsequent object-directed eye movements, although not necessarily the reaching movements themselves.

What information is and is not acquired during task performance?

Direct observation of eye movements during natural behaviour can, as we have seen, give a reasonably clear idea of what information is being provided by the eyes at each stage of the task. What these studies cannot provide, however, is an account of how extensive this information is. Is it strictly restricted to the immediate demands of the task, or are other more general features of the local environment picked up at the same time? Mary Hayhoe and her colleagues have studied this question using a virtual reality set-up in which subjects perform realistic tasks but in which changes can be made to the objects in those tasks either during saccades, when the subject is temporary blind, or when the object is in plain view.

In one paradigm (Droll et al., 2005; Triesch et al., 2003) the task was to sort bricks of two different sizes. This involved picking up each brick and placing it onto one of two 'conveyor belts' (Fig. 5.9). In 10% of the moves the size of the brick was changed between pick-up and put-down. This move was invariably accompanied by a saccade, and eye movements were monitored to determine whether the change coincided with a saccade. The question was, 'Under what circumstances will the change be noticed?' The subjects were not told specifically to look for size changes but were instructed to report if anything odd happened. There were three conditions: (1) 'Pick up the bricks in front to back order and place them on the closer conveyor belt'. Brick size is irrelevant here for both pick-up and put-down decisions. (2) 'Pick up the tall bricks first and put them on the closer conveyor belt. Then, pick up the smaller bricks and also put them onto the closer conveyer belt.' For this condition, size is important during the pick-up phase but not the put-down. (3) 'Pick up the large bricks first and put them on the closer conveyer belt. Then pick up the small bricks and put them on the distant conveyor belt.' Here brick size is relevant for both pick-up and put-down decisions.

The first conclusion was that the number of times a size change was reported at the time increases from about 2% in Condition 1 to 20% in Condition 2 and to 45% in Condition 3. This suggests that changes are noticed in proportion to their importance in the performance of the task. When they are not relevant, the changes are simply not noticed. Remarkably, there were even occasions when the size change was made while the subjects were looking directly at the brick, but nevertheless they failed to notice or report the change. Similar detection failures during fixation have also been seen in audiences at magic shows when their attention has been deliberately misdirected by the magician (Chapter 9). The second conclusion was that when a change was noticed, fixation times on the brick increased by about 300 ms, irrespective the condition being tested. Unnoticed changes produced no increase in fixation times. These extended fixations must have been the result of the engagement of attention, not the changes in the retinal image. The overall conclusion of the Triesch et al. (2003) is summed up by

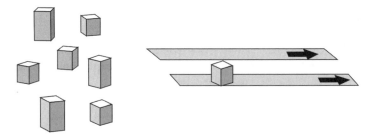

Fig. 5.9 Virtual work space for the brick sorting task. Subjects sort bricks of two different heights onto two 'conveyor belts' (right) according to different rules that vary the points at which brick height is relevant to the task. Based on Triesch et al. (2003).

the title, 'What you see is what you need' of their article. We can probably infer from this that during the performance of a task, very little visual information is taken in that is not flagged up as being of immediate use.

Shinoda et al. (2001) had already reached a similar conclusion in a virtual reality study of the detection of Stop signs while driving. Stop signs were rarely detected when they appeared mid-block – where they would not be expected – but were invariably noticed at intersections. Thus even highly salient stimuli were detected only if they were relevant to the task at the appropriate time. They proposed 'that vision involves the dynamic application of specialized routines initiated by the observer, whose current goals specify the information that is extracted from a scene and the time it is extracted' (p. 3544).

Finding the right information for eye and limb movements

In driving, ball games, and many everyday activities the main function of vision is to supply the motor system with the various kinds of information it needs to carry out the task it is engaged in. In most cases this involves directing the foveae to some specific region of the environment, which, at the time, contains the most useful information. Thus in driving it may be the nearside lane marking one moment and a road sign the next (Chapter 7); in cricket it may be the bowler's arm or the bounce point of the ball (Chapter 8); and in food preparation it may be the handle of the kettle or the carton of milk. Clearly, before it can help the motor system, the gaze and visual systems need to know when to look, where to look, and what to look for. We have seen that, for familiar tasks, there is surprisingly little uncertainty about this: the eyes go to the appropriate object, in the right place, usually during the second before the associated action begins. Extensive searches are very uncommon in familiar tasks. However, finding the next object in the action sequence is far from simple. The object must be recognized either when it is in the visual periphery or after the fovea has fixated it. In either case an appropriate recognition template or 'search image' must be activated. Positional information can come from two sources: memory and immediate vision. In many instances, during tea making, a subject would make an appropriate turn to the location of an object that was out of sight on the other side of the room, and it is a good assumption that the object's position was established in an earlier phase of the task (in a 'locating' or 'look-ahead' fixation). Often locating an object was clearly a two-stage process. For example, there were several occasions when an object was fixated a minute or more prior to its ultimate use, and when it was time to fetch the object, a 'memory' saccade took gaze to within 10 to 20° of it. This was then followed by one or two visually guided saccades, finally resulting in fixation (Land et al., 1999). There were also many examples of single accurate saccades to objects up to 50° away, suggesting that visual recognition could be effective even in the far periphery: at larger angles the initial saccade was nearly always followed by one or more secondary saccades, implying a two-stage process. Object acquisition thus involves a complex interplay between spatial memory, direct vision, and object recognition.

The control of events involved in an object-related action

In the analysis of tea making we defined a unit of behaviour, the 'object-related action', as a basic building block of goal-directed action sequences. Whilst not claiming that this is the only mode of visuo-motor activity, it nevertheless provides a useful way of parsing a great deal of complex action. Figure 5.10 is an attempt to put into an information flow diagram the various operations that must occur during the performance of an object-related action. Its structure is based on the scheme in Fig. 1.1. We assume that the 'script' of the task provides a succession of 'schemas' that define successive actions (Norman and Shallice, 1986). These are roughly equivalent to the 'routines' discussed by Hayhoe (2000). Each schema specifies the location and identity of the object to be dealt with, the action to be performed on it, and the monitoring required to establish that the action has been satisfactorily executed and completed. First, the gaze control system is instructed to locate the next object. At the same time, the visual system is primed to identify the object and the motor system informed about which action to perform. If the object is initially out of the field of view, the first action in locating it will be a movement of the body involving the trunk and feet. Although it is performed by the lower body, this movement is functionally part of gaze control, which is why in Fig. 5.10 the command is routed through the gaze control system. The eyes and head can then be directed to the object, either from memory or with direct input from vision, or a combination of the two. Vision then confirms that the right object has been found. If this process fails to locate the object then the gaze system can go into a repetitive search mode until it is found. The hands can then be directed to the object either under direct visual control or via coordinates already obtained by the gaze system. The manipulative operations of the hands can then begin, and the action is monitored and guided by the visual system, in conjunction with touch and proprioception. When the action is complete a further action may be performed on the same

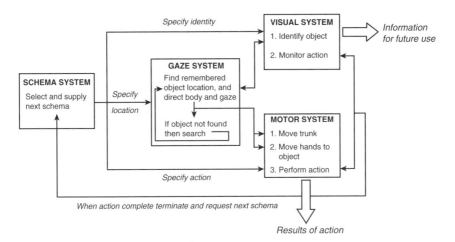

Fig. 5.10 Information flow diagram of the events involved in an object related action. Description in the text. From Land (2009).

object (e.g. lift milk jug, pour milk into cup, set down jug), or if no further actions are involved the schema system is informed, the present set of instructions is abandoned, and the next schema in the script is initiated. Look-ahead fixations do not involve immediate action, and these are represented in Fig. 5.10 by the 'Information for future use' arrow from the visual system.

Errors and schema selection

The question of what releases the next schema in a task sequence is unresolved. At one extreme this could just be a matter of supplying it from a pre-determined list or script. At the other it could be triggered in a bottom-up way by the sight of the next object that fits with the goal of the immediate task. Action sequences in food preparation tasks are generally not rigid, and the same person may perform slightly differently on different occasions. Parts of the task are more constrained than others: it does not matter much whether the sweetener goes into the mug before or after the milk, but it does matter that the water goes into the kettle before it is switched on. Errors are rare with normal subjects but become common with damage to the frontal lobes caused either by stroke or closed head injury (Schwartz, 2006). The most common error is *omission* where a step is left out of the usual sequence, implying that a schema has failed to activate. *Sequence* errors, such as spreading the jam before the butter, are also common, as are *substitutions* in which the wrong implement is used, for example, toothbrush for hairbrush. It is rare for individual acts themselves to be performed incompetently: the weak link seems to be at the schema selection stage.

Attempts have been made to model the process of schema selection. One such model (Cooper 2002; Cooper and Shallice, 2000) emulated making a cup of instant coffee and preparing a child's lunch box. Their schema structure is hierarchical, with goals (make sandwich) activating sub-goals (get bread) and ultimately individual actions (unseal bread bag, remove slices, etc.). The schemas representing these lowest-level actions are initiated when certain preconditions are met and terminated when post-conditions are met. For 'remove slices' the precondition is 'bread-bag open' and the post-condition is 'bread on table'. Thus this system involves both top-down activation from goals (or parent schemas) and the satisfying of preconditions by visual triggers. It has the merit of flexibility – for example, if the bread is already on the table the preceding schemas will not be activated and those steps are left out. By varying the amount of noise in the schema network, it was also possible to reproduce at least some of the errors (notably omissions) seen in patients with brain injury.

Summary

1. Extended activities such as food preparation consist of sequences of separate actions each involving different patterns of co-ordination between the gaze-directing, motor, and visual systems.

2. Successful production of such behaviours needs the right actions to be executed in the right order, and this requires high-level representation of the overall task.

Chapter 6

Locomotion on foot

At the heart of most of our natural behaviour is the requirement to move the body from one location to the next, from taking a few shuffling steps around a little kitchen, to a walk in the countryside. In this chapter we will consider not only the role of vision in helping us to locomote through the environment and avoid hazards but also how the eyes, head, and body work together to get our high acuity foveae to where we need them in the world to best serve our behaviour.

Control of stepping

Guiding footfalls

When walking on uneven terrain visual information is needed for placing future footfalls. Under these conditions, obstruction of the lower part of the field of view forces subjects to pitch the head downwards and proceed more cautiously (Marigold and Patla, 2008). An obvious question is how far walkers look ahead, to obtain the information they need for a safe footfall. This was addressed by Patla and Vickers (2003) who required their subjects to step on a series of irregularly spaced 'footprints' over a 10 m walkway. They found that subjects fixated the footprints on average two steps ahead, or between 0.8 and 1 s in time. We have repeated these findings in Sussex using a damaged pavement on which the subjects were instructed not to tread on the cracks (Fig. 6.1). We used an eye tracker with a second synchronized camera directed at the feet. For five subjects the average number of steps between footfall and the nearest fixation to it was 1.91 (s.d. 0.53), and the average time lag 1.11 s (s.d. 0.46 s), very much in line with Patla and Vickers' result. As can be seen from Fig. 6.1 there are roughly two fixations per step, but there is no simple correspondence between fixation points and footfalls. Typically the nearest fixation to a footfall is about 5° from it.

When walking on the level, it is rarely necessary to look at the ground ahead in order to step safely. On surfaces such as smooth paving, tarmac or mown grass walkers tended to look a few metres ahead, with gaze having no relationship to foot placement. Patla (2004) referred to this as 'travel gaze fixation', in which gaze is 'parked in front of the moving observer and being carried along by the observer' (p. 389). This implies that gaze drifts forward over the ground plane. When we recorded similar behaviour in outdoor situations, it was always associated with a modest vertical nystagmus in which smooth downward gaze movements alternated with small upward saccadic resets of 2 to 5°, indicating that the optokinetic reflex is not suppressed.

When vision is required to guide the next step, at what point in the step cycle is it deployed? This was studied by Hollands and Marple-Horvat (1996) using an intermittent light regime that denied visual information at various times during the step cycle. Subjects walked across 'stepping stones' illuminated by LEDs that could be extinguished for various periods. They found that the disruption, which took the form of a

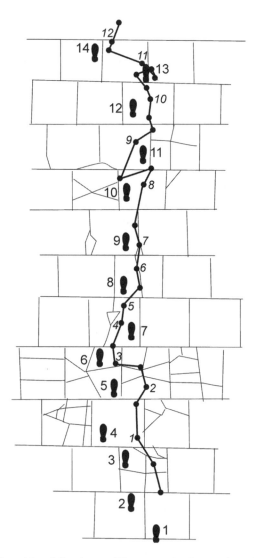

Fig. 6.1 Scan path and footfalls when walking across broken paving with the instruction not to tread on the cracks. The path of the eye is shown by the solid line; fixations are shown by dots, and the fixation nearest in time to a footfall is indicated by the corresponding number. There is typically a two-step difference between the corresponding numbers: thus, for example, Fixation 8 presumably directed Footfall 10.

delay in initiating a step, was maximal when the LEDs went out towards the end of the 'stance' period before the leg began its next step. The leg already in motion was unaffected. Dark periods of less than 300 ms had no effect, indicating that the planning system is buffered against brief occlusions. Similar results were obtained by Patla, Prentice, Rietdyk, Allard, and Martin (1999), who used a light spot to indicate the location of 'undesirable' foot placements. They found that the foot could be redirected to a new location within the duration of the preceding step and that these alternative placements were not selected at random. They were generally directed to the location that minimized the displacement of the foot from what would have been its normal footfall, thus causing the least disruption to both locomotor muscle activity and dynamic stability. The conclusion from these various studies is that footfalls are typically planned about two steps into the future (about 1 s ahead), but adjustments can be made up to the end of the stance period of the preceding step (about 0.5 s ahead), if required.

Going up steps

When ascending a regular set of steps it is important to look at the first few steps to get the placement of the feet right, but thereafter the pattern of footfalls becomes regular and predictable. In the Sussex study we found that as the stepping pattern became predictable, the delay between fixation and foot placement lengthened. In Fig. 6.2 the eyes look directly at the feet for the first few steps, and the eye–foot delay increases gradually to between 2 and 3 s by the end of each flight. As a delay of 1.1 s was typical for level but unpredictable paving, we assume that the lengthening of the eye-–foot delay beyond this period represents a progressive disengagement of vision from the

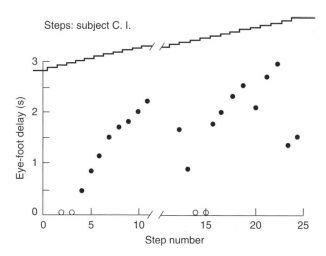

Fig. 6.2 Eye–footfall delay when walking up a double flight of steps. For Steps 2 and 3, and 14 and 15 the subject was looking directly at her feet (o). Thereafter on both flights the delay lengthened progressively to between 2 and 3 s. The steps were 38 cm deep, 15 cm high, and the distance between flights (omitted) was 2.6 m.

steps themselves, towards the condition on predictable flat ground, where gaze is directed into the middle distance rather than at future foot placements.

Changing direction

What happens when we change direction? Ultimately it is the body axis that rotates, carried by the feet, but what roles do eye and head movements play? We have seen that in walking along a straight path we tend to place our eyes about two steps ahead of our feet, suggesting that we plan our footfalls about 1 s in advance. When walking around a tight 90° corner, Grasso et al. (1998) showed similar anticipatory movements of the head and eyes. About 1 s before making the body turn, the head and eyes were turned to line up with the direction that the body would be facing after completing the turn. Interestingly, they had their participants walk around the corner in the dark also. The anticipatory lining up of head and eyes with the future direction was almost the same in the dark as in the light. This result suggest that this anticipatory lining up is not just about getting the eyes to a future target but is a fundamental part of planning the motor act of turning the corner. (We will see in Chapter 7 that racing drivers use a similar head-leading-body strategy when driving around a familiar track). In an attempt to argue that the 1-second-ahead alignment of head and gaze with future direction was an intentional part of the motor planning rather than some artefact of making a body turn, Grasso et al. also had their participants walk backwards both in the light and (frighteningly) in the dark. They found a far less-pronounced anticipation by the eyes and head and used this to argue that the head turns were not simply linked to body turning.

Hollands et al. (2002) studied walking turns by getting subjects to change direction along a travel path while wearing eye-and-head monitoring equipment (this was flat terrain, so there was no need to fixate future footfalls). The direction change was indicated either by the onset of a cue light at the new path end-point or by prior instruction about the route. The principal finding was that the turn was invariably accompanied by an eye saccade to the new destination (with a latency of about 350 ms when cued), initiated at the same time as a head movement. The eye–head combination brought head and gaze into line with the direction of the new goal as the body turn was being made (see also Imai et al. 2001). Thus gaze movements into the turn anticipate body movements, and the authors argued that pre-aligning the head axis provides an allocentric (external) reference frame that can then be used for the control of the rest of the body. Something very similar occurs when body turns are made without forward motion (Fig. 6.5) and when turning a corner in a car (Chapter 7).

Maintaining posture

An important part of successful locomotion is maintaining the correct posture and gait to ensure that the feet, legs, body, and head are all in the right place at the right time. To a large extent, this is under the control of proprioception—monitoring limb and joint positions throughout the relevant parts of the body. However, vision also plays a significant part in making sure that we get our posture right and in dealing with any unexpected perturbations. When walking on a platform that moves rather like a ship in the water, people were far less disrupted when visual information was displayed on screens around the platform than when no visual reference was available for feedback (Dobie et al., 2003). Further evidence for vision playing an important role in maintaining the correct posture was also found by looking at how disrupted people were when standing still on the platform: across a range of measures including changes the centre of pressure and critical weigh shifts (i.e. corrections to posture arising from perturbations) it was clear that postural difficulties were far more common when visual information was not available.

Visual guidance during walking

Egocentric and allocentric control

When walking along a winding path we can make use of, potentially, two different kinds of information. We might select a landmark in the near distance and aim our course in that direction, then choose another, and so on. Each landmark might simply be the farthest point along the path for which vision is not obstructed. Alternatively, we might make use of the way that objects move relative to us as we progress, making sure that the point of zero image motion (which will be in the direction we are walking) coincides with the next target on the path ahead of us (Fig. 6.3). This second alternative was the one proposed by J.J. Gibson: 'To aim locomotion at an object is to centre the flow of the optic array as close as possible to the form which the object projects' (Gibson, 1958, p. 187). Both mechanisms involve reducing the angle between our current heading and some future target. However, in the first case our current course is determined 'egocentrically', using our intrinsic knowledge of our body axis direction, whereas in the second case our course is determined 'allocentrically', from the observed location of the stationary point (focus of expansion) in the optic flow field.

The egocentric explanation seems straightforward enough, and there is plenty of evidence, for example, from pointing studies (Biguer et al., 1984), that we are able to

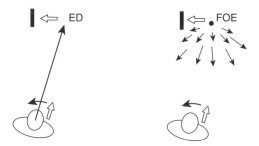

Fig. 6.3 Egocentric and flow-field accounts of visual guidance. On the left, the subject turns to minimize the angle between their egocentric direction (ED) and the target (vertical line). On the right, the turn minimizes the angle between the focus of expansion (FOE) of the velocity flow field and the target.

judge the relation between visual direction and the body axis with an accuracy of one or two degrees. The flow-field explanation seems somewhat perverse, first because at walking speeds in open terrain it seems very difficult to make out the location of the focus of expansion. Second, if we look away from our direction of motion to fixate some other object, then that object becomes the stationary point on the retina, not the focus of expansion (Regan and Beverley, 1982). Methods have been devised for recovering the focus of expansion (and hence heading) from the situation where the eye is rotating to track an eccentric object (e.g. Li and Warren, 2000), but the feeling remains that Gibson's proposal represents a particularly difficult way of going about a fairly straightforward task. To be fair to Gibson, he pointed out (1958, p. 189) that his theory referred primarily to locomotion in a medium of water or air, where proprioception is less informative about relations with environmental objects than it is on land where the limbs have contact with the substratum.

An elegant way of distinguishing between egocentric direction and focus of expansion mechanisms was devised by Rushton, Harris et al. (1998). They sfitted subjects with glasses containing wedge prisms that deviated the line of sight to the right or left and asked them to walk towards a target 10 to 15 m away in an open field. If the subjects were using egocentric information to determine their heading, then when they tried to align their body axis with the target they would in fact be walking at an angle to the direction of the target, by an amount equal to the deviation of the prisms. As a consequence they would follow a curved path to the target. If, however, they determined their current heading allocentrically, using the focus of expansion of the flow field, then because both the target and the focus of expansion were seen through the prisms, and thus both were deviated by the same amount, the path to the target would be straight. In fact Rushton et al. observed curved paths, consistent with the egocentric model (Fig. 6.4).

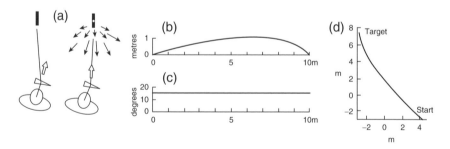

Fig. 6.4 Effect of wearing prisms on the trajectory of an approach to a target. (a) If the wearer walks towards the seen position of the target the approach will be diverted, but if they walk so that the focus of expansion (i.e the locomotor direction) and the target coincide the approach will be direct. (b) Simulated trajectory to a target at 10 m when wearing 16° prisms while walking to the seen target position. (c) If the focus of expansion is used the target – locomotor direction error remains constant during the approach. (d) Actual trajectory of an observer wearing wedge prisms when approaching a target, showing a curved trajectory like that in (b). The distances in (d) are in camera co-ordinates. Redrawn from Rushton et al. (1998).

Loomis et al. (2006) devised a virtual reality method of presenting a dynamic environment in which there were no direct (first-order) motion cues (and hence no velocity flow field), by using random-dot stereograms with single-frame lifetimes. They found that performance on tasks such as navigating a field of obstacles was comparable to the performance in the same environment when continuous motion cues were present. This shows that flow fields in the usually accepted sense are not necessary for locomotory guidance. However, this does not necessarily mean that such cues are never used.

Warren et al. (2001) repeated the prism experiment using a virtual reality simulator in which the amount of texture in the surroundings could be varied. They found that in a textured environment much straighter paths were taken when using prisms and concluded that optic flow information could at least contribute to the visual guidance of locomotion. Crucially, the relative extent to which people appeared to rely on egocentric direction or optic flow varied quite consistently with the information available. When walking in an environment with only ground plane grass-like texture, only weak optic flow cues were available, and egocentric direction dominated the guidance of walking. When walking through highly textured environments with doorways, optic flow cues were prevalent, and people used these cues. In an intermediate environment, the utilization of egocentric direction and optic flow was also intermediate. The authors argued that having both egocentric and optic flow mechanisms available provides robust locomotor control under a variety of environmental conditions. Moreover, this is a nice demonstration that our visual systems are adept at utilizing whatever information is available for the situation at hand.

Fajen and Warren (2004) also examined the task of intercepting a moving target on foot. They found that their subjects did not adopt a pursuit strategy, in which the interceptor always heads in the direction of the target but a true interception course in which the target is held at a constant angle to the current heading. This is essentially how navigators know whether a collision will occur at sea, when another ship remains for some time on the same bearing. Interestingly, they found no evidence of the use of flow-field information and concluded that the strategy is based on the egocentrically determined direction of the moving target.

Dealing with hazards while walking

Now we have some idea of how the behaviour of the eye–head–body system during walking, we can consider how this is put to use for dealing with potentially hazardous situations in real or virtual environments. Here we shall deal with two common situations that we face in our everyday lives: crossing busy roads and avoiding colliding with other pedestrians.

Crossing the road

Sometimes we find ourselves in a situation where me must cross a busy road without the aid of a signal-controlled pedestrian crossing. Logically we might assume that in this situation we have to gather information about oncoming traffic, such as its distance and speed, often for traffic coming from opposite directions; process this information to make a decision about when is safe to cross; monitor danger while crossing; and get safely to the other side of the road. Not only is this a lot to deal with but also the potential risk of getting one of these judgements or tasks wrong is high. Geruschat et al. (2003) recorded eye movements of participants as they crossed two busy intersections: a 'plus intersection' (with four roads meeting at right angles) and a roundabout (with three exits). Participants were led up to the crossing points with eyes closed and so had no prior information about the road before they were asked to cross it. At one of the two intersections there was a signal-controlled crossing, but because people were asked to cross before the signals stopped the traffic, they were free to choose to cross then or wait for the lights to change. Reassuringly, people tended to look both ways before crossing the road at both junctions. When crossing either the plus intersection (before the lights changed to 'safe'), or the roundabout, people tended to look mainly at the traffic before starting to cross. In contrast, those who decided to wait for the signal to cross at the plus intersection directed most fixations to the signal lights. Thus before crossing, the allocation of fixations correlated well with what would be expected for the chosen crossing behaviour (crossing before the lights or waiting for the lights to change). Somewhat unexpectedly, while the participants were actually crossing the roads, few fixations on the cars were made and this was true whether or not they waited for the signal to cross – that is, whether or not the traffic was still flowing when they stepped out into the road! Instead, while crossing, most fixations were directed to elements such as the curb, crossing markings and bollards, or to the general surroundings. Presumably, rather than constantly monitoring moving traffic while crossing the road, people make their decision about whether it is safe to get the whole way across the street before they set off.

Avoiding other pedestrians

We are very good at not colliding with other pedestrians when walking in busy towns. Most people are well-behaved and keep out of the way, but others, for a variety of reasons may be less thoughtful and so pose the threat of potential collision if not avoided. Jovancevic and her colleagues have explored how we monitor potential colliders when walking either in a virtual or real environment. In both environments participants walked along a path that followed a route around a central structure, which meant that oncoming pedestrians did not appear until they were at a maximum distance of 6 m (in VR) from the participant.

In the virtual environment (Jovancevic, Sullivan, and Hayhoe, 2006), some pedestrians ('colliders') would suddenly take a course toward the subject, whereas others did not. Potential colliders attracted more fixations than ordinary pedestrians, but the difference was only 20%, and many potential colliders were missed, suggesting that their 'looming' effect was not an especially powerful stimulus. However, after an encounter with a collider, the amount of time spent fixating on all pedestrians increased, suggesting that a potential collision increases the subject's vigilance. When instructed to follow a virtual leader, subjects' fixations on other pedestrians decreased substantially, and the difference between the monitoring of colliders and non-colliders disappeared. These observations indicate that the priorities assigned to the monitoring of other pedestrians change as other tasks (following a leader) require attention, and that monitoring behaviour is affected by immediate past experience.

In a subsequent study using real people as the oncoming pedestrians (Jovancevic-Misic et al., 2007, Jovancevic-Misic and Hayhoe, in press) different oncoming pedestrians were given different roles: one always took a collision course with the participant ('rogue'), one took a collision course 50% of the time ('risky'), and one never took a collision course with the subject ('safe'). The subjects rapidly learnt who was likely to pose a threat and adjusted their viewing behaviour accordingly: they were more likely to look at the rogue than the safe oncomer and the probability of fixating the risky oncomer fell between these two extremes. As the experiment progressed over a number of laps, so the allocation of fixation between the three oncomers changed: in the first four laps subjects spent roughly the same amount of time looking at each of the oncomers but by the final 4 laps (of 12) more time was spent looking at the rogue and least time was spent looking at the safe oncomer. If the 12 laps were then repeated, but the roles of the rogue and safe oncomers reversed, allocation of attention initially matched that at the end of the first 12 laps, but subjects soon learnt to switch to looking at the now-rogue (previously safe) oncomer more than the now-safe (previously rogue) oncomer. These results not only replicate and extend the previous findings in virtual reality but they also demonstrate that we can quickly learn the behaviour of others and adapt our visual strategies for monitoring our environment accordingly.

Co-ordination of eyes, head, and body

In natural behaviour the relocations of gaze that are crucial for our visual interactions with the world can be made with eye movements alone, but more commonly they involve combined eye and head movements, or even movements of the eyes, head and trunk. In such vigorous activities as playing tennis it is often necessary to look in one direction whilst rotating the trunk in another, and so there can be no simple rule of thumb that specifies the rotations of the different moveable parts in a gaze rotation of a particular size. In this Section we will consider how such flexibility is achieved.

Which combination of eye, head, and trunk movements occurs depends in part on the size of the gaze rotation required. In the horizontal plane the eyes can rotate up to a maximum of about $\pm50°$, although head movements typically accompany eye movements for gaze rotations larger than a few degrees. For gaze movements within the eye movement range, the contribution of the head is typically about one-third of the total (Goossens and van Opsal, 1997; see also Fig. 9.3). The neck can turn the head through about $\pm90°$. Thus, for gaze rotations greater than 140° the trunk must also become involved. With freely moving subjects, especially during forward locomotion, trunk turns can occur with gaze rotations of any amplitude. The eyes rotate faster than the head, which in turn rotates faster than the body. This means that there are potential co-ordination problems: for example, if the eyes reach their target before the head rotation is complete, they must counter-rotate as the head catches up, and mechanisms are required to ensure that this can occur without gaze direction being perturbed. Similar considerations apply when part of the rotation is carried out by trunk rotation.

Eye and head

In the case of eye and head rotations of 10° or less Morasso et al. (1973) showed that the trajectory of the gaze is initially the same as the saccadic eye movement that would have been made with the head still; this is followed by a phase in which the eye counter-rotates as the head comes back into line with gaze (see Fig. 2.5b). This counter-rotation is brought about by the vestibulo-ocular reflex (VOR, see Fig. 2.6), which is driven by the head velocity sensors in the semicircular canals. This reflex ensures that the extent and time course of the gaze saccade is the same, whatever the head does. However, for saccades beyond the eye movement range (±50°) this will not work because the eye cannot make the whole saccade on its own. Guitton and Volle (1987) showed that during these larger gaze saccades VOR is suspended, so that at least part of the gaze saccade results entirely from rotation of the head (Figs 2.5b and 6.6a). The end-point of the gaze saccade occurs when VOR is switched on again, which happens when a pre-specified amount of gaze rotation is achieved. This is determined by internal signals that monitor head rotation (particularly the semicircular canals but possibly also neck proprioceptors or efference copy to the neck muscles) and eye rotation (efference copy or eye-muscle proprioceptors). Their sum gives the extent of gaze rotation (Guitton et al., 2003).

Head and trunk

What happens when trunk rotation is also involved? A typical situation is illustrated in Fig. 6.5. Eye, head, and trunk start to rotate more or less together (1 to 3), then when gaze reaches the target VOR is switched on, counter-rotating the eye and thus maintaining fixation (3 and 4) just as described above. During the last phase (4 and 5) the goal is in line with both eye and head, but the body continues to rotate. This means that the head must counter-rotate on the trunk until the trunk too reaches a direction more or less in line with the goal. A recording of a real turn similar to that in Fig. 6.5 is shown in Fig. 6.6a. This turn was made by a freely moving subject while turning between work surfaces in a kitchen. She wore a portable eye camera (Fig. 1.4), which provided the eye-in-head records, and the head-in-space records came from the head-mounted scene camera. The trunk angles were retrieved subsequently from simultaneous videos of the subjects' actions taken from the other side of the room (see Land, 2004). Figure 6.6a shows that the eye behaves as expected from Fig. 2.5: the saccade is made between 0.2 and 0.3 s, there is a period of 0.1 s without further motion, and then VOR recommences, with the eye returning to near the primary position by 0.5 s. The neck (head on trunk) rotates between 0.2 and 0.5s, briefly stops rotating, and then reverses direction at 0.6 s. The neck continues to counter-rotate as the trunk completes the turn, the neck rotation being a near mirror-image of the trunk rotation, and the net result is that there is little further rotation of the head in space.

Role of the vestibulo-collic reflex

What mechanism choreographs the interaction of head and trunk so that they come back into line? A strong candidate is the vestibulo-collic reflex (VCR). This reflex opposes the rotation of the head in space, which means that if rotation of the trunk

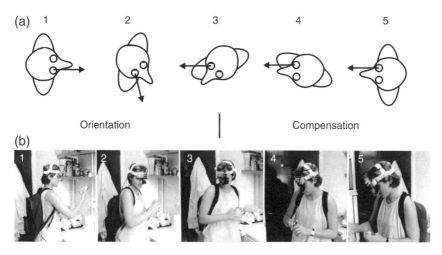

Fig. 6.5 Turns made with eyes, head, and trunk. (a) Diagram of a typical sequence of movements of eyes, head, and trunk made during a 180° turn. All three initially move together in the same direction (1–3) during the orientation phase, with the eyes reaching their target at 3. Thereafter, during the compensation phase, the eyes counter-rotate in the head (3–4), and the head counter-rotates on the body (4–5). (b) Stills from a video of a comparable sequence of eye, head, and body movements in a single large turn (from one work surface to another in a kitchen setting). A detailed record of a similar turn is given in Fig. 6.6a. Partly from Land (2004).

occurs the muscles of the neck counter-rotate the head to maintain its current direction (Outerbridge and Melville Jones, 1971; Guitton et al., 1986). Like the VOR, the VCR is driven by the semicircular canals, but differs from the VOR (which is an 'open' feed-forward system) in that it is a feedback loop in which the semicircular canals provide the basis for an error signal. The error is the desired head rotation (zero if the head rotation is to be prevented) minus the actual head rotation. This error is fed (amplified) to the neck muscles (Fig. 6.7). The result in Fig. 6.6a is that head rotation in space is reduced to near zero.

Similar to VOR, VCR can be engaged or disengaged. For the first second of Fig. 6.6a the neck and trunk move together, so presumably VCR is not engaged, or at least not used in such a way as to prevent neck rotation. It is only after 0.6 s, and for the half second after that, that the neck counter-rotates as the trunk turns through a further 60°. The first part of the turn is often referred to as the *orientation* phase, and the second half, involving counter-rotation, as the *compensatory* phase (Fig. 6.5, see Imai et al., 2001). Assuming that VCR is involved in the compensatory phase it is possible to work out the gain of the loop from the ratio of head-on-trunk speed to trunk-in-space speed, using the formula in the caption to Fig. 6.7. For the compensatory phase in Fig.6.6a, between 0.6 and 1.6 s, these speeds are 107° s^{-1} and 153° s^{-1}, which gives a closed-loop gain [$g/(1+g)$] of 0.7, and the corresponding amplification factor [g] is 2.3.

The existence of vestibular feedback does not necessarily mean that head velocity must be clamped near zero. A command to rotate the head can be injected into the input to the loop, and this will be obeyed just like a zero rotation command. The system would then be analogous to power steering in a car. Evidence that voluntary actions do make use of the vestibular feedback loop has come from a study by Day and Reynolds (2005). They modulated the usual vestibular input in human subjects using electrical stimulation of the vestibular nerves. The subjects performed voluntary

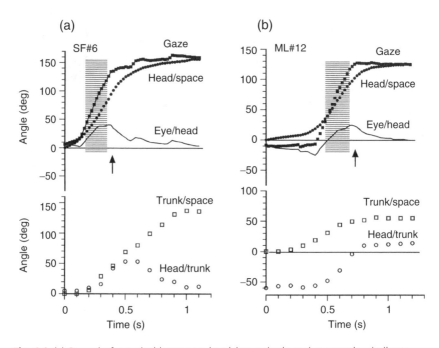

Fig. 6.6 (a) Record of a typical large turn involving a single major saccade, similar to those in Fig. 6.5. Eye, head, and trunk move together at 0.2 s. The eyes stop moving in the head at 0.3 s, indicating that VOR is not operating, but movement recommences in the opposite direction at 0.4 s, with VOR activated again (arrow) and opposing rotation of the head in space. This results in 0.2 s of gaze fixation, followed by two further small saccades and fixations. The neck (head/trunk) stops rotating at 0.5 s, but the head continues to rotate slowly up to 1 s, carried by the trunk. From 0.6 s the neck counter-rotates, largely compensating for the trunk rotation, so that head-in-space rotation is minimal. This counter-rotation probably results from the operation of the VCR.
(b) A clockwise turn in which the head starts from a position rotated 60° anticlockwise relative to the body. Eye, head-in-space and gaze follow very similar trajectories to those in (a), although the trunk starts to move about 0.3 s earlier than the eyes or the neck. The neck contribution to the turn brings the head more or less into line with the trunk, and presumably because of this there is no compensatory counter-rotation as in (a). In both records the shaded area indicates when the eyes are wholly or partially occluded by a blink. Data from Land (2004). Both records are of natural turns made during tea making.

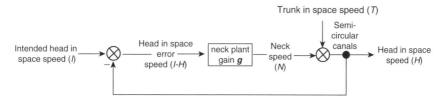

Fig. 6.7 The vestibulo-collic reflex as a servo loop. The input to the loop is a command to rotate the head at a particular speed – this is zero when the head is to be kept still. Any rotation of the head in space (H) is measured by the semicircular canals, and this is fed back to be subtracted from the command to give an error signal (I-H). This is fed, amplified by a gain factor g, to the neck muscles. These then counter-rotate the head to give neck (head-on-trunk) speed N. In this scheme the trunk movements (T) act as a disturbance to the loop, which acts to null them out. Mathematically,

$$N = gI/(1+g) - gT/(1+g),$$

where $g/(1+g)$ is the gain of the loop. As g becomes large so $g/(1+g)$ tends to 1 and $-g$ $T/(1+g)$ tends to $-T$. Thus neck speed (N) tends to $I - T$. In other words the loop obeys the command I, and opposes the disturbance T.

actions, in this case goal-directed head tilts. Day and Reynolds found that the speed and extent of the actions could be controlled by varying the stimulation as the action was occurring, indicating that vestibular feedback is continuously available during willed actions as well as more reflexive ones. A comprehensive review of the workings of the VCR is provided by Peterson and Boyle (2004).

The system is evidently very flexible in relation to head position: no two turns have to be the same. Provided it operates as a velocity rather than a position servo (as in Fig. 6.7), the VCR does not require that turns start or finish with the head in line with the body. In Fig. 6.6b, for example, the head starts 60° out of line with the body, which means that the orientational part of the turn brings it into line with the body, and no further compensation is required. In an action such as opening a door, the trunk will often start roughly at right angles to the door but with the head and eyes looking over the shoulder at the handle. Similarly, army platoons can march for some time while making an 'eyes right' with the head – although there is usually one soldier in the front row looking forwards to keep them marching in the right direction. In spite of this flexibility, most turns finish up with the head more or less in line with the body, as in both examples in Fig. 6.6. This may be due in part to another reflex, the cervico-collic reflex (CCR). This is mediated by proprioceptors in the neck, which activate the neck muscles when they are stretched, thus tending to return them to their resting length and returning the head to its primary position. Like the VCR, we would expect this reflex to be active principally during the compensatory phase of a turn, and to act in co-operation with the VCR, possibly by varying its gain. To make life more complicated, neck proprioceptors also have reflex effects on the muscles of the limbs and hence on body posture (cervico-spinal reflexes) and under certain circumstances can also drive eye movements (cervico-ocular reflex). Their relevance in everyday life is

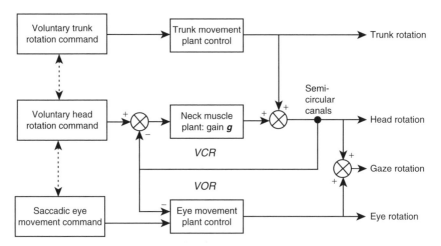

Fig. 6.8 Minimal scheme, incorporating the vestibulo-collic reflex loop (VCR: Fig. 6.7) and the vestibulo-ocular reflex (VOR: Fig. 2.6), which ensures that trunk and head can rotate independently without this affecting the direction of gaze. Voluntary rotations of the trunk, which would otherwise cause rotations of the head, are opposed by the VCR loop, so that head-in-space rotation is minimized. Voluntary head movements can be made by inserting commands into this loop. Head-in-space rotations, which would otherwise cause the eyes to rotate in space and so disturb gaze, are counteracted by the VOR, which rotates the eyes at a rate equal and opposite to the head rotation. Gaze direction can be changed by saccadic eye movements, which may also involve head movement. The dashed arrows on the left indicate mechanisms that allow co-programming of eye, head, and trunk movements, as, for example, during the first half-second of Fig. 6.6a. Note the central role of the semicircular canals, which act as input for both the VCR and VOR.

far from clear. It should be mentioned that many of these reflexes were first identified in anaesthetized or even decerebrate cats, and although they have counterparts in man it is better to think of them as tools that the nervous system has at its disposal rather than as the obligatory stimulus–response pairings that the word 'reflex' often implies.

The combined effect of the two principal reflexes – VOR and VCR – is that gaze direction can be maintained independent of rotations of the head (VOR), and head direction can be maintained independent of rotations of the trunk (VCR). Without these reflexes, head movements would mechanically cause gaze movements, and trunk movements would mechanically cause head movements. A minimal scheme showing how the reflexes work together is given in Fig. 6.8. These two reflexes permit the controlled emancipation of the different body components from the actions of the others.

Summary

1. When walking on difficult terrain, gaze leads footfalls by about a second (2 steps). When turning, the eyes and head line up with the new direction a second ahead of the body.

2. Two cues are available to navigate towards distant target: heading relative to the target and optic flow'. Which is used depends on their relative availability and reliability.

3. In potentially hazardous situations (such as crossing the road or avoiding oncoming pedestrians) allocation of gaze reflects the perceived threat of objects in the environment.

4. When moving through the environment, eyes, head, and body often share a common alignment. However, in many situations they do not, and flexible co-ordination is achieved by two reflexes: the vestibulo-ocular reflex, which allows the eyes to maintain direction independent of the head, and the vestibulo-collic reflex, which maintains head direction independent of the body.

Chapter 7

Driving

Driving is a complex skill that involves dealing with the road itself (steering, speed control), other road users (vehicles, cyclists, moving and stationary pedestrians), and attention to road signs and other relevant sources of information. It is thus a very varied task, and one would expect a range of eye movement strategies to be employed. We will first consider steering as this is a prerequisite for all other aspects of driving.

Steering

Straight roads

On a straight road without other traffic, the task is to maintain a position with the car near the centre of the lane and the driver just to one side of the centre. If the course taken leads to a departure from this position, a driver will correct the steering, making use of the visual feedback available from the road. As Fig. 7.1 shows, strong cues are available from the marker lines on the road. These are of two kinds: the location, relative to the line of travel, of the lane edges at some 'preview' distance (typically in the range 10–30 m ahead, see Fig. 7.3c) and the angles that the lane edges make with the driver's vertical (splay angle; Beall and Loomis, 1996; Riemersma, 1981). As we shall see, both cues are required for proper lane maintenance. In Fig. 7.1a the car's course (arrow) is directed towards the vanishing point and so is aligned with the roadway, whereas the driver's position is just right of centre in the left lane, which is where it should be in the United Kingdom (readers in the United States or continental Europe should imagine the figure's mirror image). At the preview distance the centre line marking is closer to the line of travel than the left-hand kerb in a ratio of about 1:2.5. The splay angles of the left lane marker and the broken centre line are approximately 55° and 30° in this instance; their exact values will depend on the lane width and the height of the driver's eye. (If the driver, whose eye height is h, maintains a horizontal distance x from a marker line, then the splay angle φ between the marker line and the vertical is given by $\varphi = \arctan x/h$.) If the driver can maintain these values, he will keep position and alignment with the road.

What happens when the vehicle departs from the alignment in Fig. 7.1a? Figure 7.1b shows the situation where the driver is veering to the left, and will eventually run off the road, although the car has not yet moved laterally in the lane. The car's heading no longer points to the vanishing point – the intersection of marker lines. Both the positions of the lane markers at the preview distance and the splay angles of the lines have changed. In (c) the car's heading is directed to the right, and if this course is maintained, the car will cross into the oncoming lane. Both the splay angles and the

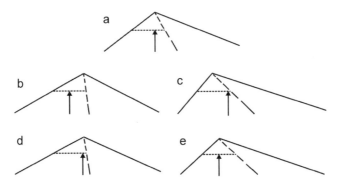

Fig 7.1 Appearance of a straight road when the driver is in different orientations and positions on the roadway (UK conditions: right-hand-drive car in the left lane). (a) Normal direction and location in the lane. (b) and (c) Course orientation to the left and right of the road direction. (d) and (e) Course parallel to road direction but displaced to right and left of the normal road position. Arrow gives the direction of the car's course. Dotted line indicates the region of gaze of the driver (preview distance). Note the similarities of lane marker angles in (b) and (d) and (c) and (e), and of the location of the car's heading at the preview distance in (b) and (e), and (c), (d).

lane markers at the preview distance are different from those in (a) and (b). In (d) and (e) the car is correctly aligned with the road, as in (a), but the position on the road is wrong: too far right in (d) and left in (e). Interestingly, the positions of the lane markers at the preview distance are the same in (d) as they are in (c) and the same in (e) as they are in (b). This means that this cue does not, on its own, distinguish unambiguously between angular (course) errors and displacement errors. The same is also true of splay angle. The splay angles in (d) are virtually the same as those in (b) and similarly for (e) and (c). However, the combination of lane marker position at the preview distance and the corresponding splay angles pattern are unique for each type of error. We can conclude that ordinary lane maintenance utilizes both cues. In practice a driver is likely first to notice the relative motion of the lane edges and make steering adjustments based on these changes. For example, a decrease in the splay angle of the centre line and a movement to the left of the heading at the preview distance (Fig. 7.1a and b) means that the car is veering to the left and a rotation to the right is needed to correct this until the pattern in (a) is restored. Displacements require two manoeuvres to correct them. Thus to return from (e) to (a) requires a rotation to the right followed after an appropriate interval by a rotation to the left. Each manoeuvre will generate its own pattern of relative movement in the lane markers that can be used to monitor the correction. However, ultimately it is the absolute values of the lane marker positions and splay angles that determine whether the driver is correctly positioned and on course.

Changing lanes involves a deliberate three-stage manoeuvre similar to the displacement correction mentioned in the previous paragraph. A turn out of lane, producing a geometry like Fig. 7.1c is followed by a period of oblique travel and then by a counterturn to restore a geometry like that of Fig. 7.1a, but in the new lane. It seems that visual feedback is particularly important in the completion of this manoeuvre. Wallis et al. (2002) came up with the curious result that when changing lanes in a driving simulator the withdrawal of visual feedback, by blanking the display, resulted in an incomplete manoeuvre. The final correction bringing the vehicle into line with the new lane was weak or absent, so that the drivers' performance was more like turning a corner than making a lane change. Some improvement resulted from providing drivers in advance with an explicit path to follow, or by using a real vehicle to give valid inertial information (Macuga et al., 2006), but this does not detract from the conclusion that visual appearance of the lane markers is the most potent source of feedback.

There are other possible cues to straight-line driving that make use of the velocity flow-field produced by the motion of the car relative to objects or contrast elements on or off the roadway. A strictly Gibsonian account of steering would have course direction determined by the driver steering so that the focus of expansion of the flow field coincided with the vanishing point of the road (see Chapter 6), and there is no doubt that heading direction *can* be obtained from flow-field information (Warren and Hannon, 1988). In principle, position in lane could be obtained from flow lines corresponding to the relative motion of objects on the lane edges. However, the lane markings themselves correspond to the lane edge flow lines, and if the markings are visibly present it would seem perverse to derive them from motion cues. A further problem with the flow-field approach is that when we track a point – a road sign, for instance – not in the direction of travel, this plays havoc with the flow field (see Chapter 6). However, as Beall and Loomis (1996) pointed out, the splay angles of the lane markers do not change their relationships to each other or to the vehicle's heading if the driver looks away from the direction of travel, and so they seem provide a better 'invariant' than any flow-field variable. Furthermore, it is often the case that neither the vanishing point itself nor the focus of expansion of the flow field is visible: if, for example, the road dips, or there is a distant bend, or there is another vehicle in front the conditions for using flow-field cues to derive course direction will be severely compromised. We conclude that under normal driving conditions where lane markers are present, there is a strong case for supposing that the geometry of these markers provides the necessary and sufficient conditions for maintaining both position in lane and direction relative to the road.

Steering around bends

Curved roads are more complicated because the lane markings are no longer straight. Keeping in the right part of the lane can still be achieved by using the splay lines in the region immediately in front of the vehicle, where the splay angles are much the same as they are on a straight road. However, as there is no single vanishing point, and the splay angles change with distance (Fig. 7.2a) it is less obvious what would be an appropriate control signal for future course control. One strategy (gaze sampling; Fig. 7.2a and b) would be to choose a point P on the future path, at a constant preview distance D of, for instance, 3 of the central marker lines, and use the horizontal eccentricity of this point (θ) to adjust the steering (Wann and Land, 2000; Wann and Wilkie, 2004). This can be done via the formula $1/r = (2 \sin \theta)/D$, easily derived from the construction in Fig. 7.2b. Here r is the radius of curvature of the car's path, and the amount the steering wheel needs to be turned is proportional to its reciprocal ($1/r$, the path curvature). The angle θ is simply the angle between gaze direction and the heading (H). The latter will correspond to the driver's body axis if he is belted in, and we can assume that the driver can estimate θ easily from physiologically available information. The distance D is perhaps harder to determine but could be obtained from the markings on the centre line or from the angle down from the horizon on a level road. As discussed in the next section, the driver can also use the tangent point (the point on the lane edge where the driver's line of sight is tangential to the marker line, just right of P in Fig. 7.2a). This does not require an estimate of distance D but does require a knowledge of the lateral distance of the driver from the lane edge. These methods, such as the use of the angle of the lane markers on a straight road (Fig. 7.2a), rely on the visual directions of objects in the field of view rather than their motions.

Figure 7.2c shows the same road but without road markers, only lines representing the paths of texture elements as the car travels over them – the flow-field. As can be seen, the geometry of the flow lines is very similar to that of the marker lines in Fig. 7.2a, and they can be used in similar ways. As Lee and Lishman (1977) pointed out, the flow line that runs beneath the driver (where it is vertical in the field of view) specifies the future path (FP) that the driver will take if his current course is maintained

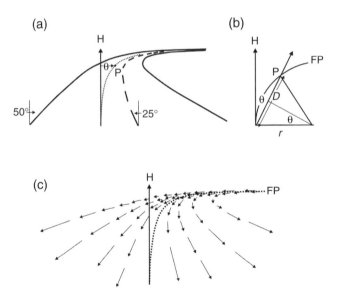

Fig. 7.2 Road geometry of a bend of constant curvature. (a) Appearance of the road from a normal driving position in the left-hand lane. Unlike Fig. 7.1a the splay angles change with distance. The bend's curvature can be assessed by observing the angle θ between the current heading H and a point P on the future path. (b) Construction showing that the curvature ($1/r$) can be obtained from ($2 \sin \theta$)/D. (c) The flow field associated with motion around the bend. The car's future path (FP) is the continuation of the flow line beneath the driver.

(Fig. 7.2c). So provided, the flow line can be discerned an appropriate course can be followed by extrapolating that line. Other more subtle cues are available from the curvature of the flow lines. Thus if a driver fixates a distant target that he wishes to pass through, the flow lines will be straight if his circular course passes through the target but curved to right or left if his course is going to overshoot or undershoot the target (Wann and Land, 2000; Wann and Wilkie, 2004). Compared with road markings, which are certainly used by real drivers on real roads, the extent to which other flow-field cues are used in real driving is less clear, but they are certainly available. Several studies suggest that the relative use of visual direction and flow information depends on their reliability and availability and the exact nature of the task (Fajen and Warren, 2003; Wann and Wilkie, 2004).

It needs to be remembered that on a gentle bend of constant curvature, simple lane position maintenance via visual feedback from local splay angles will very quickly cause the steering to adapt to the curvature of the road even without explicit esti-mates of bend curvature. It will rapidly become clear to a driver whether the curva-ture of the vehicle's path conforms to that of the lane, and appropriate adjustments can be implemented. Feed forward (anticipatory) estimates of future curvature from either road features or flow lines can supplement this but may not be necessary at moderate speeds.

Winding roads and the tangent point

Most of the suggestions in the last section applied to roads with relatively gentle cur-vatures, where the task was essentially to match the curvature of the vehicle's path to that of the road. Winding country roads are more challenging because the curvature may be changing continuously and unpredictably, making lane edge feedback on its own a rather inefficient basis for steering. Estimates of future curvature are of particu-lar value here. In the absence of any simple theory of how drivers solve this problem, David Lee and one of us (MFL) decided in 1994 to approach this problem by finding out where drivers looked under these road conditions. As we have seen in other activ-ities, people usually fixate regions that provide them with the information needed for action, and we supposed that this would also be true of driving. Earlier studies, mainly on US roads that had relatively low curvatures, had found only a weak relationship between gaze direction and steering (e.g. Zwahlen, 1993), so we were not expecting a result that was quite as startling and consistent as the one we actually got. We asked three drivers to drive the kilometre or so of Queens Drive round Arthur's seat in Edinburgh. The road is very winding but one-way and single lane, so without the dis-traction of other traffic. With all three drivers we found a quite clear relationship between direction of gaze and steering. In particular, drivers spent much of their time looking at the 'tangent point' on the upcoming bend. The tangent point (also known as the reversal point) is the moving point on the inside of each bend where the driver's line of sight is tangential to the road edge; it is also the point that protrudes most into the road and is thus highly visible (Figs 7.3 and 7.4). It moves around the bend with the car but – when curvature is constant – remains in the same angular position relative to the driver's heading. On real roads tangent point viewing on bends has been found to be a consistently used strategy (Chattington et al., 2007; Mars, 2008; Kandil et al., 2009; Land and Lee, 1994; Underwood et al., 1999;). However, this has not always been true with driving simulators, where gaze tracking results suggest that it is the future path that is viewed more frequently, more in line with the gaze sampling strategy discussed in the previous section (Robertshaw and Wilkie, 2008).

The angular location of the tangent point relative to the vehicle's line of travel (effectively the driver's trunk axis if he is belted in) predicts the curvature of the bend: larger angles indicate steeper curvatures. Thus, potentially, this angle can provide the signal needed to control steering. Fig. 7.5a does indeed show that records of gaze direction and steering wheel angle are very similar. This suggests that this angle, which is equal to the gaze angle (eye-in-head plus the head-in-body angle) when the driver is looking at the tangent point, may be translated more or less directly into the motor control signal for the arms.

The geometry of the tangent point in relation to the curvature of the bend is shown in Fig. 7.6. The curvature of the bend ($1/r$, the reciprocal of the radius) specifies the

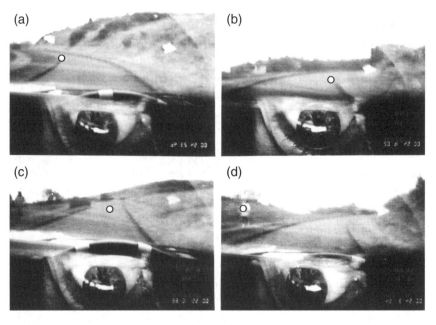

(a) (b)

(c) (d)

Fig. 7.3 Four views of Queen's Drive in Edinburgh showing sample gaze directions of the driver on (a) a left-hand bend, (b) a right-hand bend, (c) straight road, and (d) during an off-road look at a jogger. Note use of tangent points in (a) and (b), and preview distance of about 25 m in (c). Reversed from Land and Lee (1994) to give the correct (UK) driver position. Inverted eye image occupies the lower third of each view. The tape pieces on the windscreen allow the measurement of head movements relative to the car.

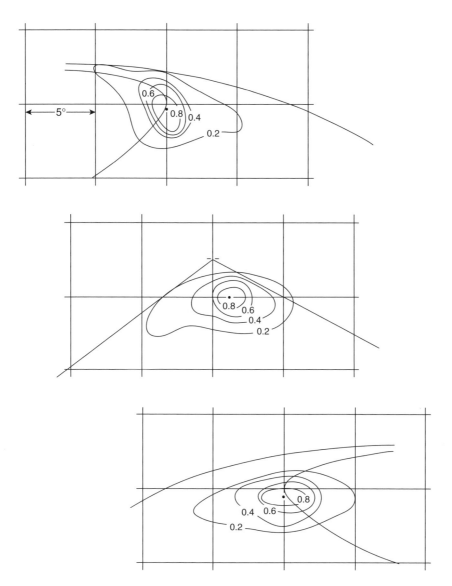

Fig. 7.4 Contour plots of the density of fixations made by three drivers when negotiating left-hand bends, straight segments, and right-hand bends during the drives illustrated in Fig. 7.3. The contour intervals are proportions of the maximum value, the absolute value of which is about 0.12 fixations per $deg^2 s^{-1}$. About 35% of the fixations are beyond the 0.2 contour and are widely spread. The car's heading has been aligned on the three figures and corresponds to the centre line in the middle figure. Bends are taken to be between the first look at the tangent point, and the disappearance of the tangent point at the exit from the bend. From Land and Lee (1994) but reversed as in Fig. 7.3.

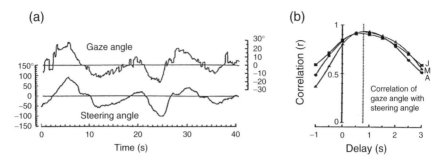

Fig. 7.5 (a) Similarity of driver's gaze angle relative to the car's heading, and angle of the steering wheel during a 40 s sequence (Queens Drive Edinburgh). (b) Cross correlation between gaze angle and steering wheel records for all three drivers, for different delays. The maximum correlation occurs when gaze leads steering by about 0.8 s.

angle through which the steering wheel needs to be turned to match the bend – at least at reasonable speeds. It is related to the gaze angle θ by the equation,

$$\cos \theta = (r - d)/r$$

However, we can use the expansion, $\cos \theta \approx 1 - \theta^2/2$, which then gives

$$1/r = \theta^2/2d$$

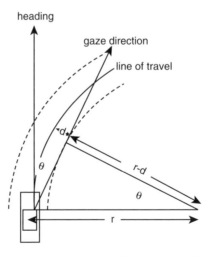

Fig. 7.6 Geometry of the tangent point. If the driver's gaze is directed to the point where his line of sight is tangential to the lane edge, then the curvature of the bend (1/r) is given by $\theta^2/2d$, where θ is the angle between the tangent point and current heading, and d is the lateral distance to the lane edge (see text).

Thus the steering wheel angle is directly related to θ^2 and inversely related to d, the distance of the driver from the kerb, or inside lane edge on a multiple lane road. Evidently, in addition to measuring the angle θ, the driver must also either measure d, possibly by the local splay angle or else maintain it at a constant value. We will return to this point later.

If a driver is using the tangent point signal, it is important that he does not act on it immediately because the part of the bend whose curvature he is measuring still lies some distance ahead. Cross-correlating the two curves in Fig. 7.5a shows that gaze direction precedes steering wheel angle by about 0.8 s (Fig. 7.5b), similar to the eye-effector delay in other activities such as walking (see Chapter 6), reading aloud, sketching, and copy-typing (Chapter 4). This is much longer than a simple reaction time (typically about 0.3 s) and so represents a planned delay. This lag provides the driver with a reasonable 'comfort margin', but it is also the delay necessary to prevent steering taking place before a bend has been reached.

The tangent point is special in two other ways. It is a near stationary point in the velocity flow field: other points on both sides of the road move laterally in the visual field and so will carry the driver's eye with them via the optokinetic reflex (Fig. 7.7). The tangent point moves only when road curvature changes and this movement, as we have seen, can be used by the driver to steer by. Second, if the view around the bend is occluded by, for instance, a fence or hedge, then the tangent point affords the longest clear view of the road ahead. These various attributes make it unsurprising that tangent points are preferentially fixated.

Experience suggests, however, that we are able to steer adequately without actually fixating the tangent point, for example when attending to road signs or other traffic. Figure 7.5a and similar records show that the eyes are indeed not absolutely glued to the tangent point but can take time out to look at other things. These excursions are accomplished by gaze saccades and typically last between 0.5 and 1 s. The probability of these off-road glances occurring varies with road curvature and with the stage of the bend that the vehicle has reached, and they are least likely to occur around the time of entry into a new bend. At this point drivers fixated the tangent point 80% of the time (Land and Lee, 1994). It seems that special attention is required at this time, presumably to get the initial estimate of the bend's curvature correct. A confirmation of this came from Yilmaz and Nakayama (1995), who used reaction times to a vocal probe to show that attention was diverted to the road just before simulated bends and that

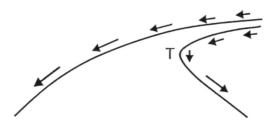

Fig. 7.7 The velocity flow field associated with points on the lane edges when rounding a bend.

sharper curves demanded more attention than shallower ones. The fewer and shallower the bends in the road, the more time can be spent looking off the road, and this probably accounts for the lack of a close relation between gaze direction and steering on studies of driving on freeways and other major roads. Nevertheless, it is certainly true that looking away from the road ahead for any substantial period of time is detrimental. According to Summala (1998), lane keeping on a straight road deteriorates progressively when drivers are required to fixate at greater eccentricities from the vanishing point. There is only a slight drop in performance by 7°, and this becomes substantial by 23° and worse again by 38°. The effect is likely to be much more pronounced on bends, especially if the curvature changes. There are probably implications here for the positioning of both road signs and in-car controls. Evidence from a driving simulator study seems to endorse this view. Wittmann et al. (2006) considered how the placement of an in-car display (quite like the satellite navigation systems that are now in many of our cars) influenced driving performance. They found that the best places were more or less in the line of sight for travel (close to where the steering wheel is). More eccentric locations were detrimental to driving performance, such as braking reaction times. What is not clear is whether the deterioration in performance results from the eyes being unable to bring to clear vision the most informative parts of the road, or whether it is the disruption of the eye movement pattern itself that causes the problem (Marple-Horvat et al., 2005).

Formal models of steering behaviour

In 1978 an engineer, Edmund Donges, showed that there are basically two sorts of signal available to drivers: feedback signals (lateral and angular deviations from the road centre line, differences between the road curvature, and the vehicle's path curvature) and feed-forward or anticipatory signals obtained from more distant regions of the road up to 2 s ahead in time, corresponding to 90 ft (27 m) at 30 mph (48 kph). Donges (1978) used a driving simulator to demonstrate that each of these signals was indeed used in steering, although he did not discuss how they might be obtained visually. A version of his steering model is shown in Fig. 7.8. It now seems that we can begin to identify the feed-forward and feedback elements in the Donges' scheme with the far-road (tangent point, future path point, vanishing point) and near-road (lane edge marker) visual inputs already mentioned. It is not difficult to see why both are required. The far-road signal may provide excellent curvature information, but if the car starts out of lane, it will stay that way, however well it follows road curvature. One might think that lane-edge feedback on its own would be sufficient, but visual processing and mechanical delays mean that the feedback loop becomes unstable at even moderate speeds (as, for example, when driving in fog with no far-road input). Matching road curvature takes the pressure off the near-road feedback loop, and it means that it can operate faster at much lower gain and thus be much less prone to instability.

Studies on a simple simulator (Fig. 7.9) have shown that feed-forward information from the distant part of the road is not on its own sufficient to give good steering (Land, 1998; Land and Horwood, 1995). When only the farthest region of the simulated road

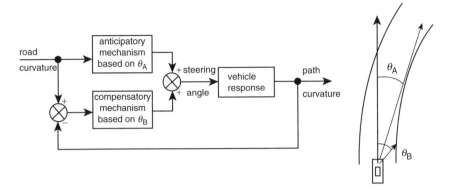

Fig. 7.8 Control diagram of steering incorporating feed-forward information from distant parts of the road (θ_A) and feedback information from the near lane edges (θ_B). Based on Donges (1978).

was visible, curvature matching was still accurate, but position-in-lane control was very poor (a). Conversely, with only the near road region visible (c), lane maintenance was quite good, but curvature matching was poor, mainly because of rather wild 'bang-bang' steering induced by the short time (<0.5 s) available for reaction to the movements of the road edges. Although it would seem from (b) that somewhere in between, about 5° down from the horizon, gives a good result on both criteria, it turned out that the best performance was obtained when distant (a) and near (c) regions were combined. This was better than having region (b) on its own and was indistinguishable from having the whole road visible. Interestingly, the near part of the road was rarely fixated compared with the more distant region, but it was certainly seen and used; it is typically about 5° obliquely below the typical direction of gaze.

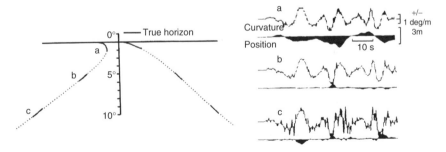

Fig. 7.9 Performance on a simulator when different 1° vertical segments of a winding road were visible (a-c, top). Records show curvature of road and car's track, and position of car relative to the midline of the road. Inaccuracies – discrepancies between the road and car track – show up in black. More distant parts of the road (a) allow road curvature to be matched accurately but are very poor at keeping the car in lane. Near regions (c) are better for maintaining lane position but cause the steering to go into 'bang-bang' mode. From Land and Horwood (1995).

Mourant and Rockwell (1970) had already concluded that lane position is monitored with peripheral vision. They also argued that learner drivers first use foveal vision for lane keeping, then increasingly move foveal gaze to more distant road regions, and learn to use their peripheral vision to stay in lane. Summala et al. (1996) reached similar conclusions. The principal outcome of these studies is that neither the far-road input (from tangent points or elsewhere) nor the near road lane-edge input is sufficient on their own, but the combination of the two allows fluent accurate driving (Land, 1998).

An explicit model of steering control has been put forward by Salvucci and Gray (2004): the 'two-point visual control model'. It differs from the tangent point or gaze sampling schemes outlined above but, like them, still incorporates contributions from both near- and far-road inputs. Salvucci and Gray proposed that drivers select two points on the road, one at a near distance in front of the car convenient for viewing the lane edges and a second at some distance up the road. The attractive feature of this particular model is that the exact location and identity of the distant point is not important: it might be the tangent point, or a car in front, or the vanishing point. The reason for this flexibility is that it is only the angular velocity of this point, not its location, that is used as a control variable. This means that any salient distant point can be used. These include points off or on the road. For the near point both angular position and velocity are important. The control equation thus has three terms: near-point location (θ_n), near-point angular velocity ($\dot{\theta}_n$), and far-point velocity ($\dot{\theta}_f$). Between them they control the rate of change of car direction ($\dot{\varphi}_n$) which, at any one speed, will be proportional to the steering wheel angle:

$$\dot{\varphi}_n = k_f\,\dot{\theta}_f + k_n\,\dot{\theta}_n + k_1\theta_n$$

In this equation the ($\dot{\varphi}_n = k_1\theta_n$) part of the equation describes a simple tracking loop that keeps the car heading towards the near point on the road ahead. The two angular velocity terms act to stabilize the system by minimizing the angular motion, relative to the car, of both far and near points. Salvucci and Gray were able to show that, with suitably chosen values for the constants, this control system was able to duplicate the results of Land and Horwood (1995) on steering with only parts of the road visible (Fig. 7.9). It also reproduced a series of recovery manoeuvres, studied by Hildreth et al. (2000), in which human drivers corrected for imposed deviations from the centre line. It could also successfully model the time courses of lane-change manoeuvres (Salvucci and Liu, 2000) by switching near and far points from the current lane to the new lane.

The success of the Salvucci and Gray's two-point model does not necessarily imply that other sources of information are unused. Systems based on tangent point direction (Fig. 7.6), rather than its angular velocity, also model steering competently (Murray et al., 1996). Although the tangent point is fixated consistently by drivers, it is not possible to say whether the information derived from it concerns its position or its angular velocity (or both), and it will be hard to establish this in real driving conditions. Exactly what mix of potentially useful control variables contributes to steering may well vary with the nature of the task and the road conditions (Wann and Wilkie, 2004).

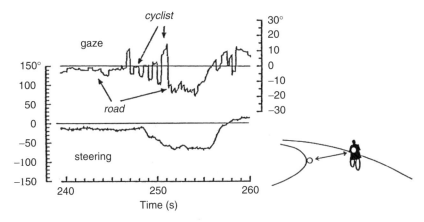

Fig. 7.10 Gaze movements when simultaneously steering around a bend and monitoring the behaviour of a cyclist. Gaze moves between tangent point and cyclist at roughly half-second intervals. Steering is related to the movement of the road edge and is (fortunately) suspended when gaze is transferred to the cyclist. From Land (1988).

To summarize, there is universal agreement that fluent driving on winding roads requires visual information from both near and distant road regions. The near region involves feedback from the angular position and velocity of the lane boundaries. There is, however, less agreement about which features in the far road region are necessary or sufficient to provide prospective feed-forward information (Mars, 2008).

Multitasking

Sometimes the eye must be used for two different functions at the same time, and as there is only one foveal direction and off-axis vision is poor, the visual system has to resort to time-sharing. A good example of this is shown in Fig. 7.10, in which the driver is negotiating a bend and so needs to look at the tangent point while passing a cyclist who needs to be checked on repeatedly. The record shows that the driver alternates gaze between tangent point and cyclist several times, spending half a second on each. The lower record shows that he steers by the road edge, which means that the coupling between eye and hand has to be turned off when he views the cyclist (who would otherwise be run over!). Thus not only does gaze switch between tasks, so does the whole visual-motor control system. Presumably, while looking at the cyclist, the information from the tangent point is kept 'on hold' at its previous value in an appropriate buffer. Time sharing of this kind may be typical of urban driving (see Fig. 7.15).

How long can a driver afford to take his gaze away from the road itself when attending to traffic, road signs, or just looking at the scenery? Undoubtedly this depends on vehicle speed and on the tortuousness of the road. However, studies by Land (1998) and Hildreth et al. (2000) both showed that removal of visual feedback for up to about 1.5 s has little effect at moderate speeds but that if loss of vision lasts longer than this performance rapidly deteriorates. We have already seen that drivers impose an internal delay of about 0.8 s before acting (Fig. 7.5b), so this much information is already 'in the pipeline'. From the occlusion studies it seems that useful information remains available for about twice this length of time but not for very much longer. Clearly this has implications for the design of road signs: off road glances should not last much longer than a second.

Braking

A crucial component of driving is to know when and how hard to brake. All drivers would acknowledge that the sudden visual expansion an object in front, usually another vehicle, is a powerful stimulus for hitting the brake. Not all braking is of course this dramatic, and keeping an appropriate distance from the vehicle in front is achieved by means that barely intrude on our consciousness. Nevertheless, we are using one or more aspects of the appearance of the vehicle ahead as control variables to ensure that the appropriate speed, and acceleration or deceleration are maintained.

There are a number of things that we might monitor. The actual distance to the vehicle in front can be estimated directly from the amount of road visible behind the leading car. The visual angle subtended by the leading car (or between its rear lights at night) can be converted into distance, provided we have an estimate of the actual width of the vehicle – which we usually do. Speed can be estimated from the relative motion of the ground plane. One variable that is mathematically attractive because it requires no estimates of size or distance or velocity is time to contact (τ: Greek tau). This is the time that it will take to reach some obstacle in the path if the current velocity is maintained. David Lee (1976) showed that τ can be obtained directly from estimates of the radial velocity (on the retina) of elements in any part of the plane containing the obstacle. The ratio of the angular distance of some element in the obstacle plane from the direction of heading (or centre of expansion of the flow-field) to the radial angular velocity of the same element gives the value of τ. In terms of Fig. 7.11, $\tau = r_1/v_1 = r_2/v_2$. Alternatively stated, τ is the reciprocal of the relative rate of expansion of the elements in the obstacle plane. A derivation of this relationship is given in Chapter 8 in the context of catching a ball. (The first use of τ seems to have been by the astronomer Fred Hoyle in his novel *The Black Cloud* (1957, p. 27), where he estimated the time to contact of the approaching eponymous cloud in the same way).

How can τ be used to control speed of approach? Clearly, if we are moving at 10 ms^{-1} (u) towards an obstacle 30 m away (s), and do nothing, we will crash into it in 3 s. We need to decelerate in such a way that the velocity (v) reduces to zero in 30 m. The equation of motion $v^2 = u^2 + 2as$, with $v = 0$, $u = 10$, and $s = 30$, gives a constant acceleration (a) of -1.67 ms^{-2} (about 0.17 g), and, using $v = u + at$, the stopping time will be 5.99 s. More generally, from the first equation, if $as/u^2 = -0.5$, the vehicle will stop exactly at the obstacle (i.e. $v = 0$). It would seem from this that a driver would have to know both his distance from the obstacle (s) and his initial velocity (u) before he can

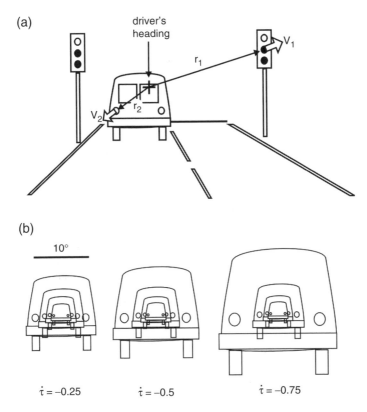

Fig. 7.11 (a) Stopping behind a stationary van at traffic lights. The time to contact (τ) is given by any of the ratios r_1/v_1, r_2/v_2, etc. for any objects or texture element in the plane being approached. (b) An attempt to visualize what different values of $\dot\tau$ would look like to a driver. They show the appearance of a stationary 2 m wide van at an initial distance of 30 m. The driver decelerates from 10 ms^{-1} to produce the values of $\dot\tau$ shown. The appearance of the van is shown at 1s intervals. A $\dot\tau$ value of –0.25 gives more deceleration than required; –0.5 will result in an exact stop at the van; –0.75 is inadequate and will result in a crash. It is not difficult to imagine that a driver could learn to use the different expansion rates as a guide to safe braking.

work out his deceleration ($-a$). He may indeed have estimates of these, but Lee (1976) first pointed out that there may be a simpler way of achieving appropriate deceleration, based on the rate of change of the optically derived variable τ, that is, dτ/dt, or $\dot\tau$. Lee showed that the visual consequence of a constant deceleration such that $as/u^2 =$ –0.5 is that $\dot\tau$ will be equal to –0.5. To be safe, it would be best to maintain a value of $\dot\tau$ slightly greater than this. Using existing data from the braking behaviour of test drivers, Lee found good agreement between their deceleration curves and the consequences of a strategy that held $\dot\tau$ at a 'safe' value of –0.425. Thus one recipe that will allow the driver to stop exactly at the obstacle is to keep the value of the optic variable

$\hat{\tau}$ constant at or just above –0.5. A study of actual braking found that drivers' perform-ance was broadly in line with this strategy (Yilmaz and Warren, 1995). However, Rock and Harris (2006) found that performance deteriorates if there is no ground plane to provide independent speed and distance information, implying that the $\hat{\tau}$ hypothesis does not provide a complete account of braking control.

Although a deceleration that produces a $\hat{\tau}$ value just above –0.5 is in some sense 'ideal', because no further adjustments need to be made once it is attained, there is no reason why a driver should base his strategy on simply trying to maintain this value. Provided he does not need to exceed the capacity of the vehicle to decelerate (Lee's estimate is a maximum of about 0.7g), there are potentially an infinite number of deceleration profiles that might be adopted. One might be to decelerate early and then ease off, another to slam the brakes on at the last minute. The crucial point is that the driver needs to be aware of what Fajen (2005) described as the 'action boundary' between being able to stop and not being able to stop. This depends on the vehicle's braking capacity, the slope, the state of the road surface and so on, as well as the vehicle's velocity and the distance to the obstacle. Whatever optical variables are used in the control of braking, acquired knowledge of the vehicle's capabilities is needed as well.

Urban driving

Negotiating urban corners

Steering around the kind of right-angled corner we encounter in cities is a rather different task from following the curves of a country road. It is a well-rehearsed, rather stereotyped task, with the amount the steering wheel has to be turned varying little from one corner to another. The following account is based on a new study in Sussex of three drivers each negotiating eight suburban right-angled corners. Each turn proceeds in two distinct phases, which, by analogy with ordinary walking turns (Chapter 6), we can call orientational and compensatory phases (Imai et al., 2001). In the orientational phase, gaze is directed into the bend by 50° or more relative to the car, with most of the rotation performed by the neck (head/car in Fig. 7.12b and c); meanwhile the eyes fixate various positions around the bend with small saccades. Once the car turn has begun, the neck stops turning, but the head continues to rotate in space for sometime, carried by the continued rotation of the car. The neck then reverses its direction of rotation (53 and 9 s in the two examples in Fig. 7.12), and the head starts to come into line with the car. This is the compensatory phase, so-called because the head rotation counteracts to a large degree the rotation of the car. As can be seen in Fig. 7.12 the car-in-space and head-in-car rotations are almost (but not quite) equal and opposite during this phase, and the head-in-space rotation is greatly reduced. This is consistent with a feedback mechanism in which the vestibular system measures the residual head-in-space rotation, and converts it, amplified, into a neck rotation command that counteracts the head-in-space rotation (this is the vestibulo-collic reflex; see Fig. 6.7 and Land, 2004). At about the same time as the neck reverses

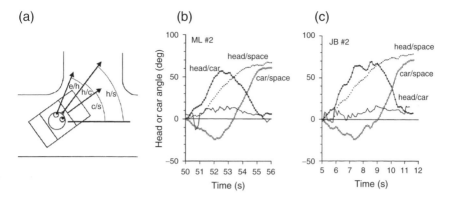

Fig. 7.12 Eye, head, and car direction while negotiating a 90° suburban corner.
(a) The four kinds of measurements that can be made from the eye-tracker and head-view cameras. (b) and (c) Records from two drivers going around the same left-hand corner (near-side in United Kingdom). The two features seen in all drivers are the large head turn into the bend during the first 2 s (head/car), followed by a return of the head to the straight-ahead position as the car turns. During this return phase the head rotates very little relative to outside space (head/space), and it is the rotation of the car that brings the body back into line with the head. Eye movements (thin line) fixate points around the road edge but contribute little to the overall changes of gaze direction, which are principally caused by head rotation.

its direction of rotation, gaze shifts from the entrance to the bend to more distant regions of the road.

What is critical in getting this manoeuvre right is the timing of the steering action, both when entering and exiting from the corner. Using the view provided by the eye tracker, it was possible to examine what timing cues were available in the half second or so before the driver began to steer into and out of the bend. The changes in the appearance of the road edge (kerb) seemed to be the only cues to provide useful timing information that also correlated reliably with the initiation of the steering action (Fig. 7.13b). In a left-hand turn (nearside in the United Kingdom) the tangent point slips leftward as the corner approaches (angle α), and steering starts when α reaches between 30 and 40° (Fig. 7.13b and c left). The cue for straightening up at the exit of the bend seems to be rotation of the nearside kerb in the visual field (angle β). Just before the end of the bend the kerb angle rotates through the vertical in the driver's view, with β going from acute to obtuse (Fig. 7.13b and c right). The change of steering direction occurred when this angle reached between 140 and 150°, about half a second after the kerb passed through the vertical in the visual field. Although these may not be the only features involved, there was little else in the drivers' field of view that was both conspicuous and reliable. Turning right (offside in the United Kingdom) is a little more difficult as there are the added problems of crossing a traffic stream and lining up with the far kerb. However, similar cues are also available for this manoeuvre.

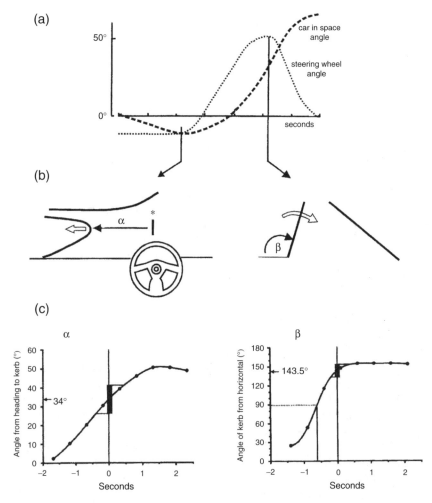

Fig. 7.13 Cues for steering round a right-angled corner. (a) Average car rotation profile and the angle of the steering wheel during a left-hand (near-side) turn. Average from a total of 12 turns by 3 different drivers. (b) The two most reliable cues for initiating the turn into the bend (left), and for deciding when to straighten up when exiting the bend (right). Coming into the bend the angle α of the kerb at the corner relative to the car's heading (*) indicates when the turn should begin. Coming out of the turn the angle of the near-side kerb (β) changes from acute to obtuse just before straightening up occurs. (c) The range of values of angles α and β at the commencement of turning and of straightening up for 12 left-hand corners. The vertical bars show ±1 s.d. and that there is little variation in these angles.

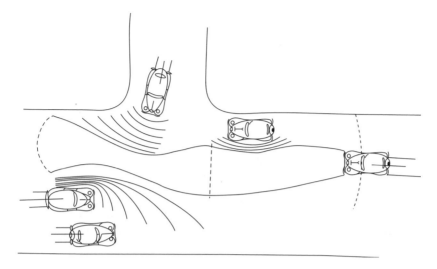

Fig. 7.14 The 'field of safe travel' for the car on the right. Modified from Gibson and Crooks (1938).

Driving in towns

In an early study trying to establish a systematic description of driving behaviour, Gibson and Crooks (1938) came up with the following definition of steering an automobile: 'Steering … is a perceptually governed series of reactions by the driver of such a sort as to keep the car headed into the middle of the field of safe travel' (p. 456). They illustrated what they meant with the splendid illustration reproduced in Fig. 7.14. Progressing safely, in their view, involves determining the shape and extent of this ever-changing field and driving within it. The form of the field is determined largely by the imaginary 'clearance lines' around the various moving or stationary objects, where the clearance lines are analogous to contour lines representing the magnitude of the consequences of a collision. The idea of a field of safe travel is straightforward and intuitively appealing. We are perhaps in a better position now than in 1938 to think about the ways the eyes might determine the boundaries of this field.

In urban driving, multitasking is even more important than it is on country roads (cf. Fig. 7.10) as each traffic situation and road sign competes for attention and potential action. To our knowledge there has been no systematic study of where drivers look in traffic, but from our own observations it is clear that drivers fixate the places from which they need to obtain information: the car in front, the outer edges of obstacles, pedestrians and cyclists, road signs and traffic lights, and so on. Figure 7.15 illustrates the visual strategy of a driver (MFL) negotiating a rather typical urban situation in the United Kingdom. Like many towns, the High Street in Lewes in Sussex is relatively narrow, has parked cars or delivery vans on either side, and can just manage two lanes of moving traffic. Even at low speeds, it requires considerable concentration for the driver to stay within the 'field of safe travel'. In the record in Fig. 7.15 (left) the car is travelling through the traffic at about 7 mph (11 kph). Gaze movements alternate rapidly and irregularly between the car in front (35% of the time), the oncoming vehicles on the right (42%), and the edges of the parked cars on the left (10%). Hardly any time is spent looking off road (6%) or at the road surface (7%). In the period between 10 and 20 s gaze shifts between different regions every half second, with either one or

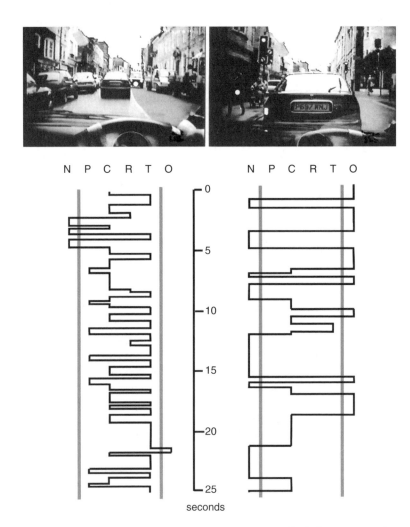

Fig. 7.15 Gaze distribution when steering through dense traffic (left, gaze is on the oncoming car) and when stationary at traffic lights (right, gaze is on a pedestrian on the left). When driving almost all fixations are on objects on the roadway; when stationary almost all are off-road. N, near-side off-road; P, parked vehicles on near-side; C, car in front; R, on or above open roadway; T, oncoming traffic; O, off-side off road. Grey lines are edges of roadway (kerbs). Each 'look' at a particular region usually involves more than one fixation.

two fixations on each region. In Fig. 7.15 (right) the car is stationary at traffic lights, and the fixation pattern is completely different. Most of the fixations (75%) are off-road on the left or right pavements, looking at shops and pedestrians. Twenty two percent are on the car in front and 3% on another vehicle. In this situation viewing is recreational, unlike the serious vigilance apparent when driving in traffic. The leisure-liness of stationary viewing is also shown by the doubling of the time spent looking at each region (mean 1.14 s) compared with the equivalent time when moving (0.54 s). Other traffic situations produce different patterns of gaze distribution, and it is hard to make any overall generalizations. Drivers have a range of strategies to match the current driving conditions, varying between continuous two-per-second sampling of the potential obstacle field, to more relaxed road following in lighter traffic, with many more glances to the off-road surroundings.

At speeds of 30 mph (48 kph) or less on straight roads, steering is adequately con-trolled by peripheral lane-edge (feedback) information, and there is no need for far-road feed-forward information. This frees up the eyes for the multiple demands of dealing with other road users and potential obstacles. As Fig. 7.15 shows, in traffic there is a concentration of attention in the central rather than peripheral regions of the visual field. Miura (1987) has shown that as the demands of traffic situations increase, peripheral vision is sacrificed to provide greater attentional resources for information uptake by the fovea. Crundall (2005) also found that when potentially hazardous situations become visible in a video clip the ability of drivers to detect stimuli (lights) in the periphery is diminished. This effect was greater with novices compared with experienced drivers, and recovery (the time taken to re-engage peripheral detection) was also faster with the experienced group. To some extent these effects simply reflect the fact that in difficult traffic more is happening in central vision, although that does not entirely explain why peripheral stimuli cannot attract attention.

Learning to drive

In their first few driving lessons, learners have to master a great many unfamiliar pat-terns of sensory-motor coordination. These include steering (staying in lane, turning corners), braking, gear changing (exacerbated by clutch control in a stick-shift car), using the rear-view mirror, looking out for road signs, and staying vigilant for other vehicles and pedestrians. Initially all these tasks require attentive monitoring, but over the course of a few lessons many of them become at least partially automated, so that more attentional resources can be devoted to the less predictable aspects of driving, notably the behaviour of other road users.

There have been few studies of the very first stages of driving, if only because few learners are willing to add an unfamiliar eye tracker to their already onerous coordina-tion tasks. However, in a recent study (M.F. Land and C.J. Hughes, in Land, 2006) we did, with the consent of the police, use an eye tracker to examine the differences in gaze patterns between three novice drivers and their instructor, during their first four lessons. There were a number of minor differences relating to where the learners looked on straight roads; they tended to confine gaze to the ahead direction, in par-ticular, with fewer glances off the road than experienced drivers. However the most striking and consistent effect was on the gaze behaviour of the novices when turning a

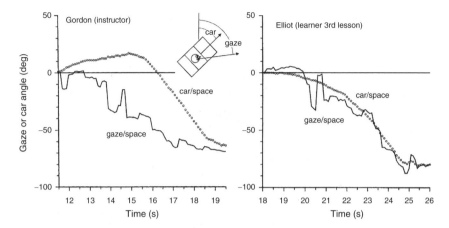

Fig. 7.16 Gaze movements of instructor (left) and novice (right) turning a sharp right-hand bend. The instructor, like other competent drivers, looks into the bend, about 50° ahead of the car's heading. This is mainly brought about by head movement. The novice's gaze hardly departs from the car's current heading.

corner (Fig. 7.16). The driving instructor, like most competent drivers, directed gaze by as much as 50° into the bend, soon after the steering wheel began to turn (see also Fig. 7.12). This was done almost entirely with a head movement; the eyes fixated various roadside objects towards the exit of the bend but rarely made excursions of more than 20° from the head axis. All three learners, on the other hand, kept gaze strictly in line with the car's heading, at least during the first lesson (by Lesson 4, two of the three were turning into the bend like the instructor, but not the third). The meaning of this change is that the novices are learning to anticipate. In Fig. 7.16, by 15 s, the instructor is already looking at a point that the car's heading will not reach for another 2 to 3 s. Presumably this allows him to plan his exit from the bend and also notice whether there are any potential hazards. The learners cannot do this to begin with, probably because the task of getting the steering right for the bend requires all their attention. The reduced functional field of view, seen in novice drivers by a number of authors (Mourant and Rockwell, 1972; Crundall et al., 1998), is presumably also related to the fact that steering itself has yet to be fully mastered.

Racing driving

We have had one opportunity (Land and Tatler, 2001) to examine the eye and head movements of a racing driver (Tomas Schekter) when driving at full racing speed round the circuit at Mallory park in Leicestershire, United Kingdom (Fig. 7.17a). Like ordinary drivers, his gaze was directed near to the tangent points of bends, but there were systematic departures from the exact tangent points that were different for each bend and were repeated on each lap. Unlike low-speed driving gaze changes were almost entirely the result of neck rotation rather than eye-in-head movements, which were of low amplitude (< ± 10°) and almost unrelated to the head movements (Fig. 7.17b). During the hairpin (D), for example, the head turned 50° into the bend,

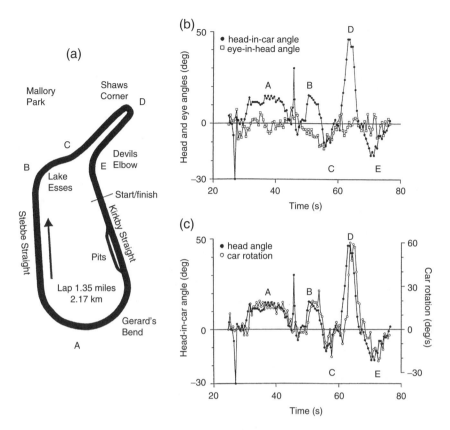

Fig. 7.17 Eye and head movements of a racing driver during one lap. (a) The Mallory Park circuit. (b) Eye-in-head and head-in-car (neck) angles, showing the correspondence between head direction and the curvature of the bend [letters correspond to the bends on (a)] and the lack of a relation between eye and head movements. (c) Very close relation between head-in-car angle and the rate of rotation of the car 1 s later. The two 'spikes' (26 and 45 s) are quick glances off-road or to the mirrors. (From Land and Tatler, 2001)

whereas the eye-in-head angle stayed close to zero. The most impressive finding, and one for which we have yet to find a convincing explanation, was that the angle of the head in the yaw plane was an almost exact predictor of the rotational speed of the car, one second later (Fig. 7.17c). Thus during the hairpin when the head turned 50°, the car rotation reached 60° s^{-1} one second later. Schekter himself believed that the head movements functioned to minimize the rotational forces on his head.

One difference between racing driving and ordinary driving is that a racing driver will have learned the circuit thoroughly. He will therefore have some stored mental model of the circuit (see Chapter 10), which can then be used to control his speed and racing line, and he probably only needs to view the tangent points to check the exactness of his line and timing rather than to provide a major steering cue as in normal driving. His ability to anticipate accurately the car's behaviour around the different bends, as evidenced by his head movements (Fig. 7.17c), also suggests that he has a very well-rehearsed dynamic representation of the circuit. At some stage it would be very interesting to see the changes that occur in eye and head behaviour as a driver learns a new circuit.

Overtaking is a crucial part of motor racing, and we were able to analyse a number of instances. There were no real surprises. Schekter's gaze alternated irregularly between the rear of the car in front, the potential gap to left or right, and, if overtaking on a bend, the tangent point.

Driving simulation

In modern driving simulators the visual representation of the world being driven through can be amazingly good, with highly realistic wide-field scene depiction and little or no delay in updating the virtual world in response to the driver's controls. Nevertheless, none of the driving simulators we have tried has provided a convincing approximation to real driving. Gentle road curvatures present few problems, but right-angled corners and roundabouts seem very hard to negotiate satisfactorily. It is also a common observation that after a few minutes of trying to steer around curves one begins to feel sick. Undoubtedly part of the problem is that the eyes and the vestibular system are giving opposite messages, with the eyes signalling that one is turning in the world, and the semicircular canals saying that the one's head is stationary. In normal locomotion, vestibular cues are used in the perception of self motion, both linear and rotational, and can also be crucial in correctly interpreting optic flow, particularly when head rotation is involved (Kemeny and Panerai, 2003). If this conflict between vision and the vestibular system is indeed at the root of the difficulties many people experience in simulators, then it seems there is little that can be done about it, short of making simulators that really rotate and translate, which rather defeats the object of the exercise. Nevertheless, in The Netherlands in particular, driving simulators are widely used in the early part of driver training as a didactic tool to establish the basics of steering and car control, although their use must then be integrated with normal on-road training (Kappé, 2005).

Summary

1. Normal driving requires maintaining position in lane and successfully navigating bends. This involves the use of both feedback information from the lane markings close to the vehicle and feed-forward information from more distant road regions.

2. An important source of feed-forward information is the tangent point of an upcoming bend, whose direction relative to the vehicle's current heading predicts the bend's curvature.

3. During urban driving, in particular, several potentially hazardous situations may require constant monitoring (other vehicles, pedestrians, etc.). In these situations

gaze switches between hazards at approximately half-second intervals. In less-demanding environments the switching intervals are much longer.

4. When negotiating right-angled urban corners, experienced drivers begin to turn their heads well ahead of the car's change of direction. This means that gaze anticipates the future direction of the car by up to 3 s. Novice drivers initially rely more heavily on feedback cues and take some time to develop this anticipatory strategy.

Chapter 8

Ball games: when to look where?

Ball sports

Ball sports such as tennis or squash probably contain the fastest feats of visuo-motor co-ordination of which humans are capable. They are so fast that there is barely time for the player to use his normal oculomotor machinery. Often the striker of the ball has less than half a second to judge the trajectory of the ball and formulate a properly aimed and timed stroke. Half a second gives time for one or at the most two saccades, and the speeds involved preclude smooth pursuit for much of the ball's flight. In cricket or baseball the accuracy required is a few centimetres in space and a few milliseconds in time (Regan, 1992; Watts and Bahill, 1990). How do practitioners of these sports use their eyes to get the information they need?

Members of both genders participate in most of the sports considered here. To avoid clumsy circumlocution, we will use the masculine throughout, with the intention that 'he' or 'him' will stand in for 'he or she' and 'him or her'.

Catching a ball

Many ball sports require players either to catch a ball (cricket, baseball, rugby football) or to intercept a moving ball with a bat, racket, stick, or foot (e.g. tennis, hockey, football in its various forms). In all these sports there are two requirements: to be in the right place at the right time and to intercept the ball effectively. In the case of catching this means running towards the point in space and time where the ball will be at catchable height and then putting the hands in a position to grasp the ball at the right moment. We will consider each step in turn.

Locating the catching point

Catching in baseball or cricket has been the subject of much work and some controversy. If a ball has been hit in a direction that could possibly result in a catch, what visual cues, and what algorithms, does a fielder use to run to the point where he will just reach it before it lands? In general this will require the fielder to move both towards (or away from) the launch point and also laterally. Taking the simpler case where the ball's direction is directly towards the fielder, but the trajectory is high and unknown, there does seem to be one efficient strategy for guiding the appropriate run. This was first suggested by Chapman (1968) who analysed the visual information available to a baseball player catching a fly ball. He concluded that if the trajectory is parabolic and the fielder runs at constant speed the angle of elevation (α) of the ball, during its flight relative to the catcher, will be such that the acceleration of the tangent of α will be

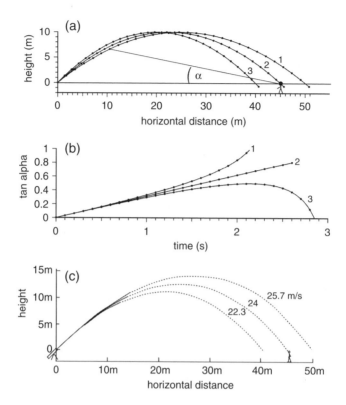

Fig. 8.1 Cues available to a fielder deciding whether to run forward or backward.
(a) Three balls with trajectories of the same height but slightly different launch angles.
(b) The value of tan α, as seen by the fielder, for the three trajectories in (a). He has to
decide whether the rate of change of tan α is increasing (1: go back) decreasing
(3: go forward) or constant (2: don't move). (c) Three trajectories with the same launch
angle but different velocities. The end of the full lines shows the point at which fielders
started to move forward or back. This typically occurred about 0.8 s into the ball's
flight. Comparison with (b) shows that the differences in tan α at this point are very
small. (c) is redrawn from McLeod and Dienes (1996).

zero, that is, $d^2(\tan \alpha)/dt^2 = 0$. An equivalent way of putting this is that the rate of
increase of tan α will be constant (Fig. 8.1a and b). If this condition is met, then the
fielder and ball will arrive at the same place at the same time. Michaels and Oudejans
(1992) found that fielders did indeed run in such a way that the tangent of α increased
with approximately constant velocity as the fielders moved to make the catch. This
result indicates that the fielders were doing the right thing, but it does not indicate
how they managed it.

The Chapman formulation, where the fielder moves at constant velocity, requires
that this velocity is worked out very early in the ball's trajectory and then maintained.
McLeod and Dienes (1996) pointed out that this is unrealistic, given that the differences

in trajectory visible to the fielder are tiny at the time they start to move (after about 840 ms; Fig. 8.1b and c). They found that fielders do start moving in the right direction (backwards if the ball will land behind their present position and vice versa) at about this time, but their velocity is not directly related to landing position, and furthermore it varies throughout their run, as though under continuous control (Fig. 8.2). Like Michaels and Oudejans, they found that fielders did keep closely to the $d^2(\tan \alpha)/dt^2 = 0$ rule but seemed to be using departures from this condition (or from constant velocity of $\tan \alpha$) as an error variable with which to control their speed. They also showed that simpler strategies, such as maintaining constant α, or constant velocity of α ($d\alpha/dt$ rather than $d(\tan \alpha)/dt$), will not guarantee a successful catch. However, they pointed out that in a system that uses continuous feedback it is not necessary to adhere strictly to Chapman's zero acceleration of $\tan \alpha$ rule. All that is required in practice is to keep the angle of elevation of gaze to the ball increasing, at a rate that decreases with elevation (this is because $\tan \alpha$ increases faster than α, reaching ∞ at 90°. Thus, if $d(\tan \alpha)/dt$ is to remain constant, $d\alpha/dt$ must be reduced at high values of α). Whatever the exact nature of the measurements made by the fielder, it is clear that both angle of

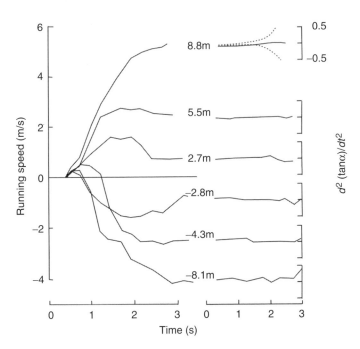

Fig. 8.2 Running speeds of a fielder intercepting balls whose landing positions would be in front of (positive values) or behind the initial position of the fielder by the distances shown. Note that the running speeds are not constant, implying that adjustments are made continuously throughout the balls' flight, not just at its beginning. Graphs on the left show that the acceleration of $\tan \alpha$ is kept nearly constant throughout the flights. Dotted lines (top right) show the values the fielder would have seen had he run at constant velocity and missed the ball by 2 m. Redrawn from McLeod and Dienes (1996).

elevation and its rate of change have to be determined. The simplest way of doing this would be to track the ball with eye and head – which catchers do – and measure the extent and rate of the tracking effort (Oudejans et al., 1999; Tresilian, 1995).

Fielders will also have to move laterally to intercept balls that are not coming straight towards them. To establish the initial running direction the fielder only has to see whether the ball moves to the left or right of the direction of the launch point – or alternatively he has to notice which direction his gaze is turning as he tracks the ball. For the fielder to reach the ball his lateral velocity, relative to a line joining him to the ball's launch point, must on average be the same as the ball's lateral velocity, relative to the same line, by the time the ball falls to catching height (Fig. 8.3). This can be achieved in various ways: by accelerating early to get into line with the ball's trajectory, running at a constant lateral velocity to arrive at the plane of the trajectory as the ball reaches hand height, or running fast initially to get ahead of the trajectory and then slowing down. In practice all three strategies are observed (McLeod et al., 2006). What all successful strategies have in common is that in the later stages of the run, the rate of rotation of the fielder's gaze ($d\delta/dt$; Fig. 8.3), as he tracks the ball, is kept constant. If it accelerates the ball will hit the ground ahead of him, and if it decelerates he will overshoot it. Whether the gaze rotation velocity is positive, negative, or zero will depend on the strategy initially adopted and the lateral speed of the ball. Although fielders differ in the strategies they use, all keep gaze rotation velocity constant for the last second or more of the run. McLeod et al. (2006) proposed that fielders operate as servo mechanisms in which departures from constant gaze rotation velocity result in increases or decreases in lateral running speed, so stabilizing gaze rotation speed, which is the condition for interception.

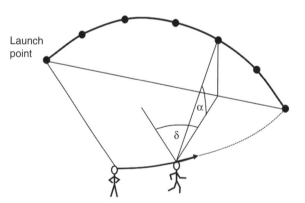

Fig. 8.3 Running to catch a ball whose trajectory is not in line with the fielder. According to McLeod et al. (2006) the crucial feature of the fielder's run that allows him to intercept the ball is that in its later stages the rate of rotation of gaze ($d\delta/dt$) is held constant. The fielder adjusts his speed to maintain this constancy. He must also keep the acceleration of $\tan \alpha$ constant, as with an in-line ball. Based on McLeod et al. (2006).

To summarize, intercepting a high-flying ball involves two strategies—one dealing with motion towards or away from the launch point and a separate strategy for lateral motion towards the plane of the trajectory. The first involves tracking the ball as it rises and moving so that the rate of vertical rotation of gaze decreases with elevation angle. The second involves moving laterally so that the rate of horizontal rotation of gaze is constant during the later stages of the run. These two strategies, which are independent of each other but generally operate simultaneously, have been described as 'the generalized optic acceleration cancellation theory of catching (GOAC)' by McLeod et al. (2006). There is a rival theory, the 'linear optic trajectory (LOT)' theory (McBeath et al., 1995; Shaffer et al., 2003) in which the fielder runs in such a way that the ratio of the vertical angle of the ball (α) and horizontal angle between the fielder, the ball and its starting point (β) remains constant. Thus in the GOAC theory vertical and horizontal ball angles are dealt with separately, and in the LOT theory they are controlled jointly by keeping their ratio constant. Both theories can be used to generate simulations, and both provide reasonable approximations to the paths taken by real fielders, although McLeod et al. (2006) claimed that the GOAC simulations are more accurate. They also pointed out other problems with the LOT model, for example, when the ball comes straight towards the fielder the ratio α/β becomes infinite, and for the same reason LOT theory cannot deal with the situation where a catcher moves into line with the ball and waits for it, as often happens. As these situations produce no special problems for fielders, it seems that a theory that separates vertical and horizontal mechanisms is the more plausible.

Timing of hand closure

During the last stages of a catch attempt, the hands need to prepare to close around the ball. As well as being in the right place, they need to have information about the ball's time of arrival. Apart from cues derived from the trajectory, as just discussed, there are two other sources of visual information available when the ball is within about 20 m of the catcher. These are rate of looming (increase of size of the retinal image of the ball) and rate of change of disparity (the difference in the position of the image of the ball on the two retinae). Both can provide information about the time to contact of the ball (Gray and Regan, 1998; Regan and Gray, 2000).

In Fig. 8.4a time to contact (τ) = D/V, but D and V are not directly available, so we need to find an expression for D/V in terms of the directly measurable quantities θ and its rate of change, $d\theta/dt$. Consider the right-angled triangle with sides r and D. This is similar to the small triangle with sides δD and δr, so that $\delta r/\delta D = r/D$. Hence $\delta r = r$ $\delta D/D$. But $\delta\theta \approx \delta r/D$, hence $\delta\theta = r\delta D/D^2$. However, r/D is the angle θ (in radians), hence $\delta\theta = \delta D.\theta/D$. Dividing by δt gives $\delta\theta/\delta t = \theta/D. \delta D/\delta t$. Rearranging, and substituting V for $\delta D/\delta t$ gives,

$$\theta/(\delta\theta/\delta t) = DV = \tau$$

Time to contact is thus the ratio the angular size of the ball to the rate of expansion of its edges. The derivation of τ from the disparity angle φ and its rate of change $\delta\varphi/\delta t$ (Fig. 8.4b) is analogous, and leads directly to $\tau = \varphi/(\delta\varphi/\delta t)$. The use of τ as a control variable in behaviour was first proposed by David Lee (1976). See also 'braking' in Chapter 7.

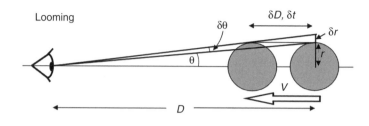

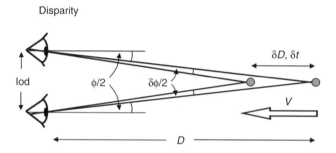

Fig. 8.4 Determination of time to contact (τ) of an approaching object from the rate of increase in angular size or from the rate of change of disparity. For looming $\tau = \varphi/(\delta\varphi/\delta t)$, for disparity $\tau = \phi/(\delta\theta/\delta t)$. Details in the text.

The relative contributions of looming and disparity change in catching were studied by Rushton and Wann (1999). They pointed out that for large balls such as footballs looming gives the better estimate, whereas for objects such as table tennis balls which are smaller than the inter-ocular distance (Iod, Fig. 8.4b) disparity is more useful. One might therefore expect different weightings to be given to the two cues depending on the circumstances. They used a virtual reality task in which subjects caught approaching tennis balls. Subjects could do this accurately, with grasp being initiated on average 146 ms before the ball arrived, when approach cues were normal. They could manipulate the looming and disparity cues separately, so that one led to an earlier time-to-contact estimate than the other, or one provided a normally decreasing estimate while the other gave an erroneously constant estimate. Rushton and Wann found that observers were always biased towards the earlier estimate of time to contact, whether this came from looming or disparity, and they were able to ignore one of the cues when it failed to provide a decreasing value for τ, or simply dropped out. They concluded that although both cues are used they cannot be simply combined additively by some fixed ratio formula, for example, $\tau = k_1\theta/(d\theta/dt) + k_2\varphi/(d\varphi/dt)$. (Here we revert to the standard differential 'd' rather than the incremental 'δ' used in Fig. 8.4). They proposed instead what they refer to as a 'dipole' model in which magnitudes and rates of change of the two variables are summed without distinguishing their origin:

$$\tau = (\theta + \varphi)/(d\theta/dt + d\varphi/dt)$$

This formulation has the implicit property that it biases its estimate of τ towards the more immediate or more effective cue. For example, if one cue drops out – say φ and $(d\varphi/dt)$ become zero – then the other cue simply takes over. This model is thus usefully flexible in the way it handles the two cues as well as having the merit of simplicity. Differential reliance on cues depending on their reliability, rather than reliance on a single cue or fixed weightings of cues, is reminiscent of the questions about whether optic flow or visual direction guides locomotion (Chapter 6). Here we see again that the perceptual system does not rely on fixed strategies for dealing with particular cues but is flexible and uses the most reliable cues for the current situation.

At what period before the catch is the information needed to perform the grasp taken in? There seems general agreement that after about 125 ms before the catch alteration of the grasp action is not possible. Preceding this, studies in which the ball was illuminated for varying lengths of time indicate that there is no one 'perceptual moment' in which sight of the ball is essential, but that the ability to catch increases when sight of the ball is made available up to about 450 ms before contact (Savelsbergh and Whiting, 1996). This is consistent with the idea that judgements of trajectory, looming, and disparity all improve over time.

Getting the hands to the ball

Catching a ball coming close but not straight towards the catcher requires a movement of hand, arm, and possibly body to intercept it. This in turn requires the catcher to assess the ball's direction, or at the least to estimate where the ball will be relative to the body when it reaches him. Figure 8.5 illustrates one way that this can be done. A ball is coming towards the catcher with a velocity V at an angle that will miss his head by a distance H, which is also the distance the hand must move to catch the ball. We need to find the value of H using information that the catcher may plausibly have available to him. In Fig. 8.5 the catcher views the ball when it is at a distance D from the potential point of capture. In a brief time δt the ball travels a distance δD, moving laterally by δh. Now by similar triangles $H/D = \delta h/\delta D$, so that $H = D\,\delta h/\delta D$. The time to contact, τ, is a variable that the catcher has presumably already obtained to time his catch, and it is equal to D/V, or $D/(\delta D/\delta t)$, Hence $D = \tau\,\delta D/\delta t$. The distance H thus becomes $\tau\,\delta D/\delta t . \delta h/\delta D$, or $H = \tau\,\delta h/\delta t$. Provided the ball is far enough away and the angle to the catcher not too large the line of sight distance to the ball will be very close to D. The angle through which the ball is seen to move in time δt will be $\delta\varphi$, where $\delta\varphi = \delta h/D$ (radians). Replacing δh by $D\,\delta\varphi$ in the expression for H gives,

$$H = \tau\,D\,\delta\varphi/\delta t$$

This is the answer: the catcher needs to know τ, the ball's distance, and its speed across the retina. The potential problem here is D, which is not obtainable directly. It could be obtained from binocular cues provided the distances are less than about 20 m, or, if it is a ball game where the player knows the diameter of the ball, then the $D =$ ball diameter / θ, where θ is the angular width of the ball on the retina. The catcher now seems to have plausible estimates of all the relevant variables, but there is still a lot to measure (López-Moliner et al., 2007).

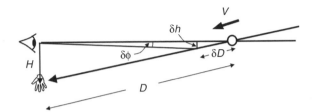

Fig. 8.5 Variables involved in catching a ball that requires a sideways arm and/or body movement to intercept it (a slip catch rather than an outfield catch). The amount the arm needs to be extended (*H*) can be obtained from $H = \tau D\, \delta\varphi/\delta t$, where τ is time to contact, derived from looming or disparity (Fig. 8.4), *D* is the current distance of the ball, derived from its apparent angular size, $\delta\varphi/\delta t$ is the observed angular speed of lateral movement of the ball. Further details in text.

A particular example where the situation is a little more straightforward is the job of being a slip catcher in cricket. This is one of the most difficult and important fielding tasks. Up to three slips stand quite close (5–15 m) behind the batsman on the side he holds his bat (off side) and their job is to catch deliveries that glance off the edge of the bat. In this situation the slip fielder knows his distance *D* from the batsman and can assume that the ball's velocity *V* is close the speed that it reached the bat. Replacing τ with *D/V* in the previous equation gives:

$$H = D^2/V.\ \delta\varphi/\delta t$$

This means that, so long as the catcher has pre-calibrated himself reasonably well for distance and ball speed, all he needs to measure, in the fraction of a second available, is the speed and direction of the ball's image across his retina. A more comprehensive account of the cues involved in catching can be found in Regan and Gray (2000).

Catching a bouncing ball

Hayhoe et al. (2005) studied the relatively straightforward case of catching a slow tennis ball that bounces once. After a little practice they found that catchers anticipated where the ball would bounce. Subjects initially fixated the hands of the thrower; they then made a saccade to just above the future bounce point, arriving at an average of 53 ms before the bounce itself. After the bounce the ball was tracked smoothly into the hands. Hayhoe et al. (2005) stated that this behaviour requires the subject to construct a dynamic model the ball's motion that can predict its trajectory before and after the bounce. They also demonstrated that the model could be rapidly updated. They did this by covertly replacing the normal ball with a bouncier one. Initially catchers were unable to track the ball smoothly after it bounced and resorted to saccadic tracking, but after three repeats their performance was back to normal. Subjects also adjusted the timing of the anticipatory saccade to the ball's new dynamics. We will see in the next section that anticipatory mechanisms of this kind are common, especially in sports that involve timing the contact with a ball.

Hitting a moving ball

In most games in which contact has to be made with a moving ball, the main problem is to work out where and when contact will be made with the ball, but in addition the player has to decide where to hit it and how hard. A further complication in tennis, table tennis, cricket, and baseball is the need both to create and to deal with spin, which alters the trajectory of the ball both in the air and when it bounces.

Anticipating the future path of the ball is essential in all sports in which the ball is struck. This requires using available visual information to determine both time to contact and the ball's position at the moment of contact. In sports such as table tennis, and usually in tennis and cricket, the ball bounces before contact – although the player must be also able to deal with full tosses in cricket and volleys in tennis where the ball does not bounce. Thus the player must determine the ball's trajectory after the ball has bounced, but because of the fraction of a second time scale involved, much of this information must be acquired before the bounce.

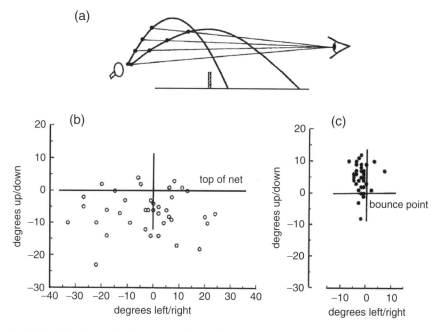

Fig. 8.6 (a) Ambiguity in the approaching ball's trajectory in table tennis. The apparent vertical velocity of the approaching ball will be similar for a long fast trajectory and a short slow one. This is disambiguated by observing the bounce point. (b) Widely spread end points of initial saccades to 38 returns relative to the top of the net. (c) Clustering of the same saccades relative to the anticipated bounce point. From Land and Furneaux (1997).

Table tennis

Ripoll et al. (1987) found that international table tennis players, receiving a ball played by the opponent, made a saccade to the expected position of the bounce as the ball came over the net. Land and Furneaux (1997) confirmed this (with more ordinary players). They found that shortly after the opposing player had hit the ball, the receiver made a saccade down to a point a few degrees above the bounce point, anticipating the bounce by about 0.2 s (Fig. 8.6c). At other times the ball was tracked around the table in a normal non-anticipatory way (this tracking almost always involved saccades rather than smooth pursuit). The main reason why players anticipate the bounce is that its location and timing are critical in determining time and place of contact for the return shot. If for the moment we ignore looming and disparity cues, the bounce point itself provides valuable information about the ball's speed of approach. Up until the bounce the trajectory of the ball as seen by the receiver is ambiguous. Very similar retinal patterns in space and time would arise from a fast ball on a long trajectory or a slow ball on a short one, just as in catching (Fig. 8.1). This ambiguity is removed the instant the timing and position of the bounce are established because a short bounce indicates a slower ball and vice versa (Fig. 8.6a). As explained in the section on cricket (below), a combination of the time from the opponent's strike to the bounce and the location of the bounce point are in principle sufficient to estimate where and when the ball will be at the time it reaches the player. Therefore the strategy of the player is to get gaze close to the bounce point, before the ball does, and lie in wait. The saccade that effects this is interesting in that it is not driven by a 'stimulus' but by the player's estimate of the location of something that has yet to happen.

Because the distances involved are reasonably short both looming and disparity cues are also potentially available for determining time to contact, as in catching. There is good evidence that updated time-to-contact information is indeed used to time the stroke, not just at its inception but also during its execution (Bootsma and Wieringen, 1990). This is the more remarkable given that during an attacking forehand drive in table tennis the ball may only spend 200 ms in the air.

Squash

In squash the path of the ball is uniquely complex because it can be made to bounce once, twice, or even three times from different walls of the court and once off the floor before being struck by the second player. Do players simply follow the ball around the court, or do they anticipate points on its future path, as in table tennis? McKinney et al.(2008) used a lightweight eye tracker to monitor the gaze movements of four skilled squash players as they volleyed balls that bounced off two walls (they did not wait for the ball to bounce off the floor before hitting it). A summary of their findings is shown in Fig. 8.7. After the ball has been played the returning player makes a saccade to the service wall ahead of the ball, anticipating the first bounce by an average of 153 ms. The player then tracks the ball smoothly for about half the distance between the first and second bounces. Then, remarkably, gaze moves not to the second wall, but to a point on the ball's trajectory *after* it has bounced off that wall, anticipating the ball's future position by 186 ms. The ball is then pursued smoothly until just before

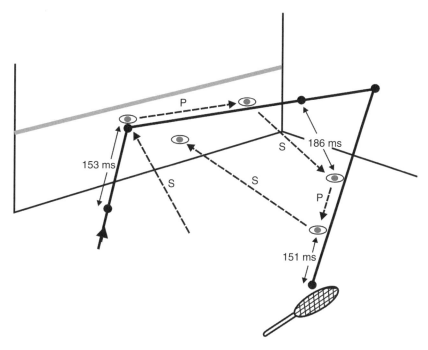

Fig. 8.7 Anticipation of the trajectory of a squash ball that bounces off two walls of the court. Heavy line is the trajectory of the ball, and dashed line the path of the player's gaze. S, saccades; P, smooth pursuit. Gaze anticipates ball position at the first bounce and after the second bounce. Further details in the text. Based on McKinney et al. (2008), and additional data kindly supplied by the authors.

contact with the racket, with gaze held still for the final 151 ms before the strike. A saccade is then made to the service wall at about the same time as the strike itself.

The anticipation of the bounce from the second wall involves much more than just moving gaze further along the current track of the ball. The geometry of the bounce will differ from shot to shot, and getting the post-bounce position correct is a far from trivial problem. Nor is this a just a rough guess: the average deviation of gaze direction from the actual trajectory was only 2.5°, considerably better than the average error of 9° for the first bounce from the service wall (although the latter was based mostly on observation of the opponent's stroke rather than the ball itself). We can conclude that the saccadic system must have at its disposal a model for generating possible trajectories based on the results of a great deal of previous experience.

Cricket

In cricket, where the ball typically bounces before reaching the batsman, there are similar problems to those of table tennis, with the complication once again being that the ball may change its lateral direction when it bounces. Thus being in a position to see the bounce point is crucial. Slow bowlers can defeat the batsman by spinning the ball so that it turns when it hits the ground or swings in the air in an unexpected manner (Regan, 1992). Fast bowlers, on the other hand, rely on sheer speed. Deliveries of speed 90 mph (40.2 ms^{-1}) are common, which means that the ball reaches the batsman only 0.4 s after it leaves the bowler's hand. As the ball usually bounces more than half way down the pitch, it leaves less than 0.2 s for the batsman to formulate his shot. According to McLeod (1987) batsmen cannot make changes to their stroke within the last 200 ms before contact with the ball (largely because of the bat's inertia). This means that the information needed to formulate the stroke must be obtained at the very latest by the time of the bounce, and even then some shots will be unplayable. If a batsman is to make a scoring shot with the 'sweet spot' of the bat, the precision required is impressive. Regan (1992) estimates that the strike needs to be timed to within 5 ms and the position of the ball on the bat to within about 5 cm (Fig. 8.8).

Coaches usually tell players, 'Keep your eye on the ball', but if taken literally this is not a good strategy when facing a fast bowler. Smooth pursuit typically has a latency of more than 100 ms, so an attempt to track will leave gaze several degrees above the ball by the bounce point. Pursuit is often accompanied by a 'start-up' saccade, which is likely to be made around the time of the bounce, making the batsman blind at the moment of most need. Fortunately this in not what batsmen do. Land and McLeod (2000) measured the gaze movements of batsmen facing medium pace (56 mph,

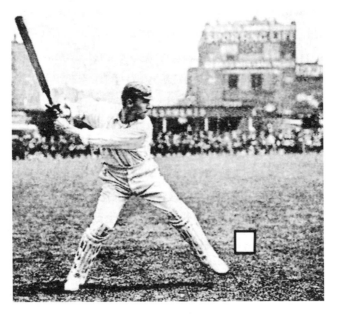

Fig. 8.8 The great batsman Victor Trumper about to make a straight drive at the Oval cricket ground in 1902. The impact between bat and ball would have occurred within the imaginary box. Modified from Regan (1992). The original photograph was taken by G.W. Beldan and is from Beldan and Fry (1905) Great Batsmen, their Methods at a Glance. Macmillan, London.

25 ms^{-1}) balls of varying lengths delivered by a bowling machine ('length' is the distance of the bounce down the pitch, from very short – closest to the bowler – to short, good length, and overpitched). With the shorter balls the batsmen watched the delivery and then made a saccade of 4 to 8° down to within a degree of the anticipated bounce point, gaze arriving 0.1 s or more before the ball (Fig. 8.9). With good batsmen

(a)

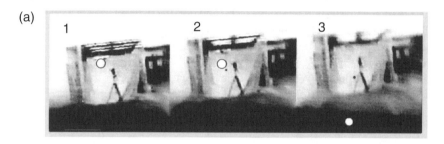

(b)

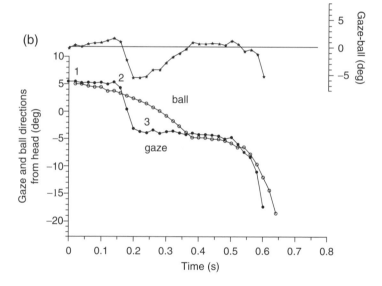

Fig. 8.9 (a) Three frames from an eye-tracker camera mounted on a batsman's head showing the point of fixation (white spot) covering the emergence of the ball from the bowling machine (1); 150 ms later when the ball (black dot) has descended about 2°, and the point of fixation has just started to move (2); 250 ms following emergence after the eye has made a 8° saccade down to the anticipated bounce point, about 5° ahead of the ball (3). Object in the distance is a camera on a tripod. (b) Complete record of the same delivery, seen from the eye-tracker camera. The eye remains stationary for 140 ms then makes an 8° downward saccade to the expected bounce point, where the ball arrives 200 ms later. Thereafter the eye tracks the ball for another 200 ms. Successful contact occurred 700 ms after delivery. Numbers correspond to the three frames shown above. Upper record shows the divergence of eye and ball after the initial saccade. From Land and McLeod (2000).

this initial saccade had a latency as short as 0.14 s from the time the ball left the bowler's hand, whereas poor or non-batsmen had more typical latencies of 0.2 s or more. This means that poor batsmen can not play really fast balls (~90 mph) because, with short balls bouncing less than 0.2 s after delivery, their saccades are either too late to catch the bounce point, or the bounce occurs in mid-saccade when they are effectively blind.

Figure 8.9b shows the oculomotor behaviour of a competent batsman during a single good-length delivery. Little happens for 140 ms after delivery, then the eyes make an 8° downward saccade, landing close to where the ball will bounce. At the same time the head begins to move down. (It is possible that with a real bowler the timing of the delivery can be anticipated earlier than with a bowling machine, and the latency of this initial saccade reduced.) When the saccade is complete 40 ms later the eyes and head counter-rotate (presumably as a result of the vestibulo-ocular reflex), so that gaze

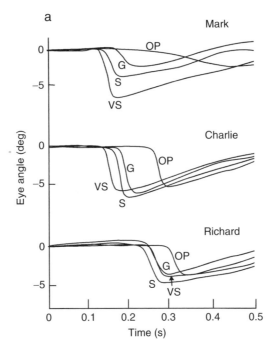

Fig. 8.10 Initial downward saccades of three batsmen of different standards playing deliveries that were very short (bouncing farthest from the batsman), short, good length, and overpitched (bouncing nearest to the batsman). Mark (professional) made strong saccades to very short balls but introduced more smooth tracking into the longer deliveries, making no saccades at all to the overpitched deliveries. Charlie (very competent amateur) always made saccades, but as with Mark they were made later for the longer deliveries. Richard (weak amateur) was almost 100 ms later than the other two in making downward saccades, and there was only a weak relationship between saccade timing and length of delivery. Each record is a mean of 5 to 7 deliveries. From Land and McLeod (2000).

remains steady for about 300 ms, through the bounce and for a further 100 ms. Thereafter eye, head and gaze all move downwards as the ball moves down in the visual field towards the bat.

There were striking differences in the oculomotor actions of different batsmen during the pre-bounce period. Land and McLeod (2000) used three batsmen, Mark (a professional), Charlie (a good amateur), and Richard (a weak amateur). Their eye-in-head movements are shown in Fig. 8.10. Mark made the largest saccades only for very short balls, which descend fastest during the latent period when gaze is stationary. For longer deliveries his saccadic latencies became longer and the saccades smaller until for overpitched balls there was no saccade at all. As the ball descended more slowly when pitched longer, it became easier to follow, and he progressively substituted smooth tracking for the saccade. Charlie always made quite large saccades, although as with Mark the latency increased as the balls were pitched longer. The striking difference between Richard and the other two was the latency of the initial saccade. Even for very short balls the latency was 220 ms, almost 100 ms later than the better players. There was also a less obvious correlation of latency with pitch length, as though he were not using the descent speed of the ball in as consistent a way as the other two batsmen. Clearly, how a batsman reads the movement of the ball after delivery is important and is related to expertise. The fact that eye movements vary with where the ball will bounce means that the batsman already has some information about the ball's trajectory, but as in table tennis this is ambiguous: at this stage slow short balls will not be easily distinguishable from fast long balls (Fig. 8.6).

What can be learned from the location and timing of the bounce? Land and McLeod (2000) showed that it can provide the batsman with the information he needs to work out where and when the ball will arrive at his bat, thereby enabling him to make an attacking shot. Figure 8.11 sets out the relevant physical parameters. The two things the batsman can have immediate knowledge of are the time from delivery to bounce (t_0) and the visual angle from the horizontal to the bounce point (φ). The two parameters that he needs for the shot are time from bounce to bat (t_1) and the vertical

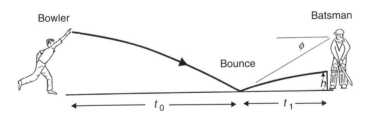

Fig. 8.11 Parameters involved in the batsman's judgement of where and when to hit a cricket ball. The batsman needs to know t_1, the time after the bounce that the ball will take to reach his bat, and h, the vertical location of the ball when it arrives. Two sources of information are readily available, t_0, the time from delivery to bounce, and φ, the angle of declination of the bounce point. How t_1 and h map onto t_0 and φ depend on such parameters as the hardness of the pitch and the height of the bowler. Typical mappings are shown in Fig. 8.12. (Modified from Land and McLeod, 2000).

location of the ball at the time of contact (h; we ignore lateral deviations for the moment; if the trajectory is straight they are relatively easy to deal with). It can be shown that t_0 and φ map directly onto t_1 and h, provided the batsman has implicit estimates of various constants: his own eye height, the height of the bowler's delivery point, and the length of the pitch (18.4 m). He also needs estimates, through practice and playing-in on the day, of the hardness of the pitch, specifically the extent to which the vertical and horizontal components of the pre- and post-bounce velocities will differ. All these parameters affect the mappings of t_0 and φ onto t_1 and h to varying degrees, but the general shape of the mappings do not change substantially. They are illustrated in Fig. 8.12.

We are not suggesting that batsmen calculate these mappings each time they face a bowler; rather we assume that they are acquired after years of practice. Although it seems a complex feat to apply a double mapping of this kind, it is no more difficult conceptually than controlling speed and steering simultaneously when driving on a winding road. In many sports actions are based on more than one variable. The tweaking of the mappings to fit the particular conditions of the day is probably achieved during the first few deliveries to the new batsman, when he tends to play defensive shots where the constraints on t_1 and h are less severe than in a scoring shot. This enables him to 'get his eye in'.

Batting against slow bowling poses quite different problems from those of fast bowling (Regan, 1992). The intention of the bowler is not to defeat the batsman by speed but to deceive him by making the ball turn when it bounces by putting spin on it. This means that it moves unpredictably (to the batsman) to left or right after the bounce, causing the ball to contact the edge of the bat rather than the middle, thus providing the near fielders with an opportunity for a catch. Where the ball bounces is crucial. If the ball bounces short the batsman has a chance to react to its new direction. If it bounces too near the batsman it will not have moved far enough laterally to provoke a miss-hit. Often the batsman will engineer the latter situation by moving up the pitch towards the ball, but then if he does miss the ball he can be 'stumped' by the wicket keeper, who knocks the bails off the stumps while the batsman is out of his crease.

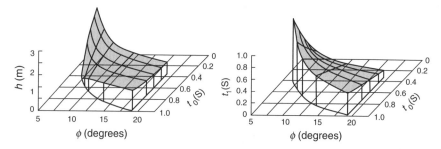

Fig. 8.12 Typical mappings of the parameters the batsman needs (h and t_1) map onto the ones he can measure (t_0 and φ). These particular mappings were calculated for a moderately hard pitch with the ball delivered from a height of 2 m. They show, for example, that small values of φ and low values t_0 produce high values of h (bouncers). See Fig. 8.11. From Land and McLeod (2000).

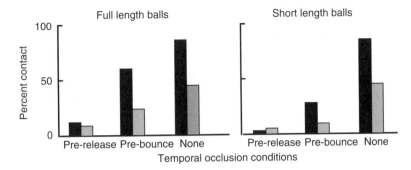

Fig. 8.13 Results of an experiment by Müller and Abernethy (2006) in which the view of batsmen facing spin bowlers was occluded from the end of the pre-release period, the end of the pre-bounce period, or not at all. Bars indicate the percentage of good shots made with the face of the bat. Black bars are for experienced, and grey bars for less experienced batsmen. Vision of the pre-bounce period is of most value to experienced batsmen facing full length balls, implying that they obtain good information from the ball's trajectory.

The question of how much information is obtained by the batsman at different stages of the delivery was addressed by Müller and Abernethy (2006). They used liquid crystal spectacles to occlude vision at different times before and during the deliveries of spin bowlers (it is not safe to use this technique with fast bowlers). They occluded vision from just before release, from just before the bounce, or not at all (Fig. 8.13). They found very little evidence of usable information from the pre-release period – although there was some evidence that experienced batsmen could at least decide whether to move to the front foot (for full length deliveries, the idea being to get as close to the bounce as possible) or the back foot (for short deliveries, to allow as much time as possible to see the path of the ball after the bounce). However, seeing the ball during the pre-bounce period did enable experienced batsmen to make a good shot with the face of the bat more than 50% of the time for full length balls but not for short length balls. The reasons for the difference are that for short balls the pre-bounce time is reduced, and also because spin deviates the ball's path much further after the bounce than with full length balls. Figure 8.13 shows that this is detected post-bounce, and the score rate rises to 90%. Less-experienced batsmen are less successful generally, as expected, but in particular they are less able to use the pre-bounce flight information, even for full length balls.

The other thing a bowler can do is to 'flight' the ball by putting backspin on it. This has the effect of directing the wake of the ball downwards, and by the law of conservation of momentum this gives the ball more lift (this is the same effect as that of the aerofoil section of a plane's wing). A bowler can use this to make a slower ball travel the same distance as a faster unflighted ball but take longer to get there. This disturbs the relationship between seen trajectory and speed and can lead to the batsman mistiming his shot. The ball can also be made to curve in the air by putting horizontal spin on it (swing bowling). This works the same way as backspin but in the horizontal plane.

The effect of the curved trajectory is to confuse the batsman as to where the ball will bounce and again provide opportunities for a miss-hit.

Baseball

In baseball the ball speeds and the distances involved are similar to cricket, but the ball does not bounce, and so the timing information derived from the bounce is not available. Bahill and LaRitz (1984) examined the horizontal head and eye movements to batters facing a simulated fastball. Subjects used smooth pursuit involving both head and eye to track the ball to a point about 9 ft from them, after which the angular motion of the ball became too fast to track (a professional tracked it to 5.5 ft in front: he had exceptional smooth pursuit capabilities). Sometimes batters watched the ball onto the bat by making an anticipatory saccade to the estimated contact point part way through the ball's flight. This may have little immediate value in directing the bat, because the stroke is already committed but may be useful in learning to predict the ball's location when it reaches the bat (the 'learning strategy'). Bahill and Baldwin (2004) suggested that in hitting a baseball the first third of the ball's flight is used to gather sensory information about the ball's trajectory and time to contact and how it is spinning, the next third to determine where and when the ball will contact the bat, and the final third in swinging the bat. For a 90 mph pitch the total time is about 0.4 s, so each phase lasts 133 ms. Making a clean hit in baseball is more difficult than cricket because the bat is round and narrow (2.75 inch diameter). the 'sweet spot' is less than 1 inch (25 mm) wide by 4 inches long. To hit a 'flyball' the batter also has to put backspin on the ball to increase lift, which means undercutting the ball by up to 1 inch (Watts and Bahill, 1990). The precision involved is formidable, particularly as the pitcher is not trying to make things easy.

The trajectory of a baseball from pitcher to batter is a generally a smooth parabola, but in spite of this the variations that can be induced by spin of various kinds have led to a wonderful variety of terms used to describe the different types of pitch (delivery). These include fastball, rising fastball, two-seam and four-seam fastball, sinker, forkball, curveball, slider, cutter, screwball, spitball, knuckleball, and bearball – the last being an aggressive ball aimed at the batter's head, analogous to a bouncer in cricket. Most of these variants rely on spin. Backspin gives the ball more lift (rising fastball), topspin directs it downwards (sinking fastball), and horizontal spin around a vertical axis results in a laterally curved trajectory (curveball). Spinning the ball around an oblique axis produces combined effects such as a sinking curveball. The effect of spin in general is to shift the wake left by the ball up, down, or to the side so that the ball receives momentum in the opposite direction. Thus backspin directs the wake downwards, providing the ball with more lift. The knuckleball is an interesting exception. Here the stitches on the seams are used in an otherwise straight flight to induce unstable eddies behind the ball which cause it to move erratically. As in cricket, a pitcher will use a variety of these trajectories to prevent the batter from developing a reliable model of what is to come. Alternatively, he will pitch consistently so that the batter does start to anticipate and then change the trajectory. Often a simple change of speed, so that the ball reaches the bat higher or lower than expected, will cause the batter to miss.

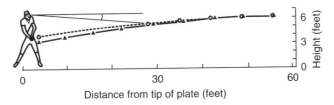

Fig. 8.14 Misperception of a high fast fastball in baseball. A slight overestimate of the speed of the ball over the first 30 ft leads the batter to believe that the ball will reach him a few inches higher (circles) than it actually does (triangles). If he takes his eye off the ball to view the contact with the bat, when the ball reappears it will seem to jump downwards. Based on Bahill and Baldwin (2004).

These changes by the pitcher can produce interesting visual effects. The ball is often said to 'break' just before it reaches the strike zone, apparently jumping upwards, downwards, or sideways by as much as a foot. Since such jumps are physically impossible there must be other explanations. Bahill and Baldwin (2004) investigated this and concluded that it results from a change in speed of the ball from the speed the batter was expecting (Fig. 8.14). If a batter estimates the speed of a high fastball to be 95 mph during the first third of the flight, based on what he sees and past experience, but the delivery was actually 90 mph, then the ball will reach him a few inches lower than he expects. (Note that the batter has no direct measure of forward speed: the future trajectory must be derived from the initial vertical and lateral seen velocities of the ball, and the estimate of time to contact, during the first 150 ms or so of the flight path.) If he keeps his eye on the ball he can probably correct this initial incorrect estimate, but if he adopts the 'learning strategy' mentioned earlier and makes a saccade to the probable contact point with the bat, then when the ball comes back into view it will be lower than he estimated. Not only will he miss it but it will appear to have jumped downwards. Similar effects can be seen with rising fastballs and curveballs.

All this makes hitting a baseball sound very difficult, and that is probably correct. One of the best batters in baseball, Ted Williams, described hitting a baseball as 'the most difficult single act in the whole of sports' (Bahill and LaRitz, 1984).

Goal-tending

Keeping goal in sports such as football (soccer) and hockey (field or ice) involves stopping the oncoming ball or puck from crossing the goal line by either catching or deflecting it. This means that this task falls somewhere between all of those that we have so far discussed.

In soccer perhaps the hardest situation for the goalkeeper is to attempt to stop a penalty kick. Here the ball is placed on a spot just 12 yards (11 m) from the goal line. The speed of the ball once kicked can vary considerably. In the fastest penalty kick on record the ball travelled at 129 kph (about 80 mph, or about 35.9 ms^{-1}), albeit that this kick was recorded indoors on a hard surface rather than on grass. If we assume that kicks can reach speeds of around 40 to 80 mph, then this will leave between

0.6 and 0.3 s between the ball being kicked and it reaching the goal line. When we consider that the goal itself is an area some 8 ft high by 24 ft wide (approximately 2.4 m × 7.3 m) the task of getting to the right place at the right time is clearly difficult. Given the need to cover such a large area, waiting until the ball is in flight to judge time to contact and direction cues would leave little time to execute the movements necessary to get to the right place in time to stop the ball. It therefore seems likely that the goalkeeper might use cues from before the ball is kicked to make a guess at what the shooter will do.

Savelsbergh et al. (2002) showed expert (regular semi-professionals) and novice (irregular recreational players) goalkeepers films of penalty kicks filmed from roughly where the goalkeeper's head would be in the goal. The participants were asked to move a joystick to indicate how they would move to save the shot. Experts were better at getting the joystick to the right location in time, but interestingly the experts and novices looked at different locations on the shooter's body as he made the kick. The experts tended to look mainly at the shooters' legs and at the ball. The novices tended to look more at the shooter's trunk, arm, and hip. Experts also made fewer and longer fixations overall. In a follow-up study, Savelsbergh, Williams et al. (2005) found that among expert goal keepers those who were more successful at 'saving' shots in their paradigm tended to delay initiating their response for longer and to spend more time looking at the non-kicking leg than experts who were less successful in the task. All of this suggests that a lot of information about the ball's flight is being predicted based on the shooter's run-up for the kick. The non-kicking leg presumably provides information on the shooter's posture and balance, which will in turn provide cues about where the ball will be directed.

A similarly demanding situation is tending goal in ice hockey. Here the size of the goal is much smaller at 6 ft × 4 ft (1.8 m × 1.2 m), but the puck is smaller and reaches speeds of over 100 mph (160 kph, 44 ms^{-1}). Panchuk and Vickers (2006) monitored eye movements as elite goal-tenders faced real shots from 5 m or 10 m. Flight times for these shots were approximately 150 ms and 200 ms from stick to goal, so again there is a clear argument for needing to base at least some of the decision about how to intercept the shot on cues from the shooter's preparation. Successful saves were associated with longer fixations on the stick (and puck) just before the shot. This final fixation on the stick/puck prior to the shot was surprisingly long given that the flight time that followed: successful saves tended to have been preceded by a fixation of about 950 ms on the stick/puck. This unusually long fixation just before the crucial event (the shot) has been referred to as a period of 'quiet eye' and has been found in other sports (see below).

Aiming sports

There are many sports in which the objective is to propel some projectile (ball, arrow, dart, bullet) to a particular goal or target. In general both the player and the goal are initially stationary or nearly so, so the difficulty of the sport arises from the precision needed in the aiming process rather than from having to co-ordinate interception with moving objects. The aiming process is generally thought to have three phases: (1) preparation, in which the required movements are programmed; (2) the impulse phase, when the initial fast phase of the limb movements occurs; and (3) the error correcting phase, when final adjustments are made to the limb movements (Abrams et al., 1990).

A universal finding of studies of aiming sports is that in the preparatory phase of an action long steady fixations are needed if the shot is to be successful (John Wayne notwithstanding). Joan Vickers (1996) first drew attention to this, and referred to it as 'quiet eye', which she defined as that portion of the final fixation from its onset to the first observable movement in the shooting action. For example, in basketball Vickers (1996) found that expert players showed quiet eye periods preceding shots at the basket that were more than twice as long as those of less expert players of (972 ms vs 357 ms for scoring shots). In billiards, Williams et al. (2002) also found a large difference in quiet eye duration not only between skilled and less skilled players, but also between successful and unsuccessful shots with both groups of player. For the latter the difference again was a factor of more than two (562 ms vs 214 ms). Similar effects have been found in golf, darts, place kicking in soccer, and goal-tending in ice hockey. It seems clear that the information needed for accurate aiming is acquired over a period of lasting half a second or more.

One challenge to the notion that a period of 'quiet eye' is essential for success in these sports comes from work by Oudejans et al. (2002). Using shutter goggles these authors occluded portions of the preparation for a shot in basketball. They occluded vision either prior to the final 350 ms before ball release or during this final 350 ms. Occluding the final 350 ms was severely disruptive, but occluding vision up until this final 350 ms resulted in performance close to that when not occluded at all. This 350 ms final viewing window is much shorter than the periods of quiet eye typically reported as being necessary for success (972 ms in Vickers, 1996) and are closer to the durations typically associated with failure (357 ms). It would seem that at least in basketball shooting, success does not require such a long period of maintained viewing just before ball release as has been suggested in some studies.

In many aiming sports there is only one object that the player needs to fixate. For free throws in basketball it is the basket or the backboard. In darts or archery it is the target. However in other sports, such as golf, there are both far and near objects that need attention: the target (the green or the hole) and the ball itself. Strategies vary somewhat but the common pattern seems to be for experts to look at the far target first to establish its direction and then concentrate on striking the ball correctly. Watching expert place kickers in rugby football it is very obvious that this is what is happening. The kicker looks at the goal for two or three seconds and then concentrates entirely on the ball. In a broadcast interview in 2002, Vickers described two types of shooters in ice hockey: the ones who look at the goal throughout ('heads up') and the others who look at the goal and then look principally at the puck ('heads down'). The latter have the advantage that their motives are harder to detect. What is interesting here is that the accuracy of the information about target position does not seem to decay, at least over a period of a few seconds.

Summary

1. Most ball sports require split-second judgements that place extraordinary demands on the co-ordination of gaze and action. The usual strategy of supplying the motor system with information a second ahead of action is no longer viable. Anticipation and prediction are crucially important.

2. Catching a ball requires the catcher to manoeuvre to where the ball will be at catching height and then to position the hands appropriately. These two processes rely on different sets of visual cues, but there is no clear agreement on which of these cues is of greatest importance.

3. In sports involving hitting a moving ball, timing of contact has to be accurate to a few milliseconds. A key feature of success in these sports is learning to predict the future position of the ball. This often involves an anticipatory saccade to a currently empty location, which the ball will occupy some tens of milliseconds in the future.

4. Making effective contact with the ball requires the learning of sophisticated mappings between visually obtained variables and motor responses.

5. In aiming sports the need to monitor both the target and the projectile requires the allocation of attention to separate locations in space. Unusually long fixations just prior to making the shot seem to increase the chances of success.

Chapter 9

Social roles of eye movements

Eyes as signals

As well as providing us with information to guide our actions, the eyes can also supply information to others about our attitudes, intentions, and emotions.

Consider the following piece of dreadful prose:

> She shot him a glance. He met her gaze and their eyes locked. 'Have we met before?' she asked. He had a gleam in his eye. 'Don't you remember?' he said. She quickly averted her eyes. She said 'You had more hair then'. Out of the corner of her eye she saw his gaze wander over her trim figure. 'You haven't changed' he said. She looked back but her eyes were downcast. 'There's a lot you don't know' she said.

Enough of this. The point is that English and other languages are full of words and expressions that imply that the eyes are used as tools in our social interactions, supplementing our spoken words. It also seems that human eyes are specially adapted for this purpose. Our scleras are uniquely white among the eyes of great apes, and we also expose more of them than other primates (Kobayashi and Kohshima, 1997). Together with the dark iris, the white of the eye provides easily read information about where we are looking and who we are looking at.

Gaze during conversation

In his pioneering book *Bodily Communication* Michael Argyle pointed out that during a neutral conversation people look at each other quite a lot of the time. The average proportion of time an individual looks at the other amounts to 75% while listening and 40% while talking. Mutual gaze (eye contact) occupies 30% of the time (Argyle, 1988, p. 159). Gaze during conversations typically occurs in roughly 3 s bouts that Argyle refers to as glances. Mutual glances are shorter, about 1.5 s. Those who look more are seen as attentive, those who look less as passive or inattentive. However, continuous gaze is distracting and uncomfortable for the recipient: in its extreme form the 'hate stare' is sometimes used as a threat. It seems that other things being equal the more people look at each others' faces the more positive and engaged the relationship, provided a subtly defined upper limit is not exceeded.

During glances to the face a number of fixations are made, especially on the triangle of the eyes and mouth (Fig. 9.1). According to Malcolm et al. (2008) different regions of the face provide different kinds of information to the viewer. The upper face around the eyes attracts more fixations when the identity of the face being viewed is in question, but the lower face around the mouth is fixated more when the question relates to the expression of anger or sadness.

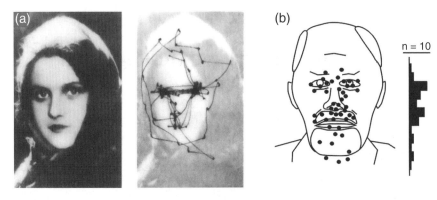

Fig. 9.1 (a) Record from Yarbus (1967) of fixations on a picture of a face. The 'knots' are fixations and the thin lines are the saccades. (b) Fixations on a colleague's face by MFL during a 30 s live conversation at a party. Inset right shows vertical distribution profile. In both cases fixations are mostly around the eyes and mouth.

Mutual gaze can vary according to the context and can serve as a signal for a variety of social factors such as intimacy (Doherty-Sneddon and Phelps, 2005). For example, the incidence of mutual gaze is higher when people are far apart than when close together (Argyle and Dean, 1965). One possible reason for this is that close physical proximity itself increases the intimacy of an interaction, and so less mutual gaze is required to maintain intimacy than when individuals are further apart. Eye contact may also vary with cognitive load: when being asked hard maths questions by an interviewer, children were more likely to avert their gaze from the interviewer than when being asked easy questions (Doherty-Sneddon and Phelps, 2005). Gaze aversion was also higher for face-to-face interviews than when the interviewer was shown on a television screen. These studies indicate that mutual gaze forms an important but quite variable component of conversational interactions.

Does the amount of mutual gaze affect another person's behaviour? It is not particularly easy to obtain reliable evidence of this, but Argyle mentions a number of studies that indicate that it does. One slightly alarming study found that confederate (i.e. stooge) job candidates with low levels of mutual gaze were less likely to be given jobs by interviewers, even though their qualifications were no different from other candidates (Argyle, 1988, p. 161).

Personality, emotion, and arousal

According to Kleinke (1986) people who look more tend to be perceived more favourably, and in particular as being competent, friendly, credible, assertive, and socially skilled. Lower-gaze levels are associated with males compared with females, and with introverts, autistic children, and most kinds of patients with mental health disorders. A consistent finding is that when people are sad they look less and look downwards.

Emotional expression is shown not so much by gaze itself as by the appearance of the regions surrounding the eyes. Most of us would agree with the observations in the following list, again taken from Argyle (1988, p. 166):

interest–excitement: eyebrows down, eyes track and look

enjoyment--joy: smiling eyes, circular wrinkles

distress–anguish: cry, arched eyebrows

fear–terror: eyes frozen open

shame–humiliation: eyes down

anger–rage: eyes narrowed

Although these facial expressions are responses to circumstances, they are also signals. For example, eyes down means that no threat is to be expected, whereas eyes narrowed means trouble.

The pupils of the eyes can provide a subtle signal indicating an individual's state of arousal. Famously, in ancient Rome and during the Middle Ages, women used atropine (in the form of belladonna, derived from deadly nightshade) to induce a wider pupil and hence appear more alluring. More recently, two versions of Richard Wiseman's book *Quirkology* (2008) were produced: both had the same photograph of a smiling woman's face, but in one version her pupils were digitally dilated. The dilated version sold far better to men but not to women!

Hess and Polt (1960) studied pupil size in relation to various stimuli. They found that for women the most effective pupil dilators were pictures of babies, mothers and babies, and nude men; men responded to nude women and, curiously, to landscapes, which actually caused a mild pupil constriction in women. The effects that Hess and Polt found were quite large, with increases in pupil area of up to 20%, certainly large enough for an interested observer to notice. The arousal that causes pupil dilation does not have to be sexual in nature. In a later study, Hess and Polt (1964) found that pupil size varied during problem-solving tasks, and others have since related dilation to the fluctuating arousal associated with various kinds of mental information processing. It is clear now that the pupil response is an indicator of a more general autonomic activation. The galvanic skin response, for example, co-varies with pupil diameter (Bradley et al., 2008).

Recent fMRI studies have suggested that specific forebrain regions are involved in generating our reactions to emotionally affecting facial expressions of others. These regions include the amygdala (fear and happiness), the right insula (disgust), and right cingulate gyrus (anger). Although there is some disagreement in the literature as to which region exactly does what, there is a consensus that different emotive stimuli are separately processed, at least initially (Blair et al., 1999). The outputs of these regions converge on the inferior part of the left ventral frontal cortex, which processes a variety of emotions.

Accuracy of gaze detection

Eye contact detection

For mutual gaze to be an effective social signal, we must be able to detect when this is occurring. How good, then, are we at judging whether someone is making eye contact with us? The answer is that we are about as good as it is possible to be. Cline (1967) asked his subjects to determine whether a trained 'looker' was looking directly between their eyes. The looker looked, via a mirror, at various points in the vicinity of the subject's face, from a distance of 122 cm. The accuracy of the subjects' estimate was taken as the standard deviation of the looker's horizontal gaze position in the plane of the subjects' face when the subjects reported that they were being looked at directly. This was 1.55 cm, which represents an angular deviation of the looker's eye of 0.75°. The corresponding linear deviation of the looker's iris is 0.18 mm, or 0.51 arc minutes in the subject's field of view. This is actually slightly better than the eye's acuity as measured with a Snellen chart. Earlier, Gibson and Pick (1963) had come up with a somewhat larger estimate of 1.1 arc minutes, but on either estimate it seems that the accuracy of the judgement of eye contact is close to the limit of visual detectability.

Estimates of direction of regard

Humans are not only good at knowing whether someone is looking at them, but they are also able to identify what objects in space another person is looking at. Anstis et al. (1969) studied this ability in adults and concluded that for objects directly ahead of both the subject and the looker (who were facing each other) acuity was as good as in the judgement of eye contact. However, when the targets of the looker's gaze were horizontally displaced the accuracy of the subjects' estimates of direction of regard decreased: subjects overestimated the displacement of the looker's gaze direction by 50% to 87%. Symons et al. (2004) repeated these observations, in this case using high resolution images of the looker and the objects being looked at, and in this arrangement they found that the subjects' resolution of direction of regard declined somewhat away from the straight-ahead condition but then improved again at larger angles of regard. They suggest that the subjects' strategies change from the use of the relative amounts of white sclera visible on the two sides of the iris to some other strategy, as one side of the sclera becomes occluded. In a study by Bock et al. (2008) the looker (sender) and subject (receiver) were 1 m apart and viewed point objects on a 30° diameter vertical ring placed between them (i.e. targets at 15° eccentricity). They used both human senders and computer-presented images of senders and found little difference in precision (standard deviations of 2.81° and 2.97°). Precision was significantly worse when the sender was monocular (but not the receiver) and was better for horizontal and vertically displaced targets than for oblique ones.

It thus seems that in the most favourable conditions the direction of regard of another can be estimated with similar precision to eye contact detection (<1° in terms of the looker's eye direction, <1 arc minute for the subject's estimate of the looker's iris position). Clearly, however, the exact conditions are important. Inevitably the estimates of gaze direction will lose precision as the distance of the subject from the looker increases, and they also decrease with increasing eccentricity.

Eye and head direction in gaze direction judgement

The location of the pupil or iris of the eye, relative to the surrounding tissues, is directly related to the direction of gaze *relative to the head* but does not specify the direction of gaze *in space*. As we have seen throughout this book, in natural behaviour we rarely move our eyes without at least some movement of the head. As such, for an observer

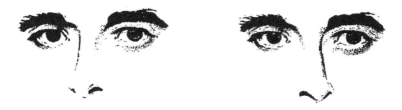

Fig. 9.2 Drawings by Wollaston (1824) showing that the interpretation of the direction of regard of identical pairs of eyes depends on the context provided by the head. The eyes on the left appear to look straight ahead (because eye-in-head and head-in-space directions are equal and opposite), whereas those on the right look to the right of the viewer.

to determine the gaze direction of another person, the direction of the head axis must be estimated as well. This was beautifully illustrated by Wollaston (1824), who showed that the gaze direction in space of two identical pairs of eyes could be dramatically altered by adding the outline of the nose to provide an indication of head direction (Fig. 9.2).

In practical terms this means that the amount of white showing on either side of the iris is only an adequate guide to where a person is looking when their head is directed straight towards the viewer. In all other conditions some independent measure of head direction is also needed. This requires the use of features that differ in depth, so that their relative left–right positions change as the head rotates. The tip of the nose relative to the eyes (as in Wollaston's drawing) is one such cue, as are the position of nose and mouth relative to the ears. The same features can also be used to estimate the vertical inclination of the head.

To what extent are eye and head directions related? Do we generally turn our eyes in the same direction that we turn our head? The questions are interesting and compli-cated, and the answers depend very much on what kind of activity we are engaged in. Figure 9.3 shows how much the head turned during gaze shifts of various sizes made by one individual towards visual targets. It shows that for gaze shifts of less than 40° the head turned through about one-third of the total extent of the gaze change (Goossens and van Opsal, 1997). For different individuals the gain (slope of the line) varied greatly, from less than 0.2 to more than 0.7, indicating that there are head-turners and non-head-turners. Even for the same individual the variation is high, as the standard deviations in Fig. 9.3 show. This suggests that, for an onlooker, head direction is not a very reliable guide to the gaze direction itself, at least for modest angles. Outside this ±40° range the head contribution necessarily becomes larger, as the eyes approach their limit in the orbit of about ±45°, and consequently head direc-tion becomes a better predictor of gaze direction. Interestingly, to auditory targets within the ±40° range, Goossens and van Opsal found that the head contribution was much greater, presumably because the ears extract positional information in head-based co-ordinates.

Of course it is perfectly possible, for modest angles, to direct one's eyes without moving the head, although it usually takes an effort of will to prevent some head movement. Equally, and more naturally, one can maintain gaze direction while

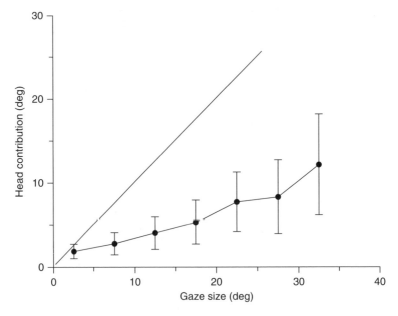

Fig. 9.3 Extent of head rotation in saccadic gaze changes of moderate size. Graph gives means ±1 s.d. for approximately 200 turns made by one subject. The head was in a variety of starting positions relative to the target. Data from Goossens and van Opsal (1997).

moving the head, as in head-shaking while fixating another person. In such cases the eyes counter-rotate in the head, driven by the vestibulo-ocular reflex (VOR). However, it is almost impossible to get the eyes and head stay strictly in line as the head rotates; nearly always the result is for the eyes to saccade through a succession of points during the scan, with VOR-stabilized fixations between the jumps. Eyes and head can also be directed in opposite directions, and this breaking of the normal same-direction coupling is sometimes done for dramatic effect by actors, comedians (notably the Marx brothers), and monarchs sitting for portraits (Goya's painting of King Ferdinand VII is a good example). It indicates that the subject is someone special, either important or just plain odd.

Gaze following

Shared attention

We have seen in the last section that we are remarkably good at detecting when someone is making eye contact with us or where they are looking. Not only do we possess this remarkable ability, but we utilize it in our social interactions. In some circumstances humans and other primates have an almost irresistible urge to look in the direction that they see others looking, in particular when pointing or similar gestures are involved. This tendency, variously known as gaze following, social attention, shared attention, or social cuing, helps co-operative action by making it possible for a group to share the same visual information. One can imagine this being of great importance to our forbears when hunting or watching out for enemies or predators. Gaze following develops early in infancy, but interestingly it requires some help to begin with; six-month infants will only follow an adult's gaze if the child's attention is first engaged by looking directly at them or speaking to them (Senju and Csibra, 2008). It has been suggested that this sharing of attention leads to a sharing of mental state – a 'meeting of minds' (Baron-Cohen, 1995). This in turn makes it possible for a child to build up, between the ages of 18 and 48 months, a 'Theory of Mind', which ultimately makes it possible to explain or predict the behaviour of others.

There have been a number of laboratory studies that have considered whether gaze direction cues trigger reflexive shifts in visual attention in the direction provided by the cue. One line of evidence comes from the use of a modified version of the Posner attentional cuing task (Posner, 1980) in which a schematic face is used to provide a central directional gaze cue immediately prior to the appearance of a peripheral fixation target (Friesen and Kingstone, 1998; Kingstone et al., 2003; Langton et al., 2000; Ricciardelli et al., 2002). In the typical Posner task, a central cue only influences attentional orienting if it is predictive of where the peripheral target will appear. However, when the central cue is a schematic face, there is a reflexive orienting of attention in the direction indicated by the face's eyes. Ricciardelli et al. (2002) compared central cuing using gaze of a face to central cuing using socially neutral arrows (Fig. 9.4). These authors found that when the gaze cue was incongruent with the location at which the target appeared, there was a high incidence of erroneous saccades away from the target and to the side indicated by the gaze cue. This tendency to make errors was not found for the arrow cue. These findings support the suggestion that following where another person is looking is a reflexive, automatic behavioural response. However, this conclusion is not without its critics. Several other groups (Kuhn and Benson, 2007; Ristic et al., 2002; Tipples, 2002) have found that well-designed arrows can be as effective as faces in inducing errors (see Fig. 9.4). Thus the efficacy of artificial faces in producing reflex orienting is still open to doubt.

Cues for shared attention in more realistic scenes

It is interesting to note that much of the most influential work on the influence of another's gaze on and individual's attention has been conducted using schematic faces shown in the cardinal orientation and in isolation on a computer screen (Fig. 9.4). What happens when the stimuli are more like those we encounter in our everyday life? Some insights into this can be gained from considering how observers explore social scenes when being asked to make judgements about where the people in the scenes are attending. One such study (Smilek et al., 2006) found that while the observers reported that they based their judgements on body postures and the context of the scenes, eye movement recordings revealed that they spent much of their time fixating the eyes and heads of the people depicted. This study certainly highlights the importance of gaze direction cues in social scenes but does not directly address the effectiveness of such

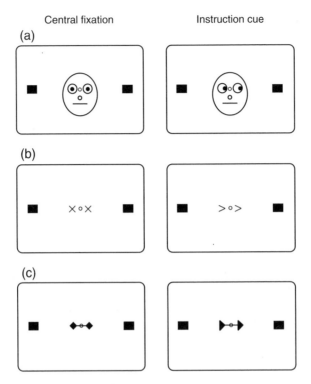

Fig. 9.4 Stimuli used in typical gaze cuing variants of the Posner task, showing both the pre-trial neutral arrangements (left panels) and the directional cues (right panels). The small circles in the centre of each display indicate the markers participants were instructed to fixate. (a) Schematic of gaze cuing condition. Initially, gaze is oriented straight ahead at the observer. The directional cue involves shifting the pupils to that the eyes appear to point toward one side of the display. Note that in some experiments, schematic faces such as those shown here are used (e.g. Kuhn and Benson, 2007), whereas in others, photographs of real faces are used (e.g. Ricciardelli et al., 2002). (b) Arrow cues used to indicate direction in Ricciardelli et al. (c) The arrow cues used by Kuhn and Benson, which they argued were better matched to the gaze cues and were more like arrows typically encountered in our everyday experiences.

cues in triggering attentional orientations to the locations cued by the gaze of the people in the scenes. Moreover, we remain some way from the natural setting of a social interaction, where these use of these gaze cues ought to be most prominent.

Gaze cuing during conversation

Although there is relatively little research on how powerful gaze cues are in triggering reflexive orienting to the cued locations in real-world social settings, some interesting insights can be found in studies of gesturing during conversation. Work using artificial avatar speakers found that observers tended to spend much of their time fixating the gestures of the avatar (Nobe, Hayamizu, Hasegawa, and Takahashi, 2000).

However, in live one-to-one conversation, 96% of viewing time was spent looking at the speaker's face, with only 0.5% of fixation time being allocated to gestures (Gullberg, 2002). Within the time spent looking at gestures, there was a difference according to whether the speaker was looking at their own gesture: 23% of gaze-cued gestures were fixated by the listener. In contrast, only 7% of gestures that were not gaze cued by the speaker were fixated by the listener. Thus we can use this result to argue in favour of the speaker's gaze direction being a cue for orienting the attention of the observer; however, the magnitude of this effect is very small, with most gaze-cued gestures not receiving direct fixation by the observer. Interestingly, Gullberg's work also nicely illustrates the importance of the natural social setting in how the oberver allocated their attention to the listener. Gullberg compared the observer's gaze behaviour when engaged in a live one-to-one setting with the speaker to a setting when watching a video of the same speaker telling the same story. In the latter case, the time spent looking at the speaker's face decreased slightly (to 91%), and the tendency to follow the gaze of the speaker when looking at their gestures also decreased (only 8% of gaze-cued gestures were fixated). This result demonstrates that the effectiveness of gaze as a cue to orient another individual's attention may well be at its strongest when engaged in real interaction with people rather than the more artificial viewing conditions that are often used to evaluate social attention. The importance of the social setting in regulating our behaviour can also be seen in Gullberg's work: the observers were more likely to fixate 'socially unacceptable' locations on the speaker when watching the video (57%) than when watching the live speaker (35%)!

Gaze judgements of autistic children

The well-known failure of autistic children to follow the gaze of others might be owing to either a disinclination to follow eye direction or an inability to detect the gaze direction of others, and so respond to it. Leekham et al. (1997) devised two tests to distinguish these possibilities. The first *gaze monitoring* test provided a measure of a child's spontaneous tendency to follow the gaze direction of someone else when they altered their eye and head direction. In the second *visual perspective taking* task the child was instructed to work out, from their gaze direction, what a second person was looking at. Normal children, and children with Down's syndrome, were successful in both tests. Autistic children, however, did not spontaneously follow the gaze of others, but they were essentially normal when asked to assess the gaze direction of a second person. Thus the ability of autistic children to work out gaze direction is not impaired: it is the social significance and use of gaze following that seems to be the problem.

According to Klin et al. (2002) the best predictor of autism, in terms of gaze behaviour, is reduced fixation times on the eye regions of people in social situations, with increased viewing of mouths, bodies, and objects. Increased viewing of mouths, rather than objects, was associated with improved social adjustment. (Klin et al. used Edward Albee's 1967 film *Who's afraid of Virginia Woolf* in this study, because of the intense interactions of the four protagonists.)

Much work has been done trying to pin down neural correlates of autism and Asperger Syndrome. Impairment of the 'social' brain seems to be particularly associated with decreased activity in the amygdala. For example, Ashwin et al. (2007) used pictures of faces with fear-inducing threatening expressions in an fMRI study of various social brain regions. They found decreased activity in the left amygdala and left orbito-frontal cortex in autistic subjects compared with controls but more activity in the anterior cingulate gyrus and the superior temporal cortex. Interestingly, the control group showed varying responses to different intensities of fearful expression, including differential activations in the left and right amygdala; this differential response was absent in the autistic group.

Gaze following in other species

The list of species that show gaze following has been growing steadily in recent years, and now includes chimpanzees, macaques, dogs, seals, goats, and ravens. What is less clear is whether this reflects elements of a Theory of Mind – an understanding that another individual has a perception that differs from one's own – or is a low-level reflex response to the other's change of orientation (Call and Tomasello, 2008). In the monkey cortex, Perrett et al. (1994) described cells in the superior temporal sulcus that responded to conjunctions of eye and head direction, and also body position, and they postulated that these can operate as a 'direction of attention detector'. Using a variant of the Posner cuing task in which attention was cued using a central image of a rhesus monkey looking to the left or right, Deaner and Platt (2003) demonstrated reflexive orienting of attention to the gaze-cued direction in both rhesus monkeys and humans. This result demonstrates that not only monkeys may exhibit a similar reflexive orienting of attention to social gaze cues, but humans are also susceptible to gaze cues from non-human faces. The gaze-cuing effect was found both for images where the entire head and eyes provided the directional cue, and from images in which only the eyes of the monkey were shown, thus demonstrating that the eyes alone are sufficient attentional cues.

Higher primates, such as humans, will look back and forth between the experimenter's face and direction of regard (check-looking), which implies that they are trying to derive some extra information about the other's knowledge, intentions, or mood. Goossens et al. (2008) found that when a human experimenter made facial expressions that mimicked those of macaques, gaze following, and check-looking were enhanced and that socially meaningful expressions (such as the Bare Teeth display) were more effective than neutral expressions. Gaze following in macaques thus appears to be a flexible behaviour with an element of social cognition involved rather than a simple orienting reflex. Of course it comes as no great surprise that other primates respond in ways similar to humans, but it is not clear whether gaze following in other animals has similar cognitive significance.

Misdirection of gaze

Disguising gaze direction

Deliberately pointing the head in one direction while looking in another can be useful when you do not want others to guess where you are looking. This may be to avoid embarrassment, as when sizing up a member of the opposite sex on public transport or covertly admiring another woman's attributes (Fig. 9.5). It may also have more

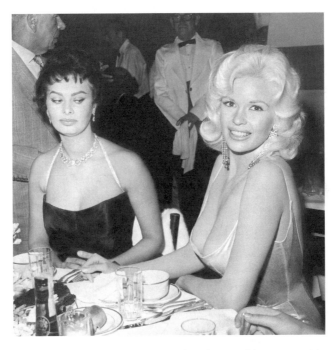

Fig. 9.5 Using head direction to disguise gaze direction. Sophia Loren and Jayne Mansfield at Romanoffs in Beverly Hills. © 1978 Joe Shere/MPTV.net.

sinister uses. Georges de la Tour's famous painting 'The Cheat with the Ace of Diamonds' (Fig. 3.1) has three of the four characters engaged in deception involving eye–head discoordination.

Misdirection in magic

Much of the magician's art consists of drawing the viewer's attention away from the place where the deceptive act is taking place, which is usually in an area of low visual interest (Macknik et al., 2008). This kind of misdirection can be physical: for example, snapping one's fingers with one hand can divert attention from what is happening in the other. Often this diversion can be enhanced by the magician directing his own gaze to the region that he wishes the viewer to attend to, thereby making use of social attention as well.

An example of this combination of physical and social misdirections is a simple trick in which a cigarette and lighter are made to disappear (Kuhn and Tatler, 2005; Kuhn et al., 2008; Tatler and Kuhn, 2007). The magician removes a cigarette from the packet and deliberately places it in his mouth the wrong way round (Fig. 9.6a). He then pretends to light the cigarette (b), which enhances interest in the cigarette region. Both magician and viewer then 'notice' the mistake and the magician turns the cigarette around while keeping his gaze fixed on the cigarette and the hand manipulating it (c).

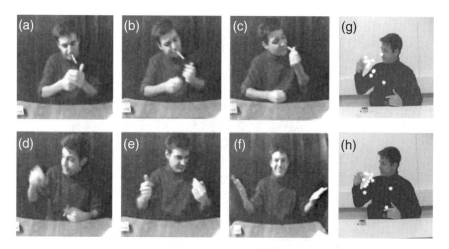

Fig. 9.6 (a) to (f). Gustav Kuhn performing the disappearing lighter and cigarette trick filmed from a camera on a viewer's head. Details in the text. From Kuhn and Tatler (2005) (g) to (h) Fixations at the time of the cigarette drop (d) for viewers who did not detect the drop (g) and those who did (h). From Kuhn et al. (2008).

During this manoeuvre the magician drops the lighter, which is in his right hand, into his lap. He then calls attention to the disappearance of the lighter by snapping his fingers and waving his hand (d), which draws attention away from his left hand, from which he then drops the cigarette from a height of about 15 cm above the table top onto his lap. This action is fully visible, but is not (usually!) seen, as attention is still with the lighter hand. He then looks at the now empty left hand (e) and opens it to show that the cigarette has disappeared too (f). The trick is surprisingly effective: of 20 participants, only 2 detected the drop on the first showing of the trick, although when the trick was repeated all of them correctly detected and explained how the trick was done.

Why is such a simple trick, in which items are simply dropped in plain sight of the view, so effective? By recording the gaze movements of viewers of the trick, Kuhn and Tatler (2005) considered whether visual factors, such as the distance between fixation and the dropping cigarette and the incidence of blinks during the drop could explain people's failure to see what should be an obvious act. In particular, these authors analysed where the observers were fixating at the time of the cigarette drop (just after Fig. 9.6d). First, blinks by the observers were unable to explain whether they detected the cigarette or not. Second, there was little difference between where people looked when they detected the drop and when they did not (Fig. 9.7). As the cigarette dropped, most viewers were fixating the magician's right hand, where the lighter had been, or his face, or the shoulder between face and hand. Interestingly, when comparing the first trial (Fig. 9.7 left panels), where most people did not detect the cigarette drop, to the second trial (Fig. 9.7 right panels), where all observers detected the drop, there is strikingly little difference in where people looked. Apart from three individuals who were looking at the cigarette as it dropped, all the others were looking roughly where they had looked on the first trial, which was about 16° from the dropping cigarette. It seems from this that there is no particular requirement to fixate on the appropriate area for detection to occur. It thus appears that what the magician is manipulating in this case is not fixation itself, but the viewer's *covert* attention.

Of course, this raises the question about how the magician can successfully misdirect his viewer's overt and covert attention. In a follow-up study, Tatler and Kuhn (2007) found that there was a strong agreement between where the observer looked during the trick and where the magician was looking. Moreover, this agreement was maximal during the crucial section of the trick, when the lighter and cigarette were dropped. Thus it seems that the magician manages to get his viewer to look where he is looking when it matters most in the trick and thus uses this strong social cue of shared attention to misdirect the viewer. It was interesting to find that this gaze-matching between the viewer and the magician still occurred even when the viewer was pre-warned to avoid being misdirected by the magician and try to uncover the secrets of the trick! It seems that even when we try to, we find it hard to avoid looking where someone we are engaged in close interaction with is looking.

We have already talked about the fact that social cues may be stronger when engaged in live interaction than when viewing an individual on a television screen. Kuhn et al. (2008) found a similar result for the effectiveness of the cigarette trick: people were

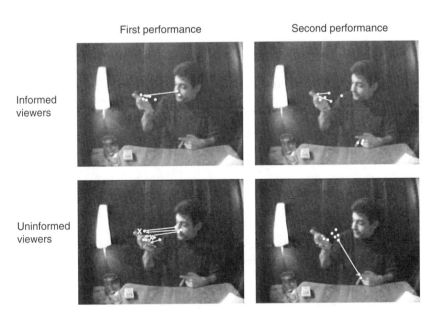

First performance   Second performance

Informed viewers

Uninformed viewers

Fig. 9.7 Fixation locations of observers during the trick illustrated in Fig. 9.6 at the moment the cigarette was dropped. Where observers were looking was not affected either by whether they were expecting the disappearance or by whether they detected the drop. Only two participants detected the drop in the first performance (fixations marked by Xs). All participants detected the drop in the second performance. From Kuhn & Tatler (2005).

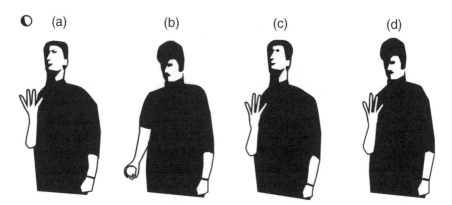

Fig. 9.8 The disappearing ball trick. (a) and b); The magician twice throws the ball up and catches it. (c) On the third throw he palms the ball but imitates the action including the upward head movement (social cuing). (d) Alternatively he imitates the throw but continues to look at the hand (inconsistent social cuing). After Kuhn and Land (2006).

more likely to detect the drop when viewing a video of the trick than they had been in the previous, live performances discussed above. What this video-based study did demonstrate, however, was that although there was little evidence for differences between the gaze allocation for observers who detected the drop and those who didn't at the time that the cigarette was dropping, differences did emerge in the seconds that followed: those who spotted the drop were faster moving their eyes to the now empty left hand (where the cigarette had been) than those who missed it. It should be noted however, that even though those who spotted the drop and looked to the left hand quicker, often stopped off for a look at the magician's face on the way.

Another trick, the disappearing ball illusion, provides a further striking example of social cuing (Kuhn and Land, 2006). In this trick the magician throws a ball into the air (Fig. 9.8a), catches it (b), throws it up and catches it again, and then on the third throw he palms the ball so that it does not leave his hand (c). The typical response of viewers was that the ball had disappeared upwards, caught by someone beyond the top of the screen in the filmed version of the trick. There were two versions of the trick. In the first the magician looks upward after the third throw (c), thus implicitly directing viewers to look there too. In the second version he remains looking down at the hand that has supposedly thrown the ball (d). In this study 68% of participants had a vivid recollection of the ball leaving the screen in condition (c), but this dropped significantly to only 32% in condition (d) indicating that social cuing had a major influence on the outcome of the trick.

When the eye movements of viewers of the trick were examined a very consistent pattern emerged. On the first two (real) throws they viewed the hand as it began the throw, then glanced to the magician's face and finally at the ball as it reached its apex above the head. On the third throw they viewed the hand and face as before, but then gaze remained close to the face, and rarely above the head. Thus, even in the viewers who were adamant that the ball had disappeared upwards, their gaze was not directed upwards. It seems that their eye movement system was not fooled by the trick, even though their percept of what had occurred was influenced by the social cuing provided by the magician's upward look. It is interesting to contrast the results of the disappearing ball trick to those of the disappearing cigarette trick. For the cigarette trick, we see that the eyes were almost always fooled by the magician and misdirected to the location cued by his gaze, but covert attention was not always misdirected in this way. For the ball illusion, the eyes were almost never misdirected to the gaze-cued location, but it would appear that covert attention may have been. Perhaps then the manner of the magician's misdirection might vary considerably for different types of tricks? These tricks seem to provide another example of dissociation between vision for action and vision for perception, consistent with the idea of dorsal and ventral cortical streams, as championed by Milner and Goodale (1995).

Summary

1. In social situations faces are preferentially fixated, in particular the regions around the eyes and mouth. A feature of autism is a decreased tendency for eye contact.

2. Eyes are potent signals for directing the attention of others, and we can judge the direction of another's gaze to within about 1°. This judgement requires not only an estimate of the position of the eyes within their sockets but also where the head is pointing. Unusual misalignments of eye and head can be used to disguise gaze direction.

3. Much of the magician's art relies on exploiting our strong natural tendency to follow another's gaze. With remarkable consistency, magicians are able to misdirect both the overt and covert attentions of their audience at crucial points in the trick, allowing otherwise highly visible events to go undetected.

Part 3

Commentaries

Chapter 10

Representations of the visual world

So far in this book we have emphasized that the main role of vision is to provide us with the information needed to guide and control our actions. The chapters of Part II have provided many examples of vision fulfilling just these functions. However, in ordinary experience this functionalist account does not quite fit with what we what we think of as 'seeing'. We have a vivid impression of the world before our eyes, and we are also able to summon up less vivid but nevertheless serviceable evocations of past scenes. In other words we appear to have internal representations of the visual world that involve both what is on our retina now, and what has been processed by our visual system in the past. In this chapter we will first explore the nature and content of these representations, and then consider how they may relate to the roles of vision in the tasks of daily life.

Retinal image and scene perception

A curious aspect of vision is the discrepancy between how the eyes gather information from the world and our internal cognitive experience of 'seeing'. Our subjective experience of seeing is complete and continuous, as if our eyes supply information much like a movie camera would. However the reality of how the eyes sample the world is far from this subjective impression. Visual sampling is not complete: high-quality vision is restricted to the small foveal region at the centre of vision (see Chapter 2). Visual sampling is also not continuous: the eyes fixate, on average, three discrete locations in each second. How does the brain reconcile the discrepancy between the input from the eyes and our subjective experience of seeing?

Perceptual continuity

Given that the saccade-and-fixate strategy of the oculomotor system results in discontinuous sampling, how is it that our percept appears continuous? At first, some assumed that perception continued during saccades (e.g. Cattell, 1900; Javal, 1878). However, a chance discovery by Erdmann and Dodge (1898) showed that this assumption must be wrong. While using a mirror to observe the eye movements of participants reading text, Erdmann and Dodge noticed that they were never able to see their *own* eyes moving. This technique remains a useful demonstration of the fact that vision is suspended during saccadic eye movements: if one looks at one's own eyes in a mirror and alternates looking between the two eyes, it is not possible to catch the eyes moving but only to see them at rest looking at either of the two positions (but if you want to defeat this suppression and catch a glimpse of your eye in motion, try the method suggested by Tatler and Troscianko, 2002). The mechanisms that underlie the suspension of vision during saccades have received considerable attention in eye movement literature and a number of possible explanations have been proposed. There may be active suppression of visual processing (Burr et al., 1994); a decrease in

(a)

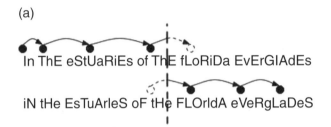

In ThE eStUaRiEs of ThE fLoRiDa EvErGlAdEs

iN tHe EsTuArIeS oF tHe FLOrIdA eVeRgLaDeS

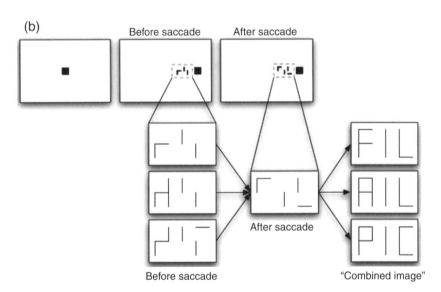

Fig. 10.1 (a) Participants read text of alternating uppercase and lowercase letters as shown in the upper line. When the eye (black circles denote fixations, the arrows saccades) passed an invisible boundary, shown by the dashed line, the case of every letter in the display was changed so that by the time the eye landed for the next fixation the text was as shown in the lower line. Participants did not notice the change and there were no measurable differences in fixation duration or saccade amplitude around the time of the change.Redrawn from McConkie and Zola (1979) (b) Participants fixated a central marker until a peripheral target appeared. When the target appeared an array of lines also appeared between the centre of the screen and the peripheral target. When the participant launched an eye movement toward the target, the lines changed to a different array. The lines were meaningless alone, but if the pre- and post-saccade lines were fused they would form one of three French words. Participants were incapable of reporting these words. Redrawn from O'Regan and Levy-Shoen (1983).

contrast sensitivity, such that vision is still possible, but only for highly contrasting stimuli (Diamond et al., 2000); backward masking of the saccade by the next fixation (Breitmeyer and Ogmen, 2000); motion blur (Nakayama, 1981) or even shearing forces acting on the rods and cones during saccades may prevent vision (Castet and Masson, 2000). Whatever the mechanisms might be that lead to vision being effectively suspended during saccades, it is clear that the apparent perceptual continuity of our visual experience is an illusion: we effectively only sample visual information during the fixation pauses between saccades.

Perceptual completeness

For some time it was thought that the pictorial contents of each fixation were fused to construct a point-by-point complete picture of the scene within the brain. The notion of an 'integrative visual buffer' as a low-level visual store in which the pictorial content of successive fixations is fused was specifically proposed and described by McConkie and Rayner (1976) and supported or at least assumed in a large number of studies (see Tatler, Gilchrist et al., 2005 for a discussion). The 'picture-in-the-mind' explanation of seeing can be traced back to philosophers including Aristotle, Crathorn and Hume (Wade and Tatler, 2005).

Despite being intuitively appealing, the evidence against the idea of a picture in the mind as an explanation for the completeness of our perceptual experience is now overwhelming. Doubts about the ability to integrate information from successive fixations surfaced in the 1970s, with a variety of studies failing to find any evidence for transsaccadic integration (Bridgeman et al., 1975; McConkie and Zola, 1979; O'Regan and Lévy-Schoen, 1983; Fig.10.1). However, despite the mounting evidence against a veridical point-by-point representation of the visual environment, it was not until the mid-1990s that arguments against this proposition found overwhelming popularity. The catalyst for the radical change in accepted understanding of the nature of visual representation was the advent of the change detection paradigm.

Changing views of visual representation

In 1991 John Grimes presented the surprising findings of a study he conducted with George McConkie in which an unexpected change was made as observers viewed a scene (later published as Grimes, 1996). Grimes found that if the change was timed such that it occurred while the observer was making a saccade, even a large change, such as swapping the heads on the main actors in a scene, would go unnoticed by the viewer. Since this landmark study, a large number of researchers have demonstrated similar failures of visual awareness with changes going unnoticed when timed to coincide with blinks (O'Regan et al., 2000) or brief artificial interruptions to viewing (Rensink et al., 1997; Fig. 10.2); a phenomenon that Rensink called 'change blindness'.

Change blindness was largely interpreted as providing a strong case against the notion of point-by-point pictorial representations (Rensink, 2002). If the pictorial content of each fixation were retained, then, it has been argued, it should be trivial to detect changes to the colour, location, or even presence of an object. The phenomenon

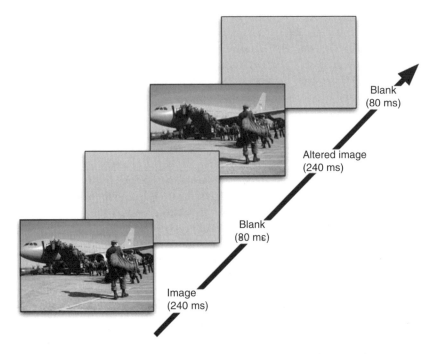

Fig. 10.2 The 'flicker paradigm'. An image is presented for a brief time, before being replaced by a blank, grey screen for about 80 ms. The image then reappears, but with one detail changed. In this case it is the disappearance of the engine on the wing of the aeroplane. This altered image is displayed for a brief time before being again replaced by a blank grey screen for 80 ms. This whole cycle repeats until the participant detects the change. Images courtesy of Ron Rensink.

of change blindness has renewed interest in the nature of scene representation and a variety of explanations of how we encode and retain information from the visual environment have been argued.

There is no representation

The first, and perhaps most extreme, suggestion was that change blindness demonstrates that we do not construct an internal representation of our visual environment at all (O'Regan and Noë, 2001). After all, why should we go to the effort of constructing a mental model of the world and access that for information about our surroundings when we can move our eyes freely and with low metabolic cost? When we need to access information about a particular location in the scene, we can simply direct our high-resolution foveae to that location and sample it visually. This viewpoint has been termed the World as an Outside Memory account of vision (O'Regan, 1992). Similar arguments against the need for internal representation have been made, famously by the philosopher George Berkeley in 1709, and more recently by Dennett (1991), Gibson (1966), and MacKay (1973).

Of course, just because an observer fails to detect a change when it coincides with an interruption to viewing, this may not mean that no representations are constructed (Simons and Rensink, 2005). A range of alternative possibilities exists: just because complete point-by-point visual representations are not constructed, this does not mean that *no* information about our visual environment is represented. Instead, higher-level abstracted forms of information may be retained but may not be sufficiently detailed to support change detection. The possibility that higher-level information is retained from scenes had been suggested by philosophers for some time: Aquinas, Ockham, and Locke all considered that mental representations need not be pictorially veridical in nature (Wade and Tatler, 2005). A variety of studies have argued that higher-level properties such as scene gist (e.g. Biederman, 1981; Intraub, 1980, 1981) and spatial layout (e.g. Gibson, 1979; Hochberg, 1968; Simons, 1996) can be extracted and retained. Furthermore, the phenomenon of change blindness cannot truly be taken as demonstrating that we do not construct point-by-point visual representations. It may be that we *do* create such detailed representations but that these are not accessible in a form that allows changes to be detected (Simons and Rensink, 2005). Although change detection studies have radically changed our views of scene representation, in themselves they cannot exclude the existence of any particular form of representation. Other schools of thought on representation, discussed below, reflect the possibility that some information is extracted from the scenes we inspect.

Attentional coherence of visual detail

Rensink (2000) suggested that some visual detail can survive interruptions to viewing, as long as it is the subject of focal attention. In this way, a limited number of *proto-objects* can be maintained as an object representation, but all unattended visual detail is lost. The attended information can be retained as a coherent object representation only for as long as it receives focal attention. Thus change detection requires attention to the changing object at the time of the change, and indeed this is the experience one has when viewing change detection demonstrations. Rensink combined this limited coherence framework with the idea of retaining more abstract and higher-level information from scenes: the attended visual details are combined with scene gist and spatial layout information to create a 'virtual representation' of the scene (Rensink, 2000; Fig.10.3).

A return to representation

A third school of thought maintains that visual representations may not only be constructed but may be far less sparse than in the scheme proposed by Rensink, or in the ideas that were first suggested in response to the phenomenon of change blindness. Using a combination of change detection and recall paradigms, a number of studies have demonstrated that object property information appears to be extracted and retained from the scenes viewed (e.g. Hollingworth and Henderson, 2002; Irwin and Zelinsky, 2002; Melcher, 2006; Tatler et al., 2003). However, opinion within this broad school of thought is divided about how the object information is represented.

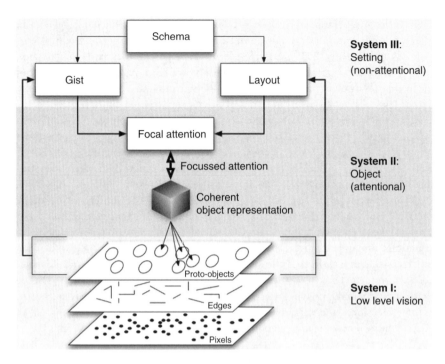

Fig. 10.3 Rensink's triadic model of scene representation. Redrawn from Rensink (2000).

One possibility is that object information is encoded into *object files* (Irwin, 1992; Irwin and Andrews, 1996; Kahneman and Treisman, 1984). The object file is temporary representation of the object, comprising a range of properties, which can be maintained across several saccades (but perhaps not indefinitely) in visual short-term memory (VSTM). In this scheme files for about 3 to 5 objects can be maintained at any time.

Alternatively, it may be that much richer representations are formed during scene viewing. Hollingworth and his colleagues have provided a compelling body of literature arguing that visual representations may be far more detailed and contain much more information than was suggested from early change detection studies (see Hollingworth, 2006). In this framework, representations combine information from both VSTM and visual long-term memory (VLTM) to construct stable and long-lasting representations of the scene.

What is interesting in both Irwin's and Hollingworth's positions is that the representations are suggested to be constructed in VSTM and so must be visual in nature rather than higher-level abstractions from the scene. In the case of Hollingworth's ideas in particular we see somewhat of a return to notions similar to those that were popular before the change blindness era: a relatively complete and detailed representation that is visual in nature and endures for long periods after the end of viewing.

Do the representations described by Irwin and by Hollingworth need to be visual in nature, or could they be more abstract? Melcher (2001, 2006) described similar accounts of information accumulation and persistence during scene viewing to those of Hollingworth but suggested that the representations are not constructed in VSTM. Rather these involve a higher-level system that he calls medium-term-memory (MTM) that acts as an intermediary on the way to long-term memory (LTM). The form of Melcher's representation is not purely visual but a more abstracted form of information from the scene. Tatler has also favoured a more abstract view of representation (Tatler et al., 2003; Tatler, Gilchrist et al., 2005; Tatler and Melcher, 2007) but one that encompasses some of the same concepts as Irwin and Hollingworth's more visual ideas. Tatler described object memories in terms very similar to Irwin's object files but in which the contents are more labile – with different properties being accumulated and forgotten in different ways and over different timescales. Thus, the object file is not a fixed set of contents but something in which different object characteristics are available depending on when they are accessed. What is interesting in the positions taken by these groups is that the reported patterns of accumulation and recall are quite similar. What differs is the manner in which these data are interpreted. Hollingworth's claim of a visually rich representation comes from the fact that his manipulations are very subtle (such as a small shift in orientation of an object). Hollingworth argued that if the representation were not visually rich, but rather abstract, such subtle differences will not be detectable. However, Tatler's interpretation is that abstract level representations can contain enough information to support such discriminations. It is hard to distinguish definitively between these two possibilities, and so the nature of the information contained in scene representations remains an open question.

Integrated representations

Spoken words can trigger short-latency eye movements to particular objects in a display when they are named (Tanenhaus et al., 1995), or even before they are named if the target of the sentence is predictable (Altmann and Kamide, 1999). Anticipating the target of a sentence in the verb that precedes it already suggests a close interplay between language and visual representations, with language activating conceptual representations that are mapped onto the affordances of objects in the visual scene (Altman and Kamide, 2007).

More striking evidence about the interplay between language and visual representation comes from paradigms in which the scene is replaced by a blank screen before the sentence is heard. In this case the participant has no visual scene in front of them as they hear a sentence that refers to the previously viewed scene. Under these circumstances, participants will still move their eyes to the locations previously occupied by objects in the scene (Altmann, 2004). For example, if faces appear and provide spoken facts, when participants are later questioned about those facts, they tend to look back to where the face that was associated with that fact had been, even though this location is now empty (Richardson and Spivey, 2000). While listening to a description of a scene participants may retrace the scene with their eyes on a blank screen or even in the dark (Johansson et al., 2006). These observations tell us that linguistic representations can index the locations of objects whether or not they are still present. We can, of course, both talk about things we see and look at things we talk about, so in some sense linguistic and visual representations are, or can be, connected.

Richardson and Spivey (2000) and Altmann (2004) have interpreted this tendency to look at previously occupied locations in the absence of concurrent visual presentation of the scene as reflecting the existence of an 'integrated representation' comprising auditory, visual, and spatial indexing information (see Richardson et al., 2009). When any part of the representation is activated there is corollary activation of all of its constituent parts. This means that when we hear a spoken reference to a previously seen object, not only do we activate the conceptual representation of that object, but we also activate the spatial index associated with that, leading to a tendency to fixate where it had been. Under normal circumstances a tendency to look back to an object when we hear spoken reference to it would be facilitatory not only in terms of activating the episodic memory trace but also by placing the eyes on the object for further visual processing.

Ferreira et al. (2008) attempted to extend the 'integrated representation' ideas proposed by Richardson and Spivey (2000) and by Altman (2004), suggesting that looking back to where an object had been actually improves memory of that object despite it no longer being there. Quite what this enhancement might mean is not clear, and at present there is no empirical support for this proposition. The idea that memory is improved by the act of moving the eyes to the old location is reminiscent of the Noton and Stark's (1971) idea that the memory of an object is actually encoded in the eye movements made when viewing it (Chapter 3), although Ferreira et al. do not go this far.

One interesting aspect of the idea of integrated language and visual representations is that these move the rather 'static' cognitive representations described in the sections above into the more dynamic setting of unfolding language. Spoken sentences are dynamic events, and as such the integrated representation represents a significant step toward a more realistic account of representation that reflects the dynamic nature of the world we operate in.

Towards a more realistic account of scene representation

One common factor in almost all of the scene representation research discussed above is that the stimuli have been static and displayed on computer monitors. This situation is of course very unlike natural behaviour in real environments in which the visual environment is immersive and dynamic. Furthermore, what is considered to be a complex visual scene varies considerably between studies: from simplified line drawings to photographs. Do the findings from static scenes, or from simplified scenes really reveal how we represent more realistic stimuli?

Levels of scene realism

We know of only two studies that have directly compared representation between different levels of scene realism. Tatler and Melcher (2007) showed that memory performance was better when recalling details of objects present in photographic scenes than in non-photographic (simplified) scenes. This benefit for photographic scenes was particularly prominent for briefer presentations times, suggesting an initial promotion of information extraction from more realistic scenes. What is interesting about non-photographic scenes such as drawings and paintings is that they can vary in how well they obey realistic scene-organizing principles (such as gravitational support). For example, the images in Fig.10.4 have all been considered 'complex scenes' in scene representation research, yet the level of realism is very varied. The realism of a non-photographic scene influenced object memory in a rather complex way: object identity showed an initial benefit for unrealistic scenes; object colour recall did not differ between realistic and unrealistic scenes; and object position showed an initial benefit for realistically organized non-photographic scenes. What this means is that we have to be very careful when extrapolating findings from simplified stimuli to the processes of representing objects in more complex scenes.

Perhaps more encouragingly, Tatler, Gilchrist et al. (2005) found that the patterns of information accumulation when viewing photographs were very similar to those when viewing real environments, although the general level of performance in object memory tests was better for viewing the real environments. Thus, it would seem that the manner of encoding representations from photographs is largely similar to that when viewing a real environment. The only differences that were found were in

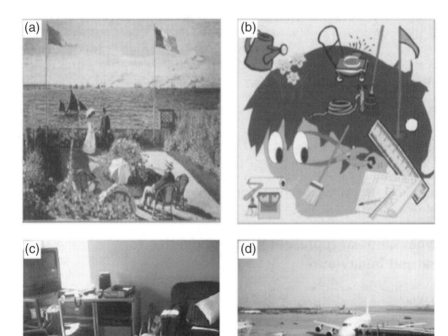

Fig. 10.4 An assortment of 'scenes' that have been used in studies of scene representation and object memory. While (a) is realistic, it is still far removed from the real world. It is hard to really classify (b) as a 'scene'. From Tatler and Melcher (2007).

the robustness of the information once encoded: different patterns of stability and transience were found for identity, colour, and position information. Although this study might suggest that we can apply findings from the lab to understand visual representation during natural behaviour, we should still be cautious. In the 'real-world' setting used by Tatler and colleagues people were asked to stand still in the doorway of each room and look around, which meant that the task remained a static and hence somewhat artificial one.

Dynamic scenes

Clearly, static scenes are not representative of real world situations and therefore dynamic scenes would be preferable. However, dynamic scenes are rarely used in scene representation research. Anecdotally, we know that people are bad at detecting things that change during an editorial cut in movies: we are very bad at detecting continuity errors in the movies we watch. This extension of something akin to change blindness to dynamic movie scenes was confirmed by Levin and Simons (1997). In fact it seems that people are even more blind to changes in dynamic scenes than in static scenes (Wallis and Bülthoff, 2000).

Editorial cuts such as those exploited by Levin and Simons are interesting because they occur frequently in film yet are often unnoticed: indeed even when asked to attend to these events and report when they occur, participants often fail to notice them (Smith and Henderson, 2008). Studies using movie scenes are an interesting step away from static scenes towards lifelike realism, but they also introduce some interesting new principles that do not match real environments. For example, the cuts between viewpoints are far more abrupt than would ever occur due to ego motion. Film conventions such as panning the camera to follow a moving target of interest also mean that when viewing a moving target in a movie the target is stationary with respect to the frame and the observer, yet the background is in relative motion; this situation is the opposite of that in real environments. How these artificial conventions of movies influence the representational and perceptual processes at work is yet to be established.

What kinds of representation are needed for natural behaviour?

In the rest of this chapter we will look at the question of representations from a different standpoint, by asking the question, 'What kinds of information about our surroundings, and the objects in them that we deal with, would be most useful in facilitating our everyday actions?'

In Chapter 1 and again in Chapter 5 we concluded that the system that directs gaze to objects that we intend to act on has access to two sources of information: what can be seen in the visual field at the time and what is available in memory about the locations of particular objects outside the visual field. This gaze-control memory must contain, as a minimum, a store of objects identified by their attributes and indexed to locations in the surroundings. Such a memory is essential even to do something as straightforward as to locate one's mug in the staff room and to identify it from (for example) its colour. Such a store will have been built up from information supplied by the eyes over various time scales. It seems reasonable to identify this object-and-location memory with a spatially extended version of the kinds of scene representation discussed earlier in this chapter.

Once the appropriate object has been targeted, the role of vision changes. The eyes now supply online information that assists the execution and completion of the task. The nature of the information required depends on what the hands are doing at the time and is closely linked to the motor actions themselves. In extended activities such as tea making, the task changes roughly every 3 s, and so too does the behaviour of the eyes. The evidence from active tasks indicates that the role of vision is usually narrowly confined to the objects being examined or manipulated, hence the three maxims discussed in Chapters 4 and 5: 'Do it where I'm looking', 'Look just in time', and 'What you see is what you need'. To the extent that it still makes sense to speak of 'representations', it is clear that during vision-for-action the representations required are different from, and more complex than, those involved in passive viewing. In what follows we will first consider the problem of locating objects in the world and then the relations between vision and action during the execution of real tasks.

Representations for navigation, object location, and gaze control

Frames of reference and scale

Most of the work discussed earlier in relation to scene representation did not involve movement through, or action in, an extended three-dimensional world. A central consideration in applying the idea of mental representation to this wider space is the question of what we anchor it to. This question has featured in many psychological and philosophical works on representation, yet is largely absent from the literature discussed above. Certainly authors have commented on the importance of space in the representations described and tested and have suggested that spatial information is extracted before more detailed object information (Aginsky and Tarr, 2000; Tatler et al., 2003). But what is the frame of reference for the 'space' referred to in these studies? We refer the reader particularly to Klatzky (1998) for a full discussion of this question.

A number of coding schemes have been put forward for representing space, but most prominent have been the ideas of encoding space either with respect to some external frame of reference (allocentric) or with respect to the individual (egocentric). Both of these coding schemes have advantages and disadvantages for the efficiency of representation. Perhaps the main difference between these two coding schemes is seen when an individual is moving around in an environment (Fig.10.5). An allocentric representation would require that the individual's position and heading in the environment is also represented and updated continuously. An egocentric representation requires no representation of the individual, but constant updating of the representations of all other elements in the environment. Which form of spatial representation

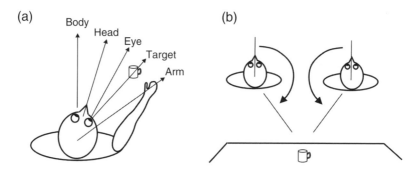

Fig 10.5 Visuo-motor transformations. (a) The required movement to grasp the mug is the angle from arm to target. This is the angle from body-to-arm minus the sum of the target-to-fovea, eye-in-head, and head-on-body angles. (b) Allocentric and egocentric angles. The egocentric turn required to pick up the mug depends on the relative positions in allocentric space of the mug and subject.

is actually used has often been debated. However, it is clear that evidence exists for both, and it seems likely that how we choose to encode a space may depend upon the task and demands of the situation. The neural bases of these representations is discussed further in Chapter 11.

Not only are there different frames of reference for spatial coding, but we can represent space at a range of different scales (Montello, 1993). According to Montello we can divide spatial scales into four categories (Fig.10.6). *Figural* spaces are smaller than the body and include pictures and objects. *Vista* space is larger than the body but encompasses only what can be seen from a single location, such as in a room. *Environmental* space includes locations that cannot be viewed from a single vantage point, but given some (considerable) locomotion could be explored fully. *Geographical* space is larger still and encompasses space that could not realistically be explored by an individual. This final category of space is unlikely to play a significant role in organizing our everyday activities, but the other three scales of spatial coding could potentially all be at work in many tasks.

Given the wealth of literature on frames of reference and scales of representation for spatial information in scenes, it is perhaps surprising that the studies discussed earlier in this chapter have not considered this issue in any detail. Most of the experiments described above used static scenes observed from fixed positions. As such, distinguishing between egocentric and allocentric coding is not possible. Moreover, the observers never occupy the space that they are representing during static scene viewing. They are viewing an image of a scene that they are not present in and being asked to remember where things were. This means that asking what frame of reference is being used may be meaningless. The question of scale is problematic here too. The participants are being asked to represent what might be thought of as vista space because they are shown a view of a scene such as a room. However, the stimulus that they are encoding occupies figural space. These two ways in which images are removed from reality may

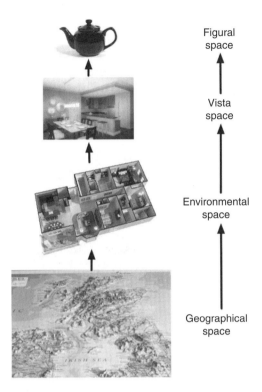

Fig. 10.6 Representational spaces, based on Montello's (1993) classifications.

make it uninformative to extrapolate any notions of spatial representations derived from static scene viewing experiments to real behaviour.

Evidence for spatial representations in natural behaviour

Earlier in this chapter we cast doubt upon the usefulness of static scene viewing paradigms for understanding spatial representation in natural environments. However, what insights can we gain from studies of natural behaviour about whether and how we might encode space? We refer the reader to Hayhoe (2008) for an excellent review of the case for spatial memory in natural behaviour, which includes additional evidence to that discussed below.

In a model-building task similar to Ballard's (Chapter 4), Aivar et al. (2005) changed the layout of the blocks in the resource area, from which each new piece is selected for building the model (Fig. 4.9). Provided the subject had sufficient time to familiarize with the layout of the environment before the first change was made, the subject launched saccades to the previous location of the next required block in the resource area. This result clearly implicates spatial memory for the layout of the blocks in the resource area.

While making tea (Chapter 5) differences can be seen in the deployment of gaze when locating objects that are looked for or used more than once. The first attempt to fixate an object typically required more search-like behaviour, involving more fixations to 'home in' on the target object. However, when relocating the same object later in the task, saccades were more direct, with fewer saccades required to fixate the object. This result is consistent with the observer retaining some information about the object from when it was previously fixated. At the very least this would involve spatial information about where it is in the scene.

A more general case for spatial knowledge of the environment being represented in tea making comes from the observation that it is possible to make a very large gaze saccade to, or very near to, an object that is about to be manipulated. This gaze saccade can be to a location that is outside the observer's field of view – gaze shifts of more than 100° were commonly observed during tea making (Land et al., 1999; see Figs 6.5 and 6.6) – and so must rely on non-visual information such as remembering where an object was placed, or at least having a rough spatial layout of the scene upon which to target these large relocations of gaze. If the object to be located lies behind the observer to the left, then the required turn is to the left, and vice versa for a rightward location. The object is in the same location in allocentric space, but because of the different starting positions of the tea maker the action required, made in egocentric space, is in opposite directions in the two cases. The conclusion seems inescapable that we use our (allocentric) knowledge of the layout of the kitchen to recall the location of the object and then translate this into egocentric coordinates in order target and retrieve the object. The spatial scale in which such turns are carried out corresponds approximately to Montello's *vista* space. In other activities, such as a racing driver storing his 'racing line' round a track, the scale of the representation is better described as *environmental* space.

The characteristics of action-based representations

As we mentioned earlier, when engaged in a motor task the deployment of vision has a seat-of-the-pants quality not observed in cognitive tasks such as scene recall. This manifests itself in a number of ways: there is more use of the world as 'outside memory', the information taken in is limited and confined to the specific requirements of the particular task, and very little is retained once a particular aspect of the task is completed.

Using the world as an 'outside memory'

As we have seen throughout the earlier chapters of this book, there is generally a close coupling between vision and action: we look at what we are currently manipulating. This is encompassed in Ballard's maxim: 'Do it where I'm looking' (see Chapter 4). This observation can be taken as favouring the arguments of O'Regan and Noë (2001) that there is no need for a visual representation and that when we require detailed information to serve our behavioural goals, we simply orient our high-resolution foveae at the informative location. However, as we will argue these findings do not mean that there is no representation during natural behaviour (see Hayhoe, 2008, for the same position).

Important support for sparse representations in natural behaviour can be found in Ballard's block copying task (Ballard et al.,1992; Ballard et al., 1995). When constructing a copy of a model using coloured blocks, all that the participant requires knowledge of for each block is its colour and where is should be placed. It might be expected that both these sources of information can be extracted in a single glance at the model before selecting a block to place on the constructed copy, and remembered until the block is placed correctly, less than 2 s later. However, the most common strategy employed by participants was to look to the model twice: once before selecting a block and again before placing the block in the constructed copy (Fig. 4.9). This was taken as evidence that different information was extracted on the two fixations of the block in the model: the first fixation served to extract the colour and allow the correct block to be selected from among the variety of blocks in the resource area; the second fixation was used to extract information about the position of the block in the model so that the selected block could be placed correctly. Thus, rather than encoding and remembering all of the information about the object that is required for the task, only the information that is required *at the present moment* is extracted. Ballard's evidence is a clear argument that representations are sparse, or perhaps even not constructed, and we use our eyes to gather information 'just in time' for when it is required (Chapter 4).

Certainly the above results imply sparse representation in natural behaviour, but these are indirect measures of representation. Tatler (2001) asked the more direct question of what information is retained and available from each fixation. Participants were interrupted in the middle of making a cup of tea by turning out the lights. When participants were interrupted in this way, they were able to give pictorially rich descriptions of what they had been fixating at the moment that the lights went out. In contrast, if asked to report where they had been fixating *immediately prior* to the moment of interruption (ideally therefore reporting the content of the fixation penultimate to the interruption), they performed very poorly. This result alone is consistent with the idea that information is lost each time we move our eyes but that for the present fixation we have access to richly detailed information. More interestingly, this study found evidence that pictorially rich information survives the end of each fixation and can be accessed until it is overwritten by information from the new fixation. Survival of information into the next fixation argues that what participants were reporting was not simply what was on their retinae, but that they were accessing stored information. The richness and precision of the reports suggest that there may be a visually rich buffer, with its contents overwritten soon after the start of each fixation (Fig. 10.7). It should be noted that this is very different from the 'integrative visual buffer' discussed earlier.

Information uptake is limited to immediate task demands

The types of information that are required for successfully completing each of the tasks we have considered in this book vary greatly. In tea making we at least require some notion of where things are and what they are. In drawing we require some storage of the information gathered from fixations on the sitter until the artist reproduces those features on the page (Fig. 4.12). For driving a racing car we must store knowledge of the

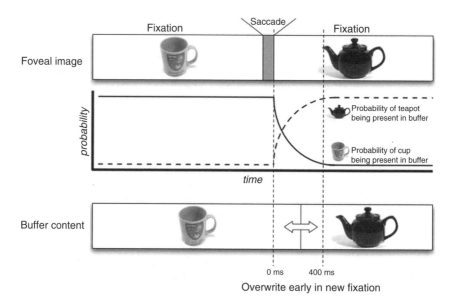

Fig. 10.7 Cartoon depicting the behaviour of Tatler's proposed richly detailed visual buffer. A veridical copy of the foveal content is retained in the buffer during the saccade that follows and remains until it is overwritten soon after the start of the next fixation. Redrawn from Tatler (2001).

ideal racing line to be driven. In cricket, the batsman must learn and represent the mappings of how the ball will behave after its bounce on the pitch (Fig. 8.12). These few examples are hard to reconcile within a one-size-fits-all approach to representation. It seems more like that the nature of represented information varies according to the task requirements.

Direct support for the notion of task-specific extraction and representation of information can be found from work by Triesch et al. (2003) described in Chapter 5. They used a virtual reality block-sorting task in which blocks of different heights had to be sorted – placing them onto one of two conveyor belts – according to different rules (Fig. 5.9). The sorting rules varied the point at which a critical feature (the height of the block) was relevant to the sorting task. In the first condition the size of the brick was irrelevant for both pick-up and set-down; in the second condition size was relevant for the pick-up decision but not the set-down; and in the third condition size was relevant for both. On 10% of trials the brick size was changed between pick-up and set-down. The change was reliably detected only in the third condition, when the height of the block was relevant to the decision about where to place the block. Of course being able to detect the change at all requires some form of represented information about its previous state and so we can use this study to infer what is being represented. The result demonstrates not only that what is retained is very task specific, but also that what is represented is constrained to the temporal dynamics of the task. If a feature is still relevant to the ongoing task (third condition), then we are sensitive to it changing – implying we have retained information about this object property. However it is important to note that if a feature is no longer relevant to the task (second condition), we are not sensitive to it changing – implying that we may no longer represent that feature. This result brings us to the question of how transiently we retain information during natural tasks.

In a similar block sorting task, Droll and Hayhoe (2007) varied the predictability of which cue would be relevant for the sorting. In this version, blocks were defined by four features: height, width, colour, and texture. For predictable blocks, there were two conditions; in both a single feature was used to cue which block to pick up, and a single feature cued the sorting (put down). However, in one condition the pick-up and put-down cues were the same, whereas in the other they were different. In the unpredictable condition a single cue was used for pick-up but the put-down cue varied randomly on each trial between the four possible features. The probability of refixating the block being carried to the conveyor belts after the put-down cue was displayed varied between conditions. In the predictable condition when the pick-up and put-down cues were the same, refixations of the block were rare. In the unpredictable condition, refixations were common. Strikingly, when the put-down feature in the unpredictable condition happened to be the same as the pick-up cue (25% chance) refixations of the block were also common. Thus when the same feature is used for both picking up and sorting the block, the probability of refixating it depends on whether it was predictable that this feature information would be needed again. This result implies that feature information is stored if we know that it will be needed again later in the task, but if a number of features might be needed later, then features are not stored and the viewer resorts to a 'just-in-time' sampling strategy.

Information obtained in a motor task is usually short-lived

In many tasks it is important that most of the information obtained for use at the time is *not* retained. When negotiating a bend in the road it is important that steering is not contaminated by the memory of the previous bend. In sight-reading music, information about the previous phrase must be discarded as the current one is executed. What happened in the last tennis shot is not useful when playing the next.

Not all information obtained during motor actions is as ephemeral as the foregoing paragraphs suggest. Occasionally during natural behaviour participants make saccades to objects that are not being used at present but will be the target of a future action in the current task. This behaviour has been explored in hand washing (Pelz and Canoza, 2001), sandwich making (Hayhoe et al., 2003), and model building (Mennie et al., 2007). Looking ahead to a future target can occur several seconds before the object is required or acted upon. These 'look-ahead' fixations cannot be explained as simply task-unrelated fixations that happen to land on objects that will be used later: if this were the case then the frequency of 'looking back' to objects that are no longer needed should be similar to the frequency of look-ahead fixations, yet look-aheads vastly outnumber look-backs (Pelz and Canoza, 2001). Furthermore, look-aheads have a measurable effect on eye–hand latencies when the target is eventually dealt with (Mennie et al., 2007). Thus it seems that these look-ahead fixations are purposeful and serve behaviour.

In the longer term still, it would not be possible to build up skills, in driving, music reading, or tennis, if nothing was retained over many repetitions of particular actions. Cricketers would not be able to build up the relationships between ball behaviour and stroke timing required to bat effectively, and racing drivers would not be able to work out and retain their 'racing line' on the track, if there were no long-term effects of visuo-motor repetition.

Within the cognitive literature reviewed at the start of this chapter, a common question has been to ask for how long the represented information is stored and accessible. Some authors argue for robust and long-lived storage (e.g. Hollingworth and Henderson, 2002), whereas others argue for transient storage (e.g. Irwin and Zelinsky, 2002). Our position is that this is most likely to be a function of how long the information is required. In some tasks we have seen that information need only be stored transiently, during a specific portion of the task where it is relevant (brick sorting); for somewhat longer where information is being collected for use in the near future (look-aheads); or for a very long time when what is required is a set of accurate parameter mappings for use in a skilled action (batting in cricket).

What does 'representation' mean in the context of action?

Motor behaviour requires a representation in the brain of actions to be performed, in addition to the representations of objects and locations that we have discussed already. In Chapters 1 and 5 we presented a scheme describing the control of component acts in extended tasks (object-related actions). Each action was initiated by a set of outline instructions (the schema) which specified three things: what object the gaze control system was required to find, what motor action was required, and what the visual system was required to monitor (Fig. 1.1). Variations of this scheme, applicable to other kinds of activity, were discussed in Chapter 4 (Fig. 4.8). If we accept this general analysis, we can then think about representations for action at two levels: the level at which an action is specified (the schema level) and the level at which it is executed (by the gaze, motor control, and vision sub-systems). Clearly we are dealing here with a fairly complex interactive system with several rather disparate components. A good deal is now known about the anatomical location and the physiology of these components, and this will be discussed in the Chapter 11. Here we will only deal with the broader questions of what is needed from representations at these two levels – task specification and task execution.

The schema system and the specification of motor actions

'Schema' in this context means the internal representation of an action or a task (Norman and Shallice, 1986), and in its simplest form the schema system can be thought of as containing a series of lists of actions that have to be executed to achieve particular behavioural ends. The Supervisory Attention System (SAS) of Norman and Shallice (1986) distinguishes between routine operations that look after themselves and non-routine operations that require supervisory intervention (Fig. 10.8). Routine actions operate via an automatic system of schema selection they called 'contention

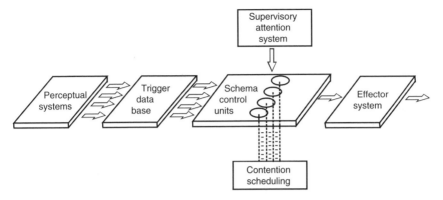

Fig. 10.8 Original Norman and Shallice model of the Supervisory Attention System (SAS). Redrawn from Norman and Shallice (1986).

scheduling'. This is a process in which different schemas compete with each other to achieve an activation level that exceeds some selection threshold. It can perhaps be argued whether the sequence of actions in a well-rehearsed task is the result of competitive selection, rather than the sequential implementation of a predetermined (although somewhat flexible) list of actions – whether this is a free market or a command economy? Whatever the mechanism, the outcome is a schema sequence that allows the smooth progress of a task.

For non-routine operations there is in addition an SAS that can override the automatic system when that is likely to lead to an undesirable result and can produce new schemas to deal with novel situations. This distinction between more routine functions (steering and adjusting speed on a country road) and ones requiring intervention and supervision (when a pedestrian steps onto the road unexpectedly) seems to correspond with our feeling that some situations involve conscious intervention and an effort of will, whereas others do not. However, this distinction between routine and non-routine does sometimes appear too rigid. If one thinks about driving there seems to be a graded series of situations in which an increasing amount of supervision is required. For example, quiet motorway driving < driving on winding country roads < low-traffic suburban driving < urban driving with traffic and pedestrians < driving during an inner-city rush hour. There seems no clear line separating the routine from the non-routine; indeed the degree of 'conscious attention' that needs to be imposed on the driver's control systems is likely to vary moment by moment. A related problem is that attention, in the sense that gaze direction is being controlled, is present at all times. For example, during tea making (Chapter 5), each new action requires attention to find the appropriate objects and to monitor each action as it progresses. All this typically happens while one is attending to the news on the radio, so the attentional commitment to the actions themselves is far from total. All that can really be said is that in some situations attention is more closely coupled to conscious awareness than in others. Bargh and Ferguson (2000) expressed a similar view: that automatic and controlled processes are not distinct and that even non-routine processes have automatic control structures at a higher level.

Schemas represent the final stages in a hierarchical decision making process that stretches from overarching strategies such as choosing a career down to opting for cornflakes for breakfast. In the original SAS model these higher-order goal-setting mechanisms were not elaborated, but a more recent model (Gilbert and Burgess, 2008; Shallice 2002; Shallice and Burgess, 1996) has sought to address this. Further 'higher-order' components were incorporated into the SAS. These include goal-setting, problem-solving, and strategy generation. The results of these operations are fed to the contention scheduler, which executes the schemas in conjunction with a special purpose working memory process. The new model also incorporates a monitoring and checking feedback process that assesses the results of schema implementation. A variety of evidence from patients with frontal lobe damage and from scanning studies indicates that the SAS itself operates from the dorsal prefrontal cortex, whereas contention scheduling is based on selection processes operating in the premotor cortex and basal ganglia.

Relations between the motor and visual systems in task execution

The representation of objects that is needed during object manipulation is not the same as the 'what-is-where' representation needed for the location of objects by the gaze system or that can be demonstrated in cognitive recall tasks. Properties such as colour and shape are now less important than attributes related to the execution of the impending action (motor descriptions). For example, if the goal is to pick up a teapot we might expect a rather different set of motor descriptions (such as grip requirements for the shape of handle; lifting force given the likely weight; arm extension in relation to proximity) than if our task is to avoid knocking it over when pouring water into it (such as knowledge of how to move in order to avoid the space occupied by the teapot; how to align the kettle spout with the shape and position of the opening in the teapot). The idea of motor-based descriptions of objects is not new. It corresponds closely to *affordances*, a word invented by Gibson (1979) to indicate the possibilities for action that a particular object offers (or 'affords'). Campbell (1993), in the more philosophical literature, used the term *causal indexical* to mean information in the form of what the individual can do with an object rather than its external physical properties. Interestingly, it has recently been highlighted that traditional approaches to object classification, based on static feature cues, may not be adequate for the emerging 'embodied cognition' viewpoint (Stark et al., 2008). Stark et al. provided a computational approach to object classification based on affordance cues. Thus their suggestion is that we classify objects using learnt affordance cues based on the functional significance of the object for action.

The required motor description of an object will vary with the action to be performed (as in the teapot examples above), and so it is presumably called for by the currently active schema at the time of manipulation, or in the half second or so between fixation and contact with the object. This does not mean, however, that it is generated from nothing. To visually assess the force needed to lift an object requires a much prior experience, just as knowledge of the behaviour of balls is essential for playing a good shot in any ball sport. Whether the action-related properties of objects are stored in the brain alongside their more conventional attributes is not yet clear.

It is interesting that recent neurophysiological studies of the cortical representation of actions in monkeys have come to conclusions quite consistent with those outlined here. Rizzolatti and Luppino (2001) proposed a scheme in which area F5 of the pre-motor cortex supplies 'motor prototypes' – outline patterns of muscle action – for various reaching, grasping, placing, and manipulative actions (see Chapter 11). Which particular action is to be activated is determined by input from parietal area AIP, which has 3D representations of the objects to be dealt with, and information about their meaning via connexions from the temporal lobe. In other words, area AIP contains the affordances that select from and shape the potential actions stored ready for use in the premotor cortex.

To summarize this section, it seems that for the performance of purposeful actions in the real-world four levels of representation are required, corresponding approximately to the four components of an action outlined in Fig. 1.1. These are a representation of goals and the means to achieve them (the schema level), of the locations of objects in the world (for gaze control), of motor actions ('motor prototypes'), and of visual representations of objects that embody the attributes needed for manipulation (affordances). There is now a considerable body of information on the brain structures involved in these representations, and we will explore some of these findings in the next chapter.

Summary

1. There is an apparent discrepancy between our subjective experience of a complete and stable world, and the discontinuous series of images supplied by the eyes. Until about 1990 the common view was that the brain constructs a faithful pictorial representation of the scene.

2. Change detection studies have suggested that much information is lost when we make an eye movement or vision is otherwise interrupted, implying that any representation of the surroundings is at best sparse. However, a range of studies now shows that certain attributes of attended objects, such as location and identity, are retained over substantial periods of time.

3. Most of our understanding of visual representation is derived from static scene viewing involving explicit memory tasks. It is not clear that such purely perceptually based representations are adequate to serve the needs of action in natural behaviour.

4. Active tasks require descriptions of objects in terms of their action possibilities (affordances) together with a robust representation of spatial layout. Task-level information must also form part of an active representation scheme.

Chapter 11

Neuroscience of gaze and action

One of the spectacular attributes of humans, compared with other animals, is their ability to engage in long complicated visuo-motor routines. Many of the examples in Chapters 4 to 9 are of this nature. Even a task as apparently simple as making a cup of tea requires 30 to 40 visually controlled and temporally co-ordinated acts, and many manufacturing crafts are very much more complex. Ideally we would like to know where and how these routines are stored in the brain, how they are made available when needed, how they access the oculomotor and limb motor control systems, and ultimately how they are acquired.

Neurophysiological research on primates, which has contributed so much to current understanding of other aspects of vision and motor control, is probably of limited help here, because other primates do not go in for these complex hierarchically planned activities to anything like the same extent as humans. Monkeys and apes do have routines involving tool use – chimpanzees use sticks to catch ants and stones to crack nuts – but these tend to be simple repeated acts without the serial complexity and forward planning typical of human activity. The other successful modern methodologies, scanning using PET and fMRI, are also of limited applicability because the physical restrictions imposed by the confined chambers of the scanners preclude much in the way of action. Nevertheless, there has been progress on at least some of these questions, and we will return to these after a brief look at the relevant brain anatomy. Mark Jeannerod's book *The Cognitive Neuroscience of Action* (1997) covers many aspects of the topic.

Anatomical basics

This section is a brief, uncontroversial, sketch of the main regions of the brain that are relevant to the visual control of action. In very broad outline the roles of the different regions of the brain are reasonably well understood. We will concentrate here on the cerebral cortex, but it is important to remember that other regions of the brain, notably the cerebellum, the basal ganglia and thalamus, superior colliculus (SC), and the nuclei of the brain stem are also involved with many aspects of visuo-motor behaviour (see Fig. 2.3). Parts of the cortex have common names, but they are also classified according to their cellular make-up (cytoarchitectonics) using the Brodmann system of numbering, and according to their functional properties using various other schemes. Because all three systems are in use, a minimal guide, for the lateral aspect of the left hemisphere of man and macaque monkey, is given in Figs 11.1 and 11.2. There are also important regions on the inner walls of the cortex (notably the cingulate gyrus

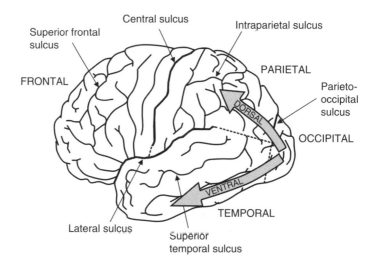

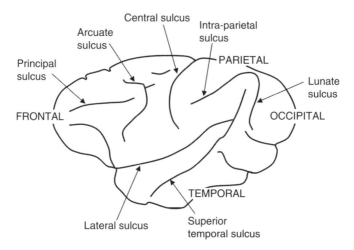

Fig. 11.1 Principal features of human and macaque cerebral cortex, showing the major sulci and the four lobes. Lateral views of left side. The dorsal and ventral visual streams are indicated on the human cortex.

in the longitudinal fissure), but to keep this section manageable these are not illustrated. Similarly little mention will be made of differences between the two halves of the cortex, although they certainly exist in activities such as tool use which, like language, is predominantly the responsibility of the left hemisphere.

The visual input

The eyes send their information via the optic nerves to the lateral geniculate nuclei of the thalamus, and thence to occipital lobes at the rear of the cerebral cortex. Part of the

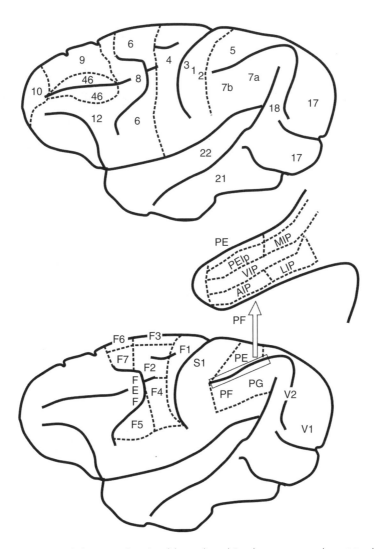

Fig. 11.2 Macaque left cortex showing (a) numbered Brodmann areas relevant to vision and motor control. (b) The numbering system used by Rizzolatti and Luppino (2001) for the motor areas (Brodmann 4, 6, and 8), and the posterior parietal region. The insert shows an unfolded view of the intraparietal sulcus and the areas contained within it.

optic nerve also supplies the superior colliculus (= optic tectum in non-mammals) in the midbrain. Almost all visual inputs to the cortex pass through the primary visual cortex (striate cortex; Brodmann Area 17; V1), which in turn projects forwards to a number of other regions in the occipital and temporal lobes where different aspects of the visual input are analysed separately: thus V4 is primarily concerned with colour, V5 with motion, and so on. These will not be considered here in detail: for a review see van Essen (2003). There is now a consensus that information from the occipital lobe

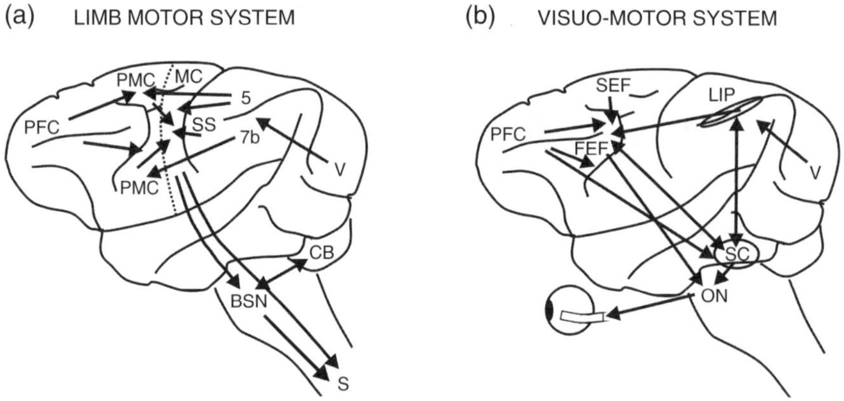

(a)   LIMB MOTOR SYSTEM   (b)   VISUO-MOTOR SYSTEM

Fig. 11.3 Principal cortical and sub-cortical structures involved in the control of the limbs and the eye movement system in the macaque. BSN, brain stem nuclei; CB, cerebellum; FEF, frontal eye field (8); LIP, lateral intraparietal area; MC, primary motor cortex (4); ON, oculomotor nuclei; PFC, prefrontal cortex (46); PMC, premotor cortex (6); S, spinal cord; SC, superior colliculus; SEF, supplementary eye field (6); SS, somato-sensory cortex (1,2,3); V, visual areas of the occipital lobe (17,18,19); 5 and 7b are Brodmann areas corresponding to superior and inferior parietal lobules. Other Brodmann areas are given in brackets.

proceeds forward in two broad, not entirely separate, routes: the ventral and dorsal 'streams' (Milner and Goodale, 1995; Ungeleider and Pasternak, 2003; see Fig. 11.1). The ventral stream is directed towards the temporal lobe and carries information about the identities of objects. Cells in the temporal lobe, for example, respond to faces, hands, and other objects. The dorsal stream is directed towards the parietal lobe and is concerned with the location of objects and their motion. The parietal lobe itself has motor as well as sensory functions and controls co-ordinated activities such as reaching and grasping. Lesions in the ventral stream lead to deficits in recognition and naming; lesions in the dorsal stream result in neglect of parts of the visual surroundings and to problems with co-ordination. In general ventral stream information is available for conscious scrutiny, dorsal stream information less so.

One interesting extension of the dorsal/ventral distinction has been the suggestion that these are associated with distinct modes of viewing scenes: an 'ambient' mode for gathering global properties of scenes such as overall layout, and a 'focal' mode for detailed scrutiny of objects (Velichkovsky et al., 2005). Velichkovsky and colleagues argue that these two modes are separable on the basis of eye movements: ambient processing is characterized by short duration fixations associated with large amplitude saccades; focal processing is characterized by long duration fixations associated with small amplitude saccades (Unema et al., 2005). Furthermore, the suggestion is that ambient processing is associated with activity in the dorsal stream, whereas focal processing is associated with activity in the ventral stream.

The motor output

The central sulcus (Fig. 11.1) separates the primarily sensory regions at the rear of the cortex from the primarily motor regions of the frontal lobe. Immediately posterior to the central sulcus is the somato-sensory cortex that receives input from the body surface and muscles in an orderly topographic array (Fig. 11.3a). Anterior to the central sulcus is the primary motor cortex (Brodmann Area 4, Fig. 11.2), which has an orderly mapping onto the musculature of the body – similar to the somato-sensory cortex – directly via the cortico-spinal tract and the motor neurons of the spinal cord and indirectly via various nuclei in the brain stem. The direct connections principally control fine movements of the distal limb segments, in particular the hands and fingers. However, there is also evidence that stimulation of parts of Area 4 evokes more complex patterns of movement that are components of the monkey's normal ethological repertoire (Graziano, 2006). The primary motor cortex receives input from other areas, particularly the premotor cortex anterior to it, about the patterns of muscular action required for the attainment of immediate goals. The dorsal and medial parts of Area 4 contain a second topographically mapped motor area, the supplementary motor area (F3 in the terminology of Matelli et al., 1991, see Fig. 11.2). This is principally involved in the control of the proximal limb segments. The premotor cortex itself (Area 6) receives much of its input from the parietal lobe, with different parietal regions mapping on to specific premotor regions. (Rizzolatti and Luppino, 2001; Wise et al., 1997). This means that the parietal lobe, responsible particularly for the visual control of hand and arm movements, has a motor output via the premotor cortex (Area 6) and its connections to Motor Area 4. The most anterior (rostral) and medial parts of the premotor cortex (F6 and F7 of Matelli et al., 1991) have input mainly from the prefrontal regions. They do not connect directly to Area 4 but diffusely to the other premotor areas and the also to the brain stem. These connections suggest that these rostral premotor areas are more concerned with the execution of longer-term plans than with the details of action co-ordination.

The eye movement system

In the cortex the main area involved in the control of eye movements is the frontal eye field (FEF). This is located towards the rear of Brodmann Area 8 and in the arcuate sulcus (Figs 11.1, 11.2, and 11.3b). It receives input from several other cortical regions. These include the parietal cortex, particularly the lateral intraparietal area (LIP) in the postero-ventral bank of the intraparietal sulcus, the visual areas MT (middle temporal) and MST (middle superior temporal), which are concerned particularly with directional motion, and the prefrontal cortex. A second frontal eye movement region, the supplementary eye field (SEF), is located in the rostral region of Area 6, in the dorsal bank of the cingulate sulcus (longitudinal fissure). Like the FEF, stimulation of the SEF will cause saccadic eye movements, although with longer latency than the FEF.

The FEF's principal sub-cortical outputs are to the superior colliculus and directly to the oculomotor-related nuclei of the brain stem. The SC of the midbrain acts as a major organizing centre for determining the magnitude and direction of saccadic eye movements and also for orienting movements of the head (Guitton, 1991). The SC has a projection back up to the FEF via the mediodorsal thalamus, and it is also reciprocally connected to the LIP region of the parietal cortex (Sommer and Wurtz, 2003). Saccadic eye movements are not prevented by ablation of either the frontal eye fields or the superior colliculus, but they are abolished by removal of both. The exact form of the neural signals to the eye muscles that produce saccades and smooth eye movements result from the interactions of the premotor cells of the paramedian pontine reticular formation (PPRF) and the motor neurons of the oculomotor nuclei themselves (see Guitton, 1991).

Executive control: prefrontal cortex

The prefrontal lobes, the most anterior regions of the cortex, are generally regarded as the highest level of the motor hierarchy, where the complex plans for goal directed action are organized (Passingham, 1993). They are conventionally divided into dorsal and ventral areas.

The dorsal prefrontal cortex, mainly Areas 9 and 46 in the sulcus principalis in macaques (Fig. 11.2), is particularly concerned with visual behaviour. It is reciprocally connected to the frontal eye fields in Area 8 and to the dorsal premotor cortex (F6 and F7, Fig. 11.2). It is also reciprocally connected to the inferior parietal lobule, particularly Area 7a that processes information about gaze direction and the spatial location of objects (Petrides and Pandya, 2002). It has a heavy projection to the superior colliculus. There is also a projection from the superior temporal sulcus in the temporal lobe, which itself has reciprocal connections with the inferior parietal cortex. Thus the dorsal prefrontal cortex is connected to both the dorsal and ventral information streams.

Lesion studies in monkeys implicate the dorsal prefrontal cortex in spatial working memory: the ability to keep in mind the locations of objects, especially during delayed response tasks (Passingham, 1993). This fits with the finding that there are neurons in the dorsal prefrontal cortex that have 'memory fields'; these are neurons that fire continuously when an object is removed from a particular location and remain active for some seconds until the object returns and a response is made (Goldman-Rakic, 1995). Fuster (1995, 2002) extended this idea to the temporal organization of behaviour more generally, pointing out that patients with large dorsal prefrontal injuries are unable to make elaborate plans for prospective action. He commented that 'the inability to plan is probably the most characteristic and least disputed of all prefrontal dysfunctions.' It is relevant that in humans the dorsal prefrontal cortex is activated in PET scans when subjects generate a series of actions at will.

A separation of function within the prefrontal cortex has been suggested by Haynes and his colleagues (Haynes et al., 2007) to differentiate the maintenance of goals during the execution of tasks from goal maintenance during preparation to execute a task. Medial and lateral areas of the prefrontal cortex were active during a delay period before task execution, in which subjects were free to pick one of two alternative ways in which to complete the task. When executing the task after the delay, prefrontal activity was more posterior.

The principal connections of the ventral prefrontal cortex (Areas 11–14) are from the temporal lobe and the amygdala. Perhaps, in view of the multimodal temporal lobe input, removal of Area 12 in a monkey causes impairment in learning what response to make, independent of the sensory modality of the cue. The connections of the ventral prefrontal cortex and the amygdala are probably concerned with reward, in the general sense of the process by which responses are selected on the basis of their success (Passingham, 1993). In the eye movement system the reward system associated with gaze strategies appears to be rather different, involving the caudate nucleus of the basal ganglia in a loop with cortical saccade-targeting areas (frontal eye fields, dorsal prefontal and intraparietal) and the superior colliculus (Hayhoe and Ballard, 2005; Kawagoe et al., 1998).

Conflict monitoring: the anterior cingulate cortex

Situated on the inner surface of the cortex between the corpus callosum and the cingulate sulcus is the cingulate cortex. The anterior part of the cingulate cortex (ACC, Brodmann's Area 24) has been implicated in conflict monitoring during complex tasks. With connections to the frontal eye fields, prefrontal cortex and parietal cortex (Posner and DiGirolamo, 1998), the anterior cingulate cortex is ideally placed for monitoring both the incoming visual information and the top-down executive control of ongoing visual behaviour.

Using electroencephalographic (EEG) recordings, error-related negativity (ERN) has been observed at the time of committing an error across a wide range of tasks (e.g. Falkenstein et al., 1995). The source of this ERN has been localized to the ACC (Dehaene et al., 1994), and it has this been suggested that the ACC plays a key role in error detection (Carter et al., 1998). However, the role of the ACC does not seem to be confined to simply signalling the occurrence of errors. Imaging studies have shown elevated ACC activation when performing the incongruent version of the Stroop task, in which colours and words do not match (Stroop, 1935), compared with the congruent version, in which colours and words do match (Pardo et al., 1990). This suggests that the ACC may be involved in overriding prepotent responses to complete the current behavioural goal. When a number of responses are available and the subject must choose in an unspecified manner, ACC activity is again elevated (Petersen et al., 1988). Both the incongruent version of the Stroop task and the tasks in which a number of possible responses are available but selection is unspecified can be seen as situations in which conflict between possible responses is high. This argument has been used to suggest that the ACC is involved in monitoring conflict during ongoing tasks, signalling to other systems, such as the dorso-lateral prefrontal cortex (DLPFC), when conflict and the potential for errors are high (Botvinik et al., 2001).

Behavioural and neural hierarchies

Roles of eye movement and limb motor systems

The picture that emerges from behavioural studies, particularly of complex routines like food preparation (Chapter 5), is that they consist of sequences of actions each of which is centred around an object or objects that require actions to be performed on them (object-related actions, Figs 5.3 and 5.4). Based on the deficits in action planning that result from frontal lobe injuries, it can reasonably be assumed that the 'script' for these actions originates in the dorso-lateral prefrontal cortex. (How the scripts got there in the first place is another matter.) The execution of these actions involves two separate but co-operating systems, roughly speaking the eye movement system and the motor system whose anatomies have been outlined above. Their roles are not the same. The eye movement system has two main functions: to locate appropriate objects in the immediate surroundings and pass their co-ordinates to the motor system, and to put the eyes in a position to provide the visual feedback required for the execution and termination of each action in the sequence. The main input for this is vision itself, supplemented by short- and long-term memory for the appearance and possible locations of objects. The motor system, on the other hand, formulates and executes the sequence of individual muscle movements required to by overall action, using visual, haptic, and proprioceptive information. The cortical outputs of these two systems are not in doubt: for the eye movement system it is the frontal eye fields, and for the limb motor system it is the premotor and motor complexes (Areas 6 and 4, Fig. 11.2a). It has to be said, however, that the way the two systems interact at different levels is less well understood.

A top-down hierarchy in the frontal lobes

One proposed control scheme is a straightforward descending hierarchy, with the prefrontal cortex determining the temporal sequence of actions to perform, the more caudal prefrontal regions working out which particular actions to perform depending on the immediate circumstances, and the premotor and motor regions formulating the execution of the individual acts. There is some evidence for this.

Using fMRI imaging in humans Koechlin et al. (2003) found a modular hierarchical organization in the lateral prefrontal cortex (LPFC). Their tasks were inevitably restricted to arrays of visual stimuli with button pressing as the output, but they demonstrated a convincing separation of activated regions according to three levels of control, which they refer to as episodic, contextual, and sensory control. At the top of the hierarchy the most anterior (rostral) part of the LPFC subserves episodic control, that is the selection of particular task schemas according to current internal goals, taking account of events that have occurred previously. The next level, located in more posterior (caudal) parts of the LPFC, involves contextual control: the selection of which particular stimulus–response combinations to activate depending on the visually perceived circumstances. The third level is the premotor level, involving the selection of particular motor acts with their associated sensory control machinery. Although this scheme maps quite nicely onto the 'script, object-related action, motor act' scheme we have derived from behavioural observations, it does not clarify the distinct roles of the eye movement and limb motor systems. Nor is it clear how the parietal cortex fits in, even though it is known to have a major role in the co-ordination of reaching and grasping, which are themselves very important components of much manipulative action. Koechlin et al. noted that the parietal cortex was active during activation of all three hierarchical levels of the frontal lobe hierarchy, but particularly during episodic (rostral LPFC) activation.

The role of the parietal cortex

Single unit recordings from monkeys and functional imaging in man have demonstrated that the parietal cortex, and in particular the interior of the intraparietal sulcus and the region around it, contain a mosaic of regions whose functions are different but related (Culham and Valyear, 2006). These regions are illustrated in Fig. 11.2. Of particular interest are areas MIP (medial intraparietal) and AIP (anterior intraparietal) that are active during reaching and grasping, respectively, and LIP that is active in saccadic eye movement generation. The equivalent area to LIP in humans (the parietal eye field) is somewhat medial to the sulcus, on the superior parietal lobule. It contains a topographic map representing memory-driven saccade direction and the direction of a pointing movement. It thus seems that all the machinery for organizing both the eye-related ('directing' fixations) and limb motor actions involved in such tasks as picking up an object is present in the parietal cortex. As noted earlier, there is no direct motor output from these parietal areas, but they project to the frontal eye fields and to the premotor and motor cortex, and hence to the oculomotor and limb motor systems. What is less clear is how the parietal reach-and-grasp system is brought into play by the action plans formulated, presumably, in the prefrontal cortex. Are they activated by direct connections, or indirectly via the premotor cortex, by subcortical pathways as suggested by Glickstein (2000), or by a combination of all three? The high level of involvement of the parietal areas – parts of the supposedly sensory rear half of the cortex – in the organization of motor actions does not quite fit in with a scheme in which task delegation proceeds in an orderly way from the front of the cortex rearwards. We shall return to this topic later when discussing the mirror neuron system.

Co-ordinate systems for vision and action

An important difference between the roles of the parietal and premotor areas involved in reaching and manipulation concerns the co-ordinate systems involved. For the eye the position of an object is specified relative to the fovea, in eye-centred co-ordinates. However, the muscles involved in manipulation are in the arms, and their activation requires a representation of the object's location in limb-centred co-ordinates. Target, eye, head, body, and limbs are hardly ever exactly aligned, which means that to get from an eye-centred to a limb-centred representation of target position requires that target-on-retina, eye-in-head, head-on-trunk, and limb-on-trunk signals must be combined (see Fig. 10.5a). The process is simplified somewhat by the fact that objects are nearly always fixated before being acted upon, which largely removes the target-on-retina step, but it still means that information about the other three stages is required for the visual guidance of limb action. Evidence from studies on macaques (reviewed by Batista and Newcome, 2000) indicates that the visual receptive fields of many premotor neurons shift to regions of space that are linked to arm position, independent of eye direction, implying that their input is fully transformed from eye-centred to arm-centred co-ordinates. Different regions of the parietal cortex contain separate functional areas with representations of space linked to different types of action (Colby and Goldberg, 1999; Scherberger and Andersen, 2003). It seems likely that in the formulation of an action it is these parietal areas that provide the required transformations, from eye-centred inputs to limb-centred motor outputs.

Egocentric and allocentric maps

To make matters more complicated, if the target is not initially visible it may be necessary to make a whole-body turn, using a memory of where the object is expected to be. The size of the turn needed requires an estimate of where the object is relative to the trunk, which in turn depends on where both subject and object are relative to each other (see Fig. 10.5b). The subject may know where the object is in the room, and his own position, in room-centred (allocentric) co-ordinates, that is to say in co-ordinates that are independent of viewpoint. To perform the appropriate turn, these have to be translated into body-centred (egocentric) co-ordinates. Only after this has been done can vision be used – in conjunction with the various transformations discussed in the last paragraph – to guide the hand to the object. As we have seen from Chapter 5, all this can be done in a single efficient and flexible operation.

There has been general agreement, since the pioneering work of O'Keefe and Nadel (1978), that the hippocampus, a curved sheet of cortex folded into the medial surface of the temporal lobe, is essential for the formation of allocentric maps of the surroundings. The rat hippocampus contains 'place cells' that fire when the animal is in a particular place in the local environment. The same place cells participate in the representation of multiple environments but with different spatial relations between the firing fields of adjacent cells in each setting. Spatially tuned cells are also found in the adjacent entorhinal cortex, but here each cell has multiple firing fields in the same environment, these fields forming a periodic triangular grid pattern (Moser et al., 2008). Moser et al. suggested that grid cell fields are generated by path integration (dead reckoning from direction and distance travelled) as the animal moves through the environment and that their activity may serve in the generation of hippocampal place fields. They conclude that between them the place and grid cells form the basis for the quantitative representation of both places and routes.

The extent to which long-term topographic information is stored in the hippocampus in humans is less certain because hippocampal lesions do not destroy all knowledge of familiar environments (Moscovitch et al., 2005). It is also not clear whether short-term allocentric memories involved in relocating objects recently seen (seconds to minutes ago) involve the hippocampus, nor is it obvious how hippocampal place information becomes available to the motor system when it is required (review by Burgess, 2006). In humans two cortical areas involved in spatial navigation have been identified from neuroimaging studies (Epstein, 2008). These are the parahippocampal place area (PPA) and the retrosplenial complex (RSC). The PPA responds strongly to complex visual scenes such as cityscapes but not particularly well to single objects. The RSC responds to familiar environments and during mental imagination of navigation through familiar environments. Patients with damage to either the PPA or the RSC have difficulties with wayfaring, but in different ways. RSC patients can identify scenes, which PPA damaged patients have difficulty with, but cannot use them for navigational purposes. Epstein suggested that the PPA is involved in the establishment of representations of local scenes that allow the appropriate 'map' to be selected in the hippocampus, whereas the RSC might specify directions to navigational goals. The RSC has strong connections with the parietal cortex, and it is a possible site of allocentric-to-egocentric translations: for example, 'you are here' to 'your goal is on the left', as in Fig. 10.5b.

The mirror neuron system

Another system that does not fit a simple rearward hierarchical scheme is the mirror neuron system. In the anterior part of the ventral premotor cortex (Area F5 of Matelli et al, 1991, see Fig. 11.2) Gallese et al. (1996) described neurons that discharge both when the monkey makes a particular action and when it observes another monkey, or human, making a similar action. The most effective actions, in terms of discharge frequency, involve grasping, holding, manipulating, and placing. The neurons do not respond just to the presence of graspable objects or to seeing an action mimed. It is the interaction between the action of the agent (self or other) and the object that is important in causing the neurons to discharge. A second population of neurons with similar properties is found in region PF of the rostral region of the inferior parietal lobule (Fig. 11.2), to which Area F5 is connected. Similar neurons, though without motor properties, are also seen in the temporal lobe within the superior temporal sulcus (Perrett et al., 1989).

The presence of these mirror neurons, which represent particular actions whether these are made or observed, raises interesting questions as to their function. There is evidence that in humans they are involved in action imitation but, as Rizzolatti and Craighero (2004) pointed out, macaques do not imitate, so this could not have been their original function. They suggested instead that what is represented is the intention, or meaning, of the action. Key evidence for this comes from the observation that if a monkey sees a particular action performed, and certain mirror neurons fire, and then when the same action is repeated, but with the final stage of contact with the target object obscured, the same neurons still fire. It is as though there were enough clues for the neurons to understand the nature of the action itself, even without its conclusion. Further evidence comes from the finding that when the same sub-actions form part of sequences that have different overall aims, there is a different pattern of firing in the mirror neurons in the inferior parietal lobule. For example, identical reach-and-grasp movements evoke different firing patterns when the goal is to put food in the mouth rather than to put it in a container (Fogassi et al., 2005). It appears that activation of the mirror neurons depends not only on the action but on the context of the action.

Action in context is perhaps what one might expect for neurons at the 'contextual' level of the Koechlin et al. (2003) hierarchical scheme discussed above. What is unexpected is that the mirror neurons respond to the corresponding actions of others. The implication is that these components of the motor system not only translate intentions into motor actions but also maintain internal representations of actions and, in the context of human imitation, actually create them. This is a function which one might formerly have considered to be the kind of high-order cognitive activity confined to the prefrontal regions. However, it now seems clear that 'understanding' – in this case action understanding – is a much more distributed cortical function. Many claims have been made for the mirror neuron system, for example, that failures of the system are involved in autism (Ramachandran and Oberman, 2006), and that, via gesture imitation, it forms a basis for language evolution (Rizzolatti and Arbib, 1998). From the more limited perspective of this book, however, it seems that the mirror neuron system shows that for the component actions of a complex routine much of the planning of the action itself, including its context and its visual consequences, is dealt with at the level of the premotor and parietal cortices, with the role of the prefrontal cortex perhaps limited to supplying the overall action script.

Co-ordinating vision and action

How do the different prefrontal, premotor, and parietal regions co-operate in the generation of a component action? A plausible scheme, embodying much of the foregoing discussion, is given by Rizzolatti and Luppino (2001). The relevant pathways are shown in Fig. 11.4. In their scheme Area F5 of the premotor cortex (which contains the mirror neurons) supplies 'motor prototypes' for various reaching, grasping, placing, and manipulative actions. Which particular action is to be activated is determined by input from parietal area AIP, which has 3D representations of the objects to be dealt with and information about their meaning via connections from the temporal lobe. It also receives direct input from the DLPFC, presumably about which actions are to be performed. The AIP can thus be considered to provide 'affordances' (the action possibilities of objects in the environment). When to make a particular move in a sequence of actions is determined by signals from the rostro-medial premotor Area F6, which communicates with F5 and in turn receives input from the DLPFC. The premotor neurons of F5 then set the action in motion via the primary motor cortex (F1). It seems that this scheme applies not only to reaching and grasping actions in monkeys, but to tool use in humans, where lesion and brain activation studies implicate very similar frontal and parietal areas in the left hemisphere (Johnson-Frey, 2004).

In terms of the Supervisory Attention System model of Norman and Shallice (1986) it seems that much of the lower-level, routine operations in the performance of a task (selecting schemata, contention scheduling; see Fig. 10.8) are dealt with by the interactions of the parietal and premotor neuron populations, with the DLPFC acting as the planner and initiator of sequences of actions, and intervening when problems arise in their execution (see Stuss et al., 1995). For the DLPFC to intervene when problems arise, an error monitoring system is required to alert the DLPFC of potential problems. Here the ACC seems to be a good candidate, and it has been suggested that there is a conflict monitoring circuit involving both the ACC and DLPFC (Miller and Cohen, 2001, see *conflict monitoring* above).

A convenient task in which to study the ongoing control of visual behaviour and in which prepotent responses must be inhibited to meet the task demands is the antisaccade task (Hallett, 1978). In this task, when a peripheral target appears, the prepotent response to initiate a saccade towards it must be suppressed and instead the subject is required to make a saccade in the opposite direction to an equidistant location in the

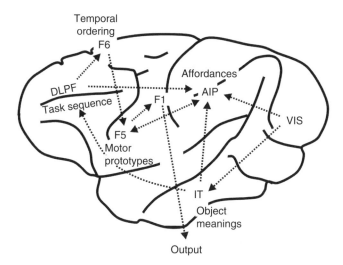

Fig. 11.4 Scheme of interactions involved in the selection and performance of an action in a sequence, based on Rizzolatti and Luppino, 2001. See text for explanation. AIP, anterior intraparietal area; DLPF, dorso-lateral prefrontal cortex; F1, primary motor cortex; F5 and F6, ventral and dorsal premotor areas; IT, inferotemporal lobe; VIS, occipital visual areas. See also Fig.11.2b.

opposite hemifield. Interestingly, when people make erroneous saccades to the peripheral target, sometimes they are aware that they have done this but other times they are not (Mokler and Fischer, 1999). Furthermore, activity in the conflict monitoring pathways is different in these two types of error: when people are unaware of making an error, there is an error-related negativity after the incorrect response. However, when people are aware of making the error the error-related negativity is followed by an error-related positivity (Nieuwenhuis et al., 2001). This suggests that there may be two separable types of error monitoring process: one for errors that we realize we are making and one for errors that we are unaware of.

Eye movements and attention

Covert and overt attention

As William James pointed out in 1890, we can with effort direct our attention to parts of the visual field that we are not fixating at the time (covert attention), but it is more usual for a shift in attention to be accompanied by an eye movement (overt attention, see Chapter 3). Attentional shifts, it seems, are closely related to the preparation of eye movements (the 'premotor' theory of attention; Rizzolatti et al., 1987). Neurophysiological evidence for this view also comes from single unit studies from areas of the macaque cortex known to be associated with saccadic eye movement initiation – the frontal and supplementary eye fields and area LIP of the posterior parietal cortex. These all contain cells that are active just before saccades are made, and whose sensitivity to visual stimuli depends on whether they lie in parts of the visual field that are relevant to the particular task to which the monkey has been trained to respond, that is, to locations where attention would be directed (e.g. Colby et al., 1996).

In an important study Corbetta et al. (1998) used fMRI scans of humans to determine whether structures involved in the generation of saccades were also active when attention was directed to the same points but without an eye movement (i.e. covert rather than overt attention). They found extensive regions of functional overlap in the posterior parts of the frontal cortex, identified as corresponding to the frontal and supplementary eye fields of macaques and also in three areas of the parietal cortex. One or more of these may correspond to the macaque LIP, which is where Colby et al. (1996) conducted their study. In addition, there was a temporal lobe region, in the superior temporal sulcus, tentatively identified with the superior temporal polysensory area in the macaque, a region also associated with attention and eye movements. Thus the data from human scans and the single electrode studies from macaques seem to match up well: the network of cortical regions associated with eye movements and attention is substantially the same in the two species. In the Corbetta et al. study there were small regions that responded only to eye movements or only to shifting covert attention, but the regions of overlap were much greater. Their minimum estimates for overlap were between 60% and 80% depending on the region, and they concluded, 'These functional anatomical data indicate that attention and eye movement processes are not only functionally related, as suggested by psychological studies, but also share functional anatomical areas in the human brain (p. 770).'

Receptive fields that shift with saccades

In the debate about why it is that the world appears to stay still when we make a saccadic eye movement (see Chapter 10), one suggestion of long standing has been that this could be achieved by a shifting the internal representation of the scene in the cortex to compensate for the movement of the image in the eye. Effectively, this means shifting the receptive fields of the cortical neurons by an amount equal and opposite to the saccadic image shift and coincident with it in time. There is good evidence that something like this does occur in the parietal cortex. Duhamel et al. (1992) found that cells in parietal area LIP update, or 'remap', the locations of stimuli when their eyes move. When a significant target appears, attracting attention and initiating a saccade, the receptive fields of the whole array of LIP neurons shift in such a way that the new target becomes the centre of the array about 80 ms before the saccade begins. This anticipatory shift only occurs if a saccade is actually made, which implies that the signal that produces the shift is a copy of the command to make the saccade (corollary discharge). The effect of the shift is to set up the LIP array so that when the saccade does occur the receptive fields are in the appropriate positions to view the newly relocated image. The remapped image is still centred on the fixation point, so it is not a transformation to a world-centred image. However, anticipation of the saccadic image shift may be part of the reason why saccades cause so little disruption to vision.

Cells with shifting receptive fields are also found in the FEFs, to which the LIP is reciprocally connected. This raises the question of where the corollary discharge is injected into the system. Sommer and Wurtz (2008) presented strong evidence for such a pathway from the superior colliculus, which organizes saccade production, to the frontal eye fields via the medial dorsal nucleus of the thalamus. Whether there is a separate pathway to the LIP, or the LIP cells are simply following the changes in the FEF cells, is not yet clear.

The route of descending attention

In our earlier discussions of how object-related actions are initiated by attentional commands from the schema system, we had assumed that the gaze, visual, and motor systems were activated more or less independently (Figs 1.1 and 5.10). There is, however, some evidence that this may not be the way descending attention is disseminated. Armstrong et al. (2006) found that microstimulation of cells in the frontal eye fields produced changes in the receptive fields of neurons in Area V4, a visual area with no direct motor connections. These responses were similar to the effects of voluntary attention. Armstrong et al. suggested that the signals that are involved in saccade preparation in the FEFs are being used to covertly select among the multiple stimuli appearing within the receptive fields of neurons in regions of the visual cortex. This could imply that in the formulation of visually controlled actions the preparation of gaze changes (where to look) and the preparation of the visual system (what to look for) are serial rather than parallel process, with the attentional instructions to the visual system routed through the gaze change system of the FEFs.

The site at which the targets of saccades are decided

A saccade can only be made to one location at a time, so somewhere in the brain there must be a spatially mapped site where the battle for the next saccade target is fought out. In Chapter 3 we discussed the factors that might influence selecting where we fixate in natural scenes. A popular contender until recent years was the idea of a low-level salience map that signals visual conspicuity across the visual field. This notion has the added appeal that it describes a topological activity map signalling the decision about where to fixate next. This has obvious neural analogies, and it is not surprising that a number of studies have been aimed at trying to uncover evidence for a neural implementation of this salience map. From these studies, a wide range of potential sites for the neural representations of salience has been suggested. The locations so far implicated include the superior colliculus (McPeek and Keller, 2002), pulvinar (Robinson and Petersen, 1992), V1 (Li, 2002), V4 (Mazer and Gallant, 2003), LIP (Gottlieb et al., 1998), and the frontal eye field (Thompson and Bichot, 2005).

What is interesting is that although the aim was to find a site where the purely bottom-up salience map might be implemented, most of the potential sites identified receive both ascending and descending connections and therefore show modulation by top-down processes. This means that any neural implementation of a map signalling where to fixate in a scene is likely to involve a combination of bottom-up visual input and descending top-down modulation. A similar observation was made by Fecteau and Munoz (2006), who suggested that a more appropriate conceptualization of the neural implementation of a mapping for saccade target selection is that of a 'priority map' receiving both bottom-up and top-down inputs. The inability to find strong evidence for neural implementation of a purely bottom-up saccade-targeting map adds further weight to our arguments in Chapter 3 that low-level models are an entirely inadequate means of describing human eye movement behaviour.

Summary

1. Visual processing begins in the occipital lobe, from which there are two distinct but interacting pathways. Perceptual processes such as object recognition are more strongly associated with the ventral pathway to the temporal lobe; the dorsal pathway to the parietal lobe is implicated in action and spatial processing.

2. Control of gaze and motor output involves a hierarchy of cortical and sub-cortical structures. In gaze control key structures are the frontal eye fields and the superior colliculus; in motor control important structures are the premotor and motor cortical areas, the basal ganglia, and the cerebellum.

3. Converging evidence suggests that the prefrontal cortex plays a key role in goal maintenance during complex behavioural sequences. Details of the execution of the component action are resolved by interactions between parietal and premotor areas. The anterior cingulate cortex monitors potential errors in action production.

4. Vision and gaze selection involve both ascending pathways from the occipital lobe and descending pathways from frontal regions, implying top-down attentional modulation of early visual processing.

Chapter 12

Attention, memory, and learning

We have argued in this book that the chief role of the brain is as the initiator and co-ordinator of purposeful action rather than just as the mediator of perception. In Chapter 1 we proposed that such action involves four major components: (1) the schema system that defines the tasks to be undertaken, (2) the gaze system that locates the objects to be dealt with, (3) the motor system that performs the required action, and (4) the visual system that has the dual role of supplying information to the gaze system and supervising the action of the motor system. The interactions between the systems were summarized in Fig. 1.1 (reproduced here as Fig. 12.1), and some of the variants of the scheme were presented in Fig. 4.8. In this final chapter we return to some of the issues raised in Chapter 1 that have not been dealt with in other chapters. In particular we will examine first the role of attention, which we supposed in Fig. 1.1 to be the means by which instructions from the schema system were conveyed to the three executive system; second, the various kinds of memory involved in the visual control of actions; and finally various ideas concerned with the way the motor system manages to operate in real time, in spite of the delays inherent in neural machinery. We conclude with a summary discussion about what we do not yet know, and where future studies might be of most value.

Top-down control: schemas and attention

Attention for action

We normally perform one action at a time. Even when 'multitasking' we alternate between actions rather than attempt to perform more than one simultaneously. At first sight the reason seems obvious: we only have one pair of hands. However, as Fig. 12.1 indicates there is more to it than that. The studies of tea and sandwich making in Chapter 5 showed that particular actions involve finding the object or objects that are to be acted upon, priming the visual system to attend to those features of the action that require visual control, and performing the action itself. These three functions – gaze control, visual control, and action – are typically activated within about a second of each other, and they are specific for a given action. These observations force one to assume that for each action there is a control programme that coordinates the three systems and specifies their duties and that for each action there is a separate programme.

In the Supervisory Attention System of Norman and Shallice (1986) the controller and generator of each action is a *schema*: an instruction set specific to that action. When activated by processes in the frontal cortex that remain poorly understood, the

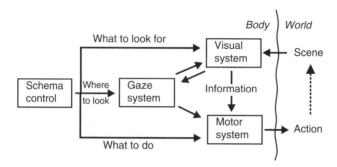

Fig 12.1 General scheme of the elements involved in a visually controlled action.

schema instructs the gaze, motor, and visual systems to perform the action. The channel through which these instructions are conveyed is likely to be the attention system. Although attention is often thought of as applying to the selection of features for object identification (perceptual selection), many authors have also emphasized its role in motor behaviour (reviewed by Neumann, 1996). Attention shifts and gaze shifts have long been associated with each other. This connection is made explicit in the premotor theory of attention, in which (covert) shifts of attention lead directly to (overt) eye movements (see Chapter 11). The idea that attention is involved with the control of action also has a long tradition. According to Neumann, this goes back to Ribot (1906), for whom attention was necessary to select the impressions from the environment that are required to control action. A similar position was taken by Allport (1989): 'Consequently some selective process is necessary to map just those aspects of the visual array, specific to the target object, selectively onto the appropriate control parameters of the action' (p. 648). Ribot also distinguished between a primitive, reflexive form of attention and voluntary attention in adult humans, which he localized in the prefrontal cortex (Neumann, 1996, p. 438). This distinction is not unlike that between the 'contention scheduling' system for handling schemas in routine actions and the 'supervisory attention system' for novel or non-routine actions, proposed in the Norman and Shallice model (see Chapter 10, and particularly Fig. 10.8). Attention has not generally been considered as the command system used to call for specific actions, but because actions and the systems that monitor them are inextricably linked, it seems logical that they should be activated by the same mechanism.

Routes of attention

So far the routes by which top-down attention reaches the gaze, visual, and motor systems are not understood in detail. There is a general consensus that the higher components of the schema system, responsible for setting the goals of action, are associated with activity in the dorsal prefrontal cortex, but this region also receives a heavy input from the parietal cortex and frontal eye fields, and activity in advance of action has been recorded in these and other areas of the cortical motor system (Passingham et al., 2005). This makes it difficult to identify the precise area where the descending signals involved in schema activation originate.

Whatever its origins, the effects of attention – conventionally, the enhancement of the representation of behaviourally relevant parts of the visual input at the expense of others – can be recorded in cells in various parts of the visual pathway. These attentional effects are often considered to be of two kinds: space-based attention, where enhancement occurs in a specific region of the image and feature-based attention in which certain attributes of the stimulus (contrast, colour, orientation, direction) are emphasized without regard to location. As an example of space-based attention, cells in V4 of monkeys can have their responses enhanced to a previously presented target in one part of their receptive field, whereas responses to a distractor in the same receptive field were reduced, as though the receptive fields had shrunk around the target (Moran and Desimone, 1985). This, incidentally, indicates that the spatial attentional bias system, wherever it originates, has better resolution than the V4 cells themselves. Feature-based attention, on the other hand, appears to operate across the whole visual field. Haenny et al. (1988) found that in monkeys primed to recognize a grating with a particular orientation more than half the recorded neurons in V4 had orientation biases that reflected the orientation that the animal was seeking. Other examples of space-based and feature-based attention are given in reviews by Desimone and Duncan (1995), Reynolds and Chelazzi (2004), and Maunsel and Treue (2006). Maunsell and Treue suggested that these two apparently different types of attentional bias may be two sides of the same coin: 'The total effect will be a population response that is no longer homogeneous, but has its highest activity in the group of neurons preferring the attended location and feature'.

When the gaze system targets an object that is visible within the field of view some process of identification, however minimal, is required to determine which of the possible candidate objects is the appropriate one. One mechanism for doing this would be for the frontal eye fields, which will initiate the gaze movement, to highlight selected regions of the retinotopic mappings in the visual regions of the cortex to determine whether appropriate features are present. There is now a body of evidence that something like this does take place.

Descending attentional selection seems to operate at many levels in the cortex, even at the level of the visual input (V1). Roelfsema et al. (1998) trained macaque monkeys to distinguish between two curves on a computer screen, one (the target curve) that passed through the initial fixation point and a second similar curve (the distractor) that did not. Both curves ended in circles. The task was to move gaze, after a delay, to a circle at the end of the target curve. They recorded from a set of 40 to 50 multiunit electrodes chronically implanted in V1. When the curves appeared, with gaze still at the fixation point, they found that electrodes responded if the receptive fields of cells near their tips contained segments of either curve. The latency of this initial response was 35 ms. However, after a further 200 ms there was an enhancement of the response but only for those electrodes whose fields lay along the target curve. This enhancement was present even if the two curves crossed, suggesting that the mechanism of selection was applied to the curve *as an object*, identified by grouping criteria such as collinearity and connectedness, rather than simple proximity. This experiment indicates that, after the initial response to the appearance of the curves, information travels forward and is compared with learned criteria. Descending information then highlights the selected curve in V1, in preparation for an eye movement to the circle at its tip.

In a later report from the same laboratory Ekstrom et al. (2008) showed that signals from the frontal eye fields enhanced responses in early visual areas (V1, V2, V3, and V4), but only if a visual stimulus were present in the congruent regions of the visual field. They used a combination of microstimulation of the frontal eye fields with fMRI scans of the whole brain. Stimulation caused enhanced activity in many of the extrastriate visual areas (MT and MST, parietal area LIP, and temporal areas TEO and STP), whether or not a visual stimulus was present. However, enhancement in the early visual areas only occurred if a visual stimulus were present. The strength of the enhancement depended on the contrast of the stimulus pattern.

Moore and Armstrong (2003) showed that microstimulation in the FEF, at an intensity that was too weak to evoke a saccade, nevertheless caused response enhancement of cells in visuotopically appropriate regions of area V4. This enhancement was of a kind consistent with the results of parallel behavioural experiments. Armstrong et al. (2006) showed that this enhancement was confined to cells whose receptive fields were aligned with the end points of saccades that would be produced from the regions of FEF stimulation. They suggested that the signals that are involved in saccade preparation in the FEFs may be being used to covertly select among the multiple stimuli appearing within the receptive fields of neurons in regions of the visual cortex.

This series of studies demonstrates that descending attentional feedback from frontal regions of the brain influences visual cortical regions at a number of levels, enhancing responses from selected areas of the visual field and reducing the responses from others. In the Roelfsema et al. (1998) study there is evidence that the enhancement is linked to a particular object. These studies mostly point to a process that precedes an eye movement to a selected object, and so are linked to gaze control. What is not clear is the location of the decision: 'Is this the correct to object to fixate?' This requires a comparison between what is visible on the retina and an internal representation of the required object, and the site of this comparison is far from clear.

Once an appropriate object has been targeted, and its image is on or near the fovea, the nature of attention changes. The task now is for the visual system to supervise guiding the limbs and managing the action. In the cortex the principal interface between the visual and motor systems is posterior parietal cortex, and for grasping movements the area AIP in particular. This area is reciprocally connected to premotor area F5 where specific movement patterns are generated (see Figs 11.2 and 11.4). Some neurons in AIP respond when a monkey observes one particular object and also when the same object is grasped (Brochier and Umiltà, 2007). This combination of visual and motor properties suggests that these neurons code for the features of visual objects that are required to make the appropriate hand configuration for grasping. Reversible inactivation of AIP results in a loss of the match between object shape and appropriate pre-shaping of the hand. Area AIP and other areas in the inferior parietal lobule also have strong reciprocal connections with certain inferotemporal areas in the 'ventral stream', responsible for object recognition (Fogassi and Lupino, 2005). It thus seems that AIP neurons have access to object identity as well as shape. Other areas of the inferior parietal lobule are active during a variety of arm, hand, face, and eye movements. Some neurons discharge selectively depending on the final goal of the action sequence of which the grasping action forms a part, suggesting that their activity reflects, to some extent at least, the intention behind the grasp. However, the decision of what action to perform in a complex sequence of actions is presumably taken elsewhere, probably in the prefrontal cortex to which the parietal lobe is strongly reciprocally connected.

Attention and working memory

Working memory was originally conceived as a mechanism for explaining how comprehension emerges from written or spoken language (Baddeley and Hitch, 1974). It is conceived as a powerful process that holds a limited amount of information for periods of a few seconds. It can integrate current sensory information with information from short- and long-term memory stores, and after evaluation can use this information for planning and making decisions. Many of these features make working memory an attractive candidate mechanism for controlling actions that take place over a short timescale.

It is important to try to pin down the functions that a working memory-like system might fulfil, particularly in the context of the visual control of action. Baddeley (2007) suggested four component processes for the central executive of the working memory system: the capacity to focus attention, to divide attention, to switch attention, and to provide a link with long-term memory. In the scheme in Fig. 12.1 the capacity to switch attention is the function of the schema control system, which contains the job lists for different tasks, and the capacity to focus attention is the mechanism by which the schema system instructs the visual, gaze control, and motor systems. The schema system thus embodies two of the suggested tasks of the working memory executive.

It is not always easy to distinguish division of attention and switching of attention, and the distinction may simply be one of time scale. Our studies provide numerous examples of multitasking, where two or more tasks occur together and gaze alternates rapidly between the key parts of the scene. Pianists take their eyes from the music for a few hundred milliseconds to check the positioning of the fingers on the keyboard (even expert pianists do this while sight-reading). Remarkably, this usually has no disrupting effect on the passage of gaze across the music (Fig. 4.6), implying a very precise short-term ability to reinstate gaze position across saccades. In driving it is common to alternate gaze between the road, the traffic, pedestrians, and road signs. An example of this is seen in Fig. 7.10, where a driver is keeping an eye on a cyclist while steering round a bend and moving his eyes every half second. More complex examples of multiple monitoring are seen in urban driving (Fig. 7.15). In all these cases the shift in attention is overt – that is, the eyes move. In other situations, for example, driving on a winding road, two processes may be occurring together but only one is monitored directly by the fovea. The relative motion of both far and near parts of the road is involved in the control of steering, but foveal gaze is directed only to the more distant region. Arguably, the near road can be observed with very little recourse to overt attention, but it is being monitored nevertheless.

Whether these various tasks can be corralled into a single system called 'working memory' is debatable. There is a danger in putting too many functions into a single conceptual unit. As Baddeley put it (2007, p. 12):

> One problem in having an executive that comprises general processing capacity is that it is potentially able to explain any result. This excessive flexibility means that it is not empirically productive in generating experiments that tell us more about how the system works.
>
> (Baddeley, 2007, p. 12)

Rather than considering working memory to be a single entity, it might be better to think of the functions that have been attributed to it (such as the link to long-term memory) as distributed among the various sub-systems that require them.

Bottom-up attention

In a recent review of attentional mechanisms Knudsen (2007) restricted 'salience' (in its image-driven sense) to surprising events, rather than applying it generally to the sum of the outputs of retinal and cortical filters which, according to the scheme of Itti and Koch (2000), lead to a winner-takes-all targeting of particular features in the image (Fig. 3.6).

'Typically, salient stimuli occur infrequently in space and time, for example, a sudden sound, a flash of light, a red dot on a field of green dots'.(Knudsen, 2007, p. 64). Indeed, Itti and Baldi (2006) have argued a similar position to Knudsen and constructed a computational account of surprise based on the same features as implemented in Itti's original salience map model. This account is certainly a step towards a computational account of the notion of surprise but is still in its early stages.

In Chapter 3 we gave many reasons for rejecting the idea that salience, in the sense that some features of the image are more eye-catching than others, had any real relevance to the deployment of attention during purposeful action. The overriding reason for this view is that target selection by such a mechanism would simply get in the way of whatever we are trying to do. However, there are stimuli that are so strong that they distract us from the task in hand. This fits with our common experience that attention to a task is sometimes usurped by extraneous stimuli, for example, by someone coming into the room, and for a while a new behaviour takes over from what we were doing before. However, like Knudsen, we would classify these as rare and intrusive events, rather than the normal way that our visual system deals with the surrounding world. We also feel that the notion of surprise may not be as 'primitive' or bottom-up as implied by recent authors. An important consideration in whether an event 'intrudes' is the context of our current behaviour. If surprise is purely a bottom-up process then an event should be equally distracting independent of what the observer is doing. However, this seems anecdotally unlikely. Consider a car suddenly pulling out from a line of queued vehicles and driving on the wrong side of the road. This event is certainly surprising, yet is likely to show far more 'intrusion' for a pedestrian considering crossing the road, than one who is not. It therefore seems hard to construct a notion of surprise that is divorced from high-level task contexts.

The challenge for the future is to work out how the normal machinery of the striate and prestriate visual cortex, with its various abilities to analyse different attributes of the visual scene, is put to use during the identification of objects and the control of manipulation. There is strong evidence, some of it discussed above, that the early visual regions can be addressed, via attention, by higher regions. Perhaps the interesting question now is: having been addressed, what sort of information do the early cortical regions now send back, and to where?

The roles of memory in gaze control and interaction with objects

Visible and remembered locations

Objects that we need to retrieve in the course of our actions may be plainly visible, but many times they are not initially in our field of view. There were many examples of the latter in the tea-making study (Chapter 5), where finding an object required a large turn and sometimes a few steps before it could be brought into the field of view. The memory of an object's location may initially be in the form of an allocentric representation, a map of space that is independent of the subject's current orientation. But for the object to be retrieved this must be then be converted to muscular instructions in an egocentric framework. This conversion requires a working out, in allocentric space, of the direction of the object relative to the subject. In Chapters 10 and 11 there was some discussion of the possible sites of these representations and of their interconversion.

Even when an object is present in the visual periphery, it may not be possible to make out what it is, because the resolution is too low (see Fig. 2.1), in which case it may be more efficient to locate it from memory than to search for it visually. In a hand-targeting task, Brouwer and Knill (2007) found that both vision and position memory influenced the movement of the arm to objects in the visual periphery, but the relative weightings depended on the target's visibility. The arm had to move to allow the index finger to pick up and move two neighbouring virtual targets into a trash bin. As the first target was being transported, the position of the second was shifted slightly. Although the second target was visible, approximately 33° away from the current gaze direction, the initial direction of the arm movement when picking it up was affected by its remembered position. From the deviation of the trajectory it was possible to work out the relative weights attributable to memory and vision. Brouwer and Knill found that for high contrast targets these were 0.33 for memory and 0.67 for vision, but for low-contrast targets the weight for memory became higher than for vision. For peripheral targets that have been viewed recently it appears that memory and direct vision are to a degree interchangeable.

Similar recourse to memory can be seen in saccade targeting. Aivar et al. (2005) demonstrated this using a 3-dimensional virtual model-building task similar to that devised by Ballard et al. (1992) illustrated in Fig. 4.9. This involved making a copy of a block model out of coloured blocks obtained from a source area on the right. The blocks were transported 20° to 30° from the source area to the copy. Occasionally, while gaze was on the copy, the blocks in the source area were rearranged by the experimenter. When subjects made a saccade back to the source area to pick up a block, on about 20% of occasions their gaze was directed back to the old location of the block they needed, and this was typically followed by a corrective saccade to the new location. The precision of these memory saccades was about 2°, or about 10% of the saccade distance, which is comparable with those made under visual control.

Just-in-time fixations and trans-saccadic memory

The position memory demonstrated by Aivar et al. (2005) contrasts with the conclusions from change blindness studies, which find that observers are very insensitive to changes during an eye movement, a brief mask or a film cut. The exception is when an object has already been attended to, in which case the change becomes visible. That was presumably true for the blocks in the experiment of Aivar et al. as their positions had been previously noted.

Memory use also contrasts with the 'just in time' strategy of Ballard et al. (1995) discussed in Chapter 4. Subjects looked at the model to determine the colour of a block, picked up a suitable block from the source area, and then returned to the model to determine its location for placement in the copy. Here it seems that the use of memory was limited to just one attribute of the block (colour or position), and only for the half second of the gaze movement from model to block. A similar lack of memory for object attributes was found by Droll et al. (2005) during a brick-sorting task (Fig. 5.9). Changes in brick size were only noticed when size was relevant to the action being performed at that moment, hence the maxim 'What you see is what you need'.

We have to conclude that although visual short-term memory is available during task execution, it is made use of sparingly. Droll and Hayhoe (2007) found that as memory load increased or the task became less predictable, subjects made more just-in-time fixations, and they could switch flexibly between making a fixation and retaining information in working memory. As Mary Hayhoe put it,

> In making tea or sandwiches, subjects invariably fixate the objects they are about to grasp. During this fixation the subject must compute information to control reach direction and plan the grasp, including the position, orientation, and size of the object, and perhaps information about surface friction and weight to plan the forces. Given the complexity of the information that might be required from the visual scene, it is not too surprising that much of it needs to be extracted on the fly, and it is clearly efficient to compute only task-relevant information.
>
> (Hayhoe, 2008, p.125)

The time scales of memory deployment

Memory processes have long been divided into short and long term, the former lasting for seconds to minutes and assumed to result from continually refreshed neural activity and the latter lasting up to a lifetime and brought about by consolidated molecular changes at the synaptic level. However, this classification, based on decay times, ignores the functional differences between different memory systems. There can be memories for objects as entities, for particular properties of objects such as size or colour or location, for the gist of whole scenes, for particular places and their geographical relationships, and episodic memories for particular events. There are also the sensory-motor memories that are drawn on in the performance of actions;

for example, the specific relationships between visual events and limb action when catching a ball or steering a car. Such memories also include affordances – the uses to which objects can be put. Some of these memory systems were mentioned in Chapter 10 and are discussed from many angles in Brockmole (2008). We will not attempt to explore the differences between these types of memory here but concentrate on the time scales over which they operate.

Many activities involve processes that operate continuously and have a throughput time of about a second. We have likened these to a production line (Fig. 4.8b), and they include reading aloud, typing, and sight-reading music (Figs 4.4–4.7), walking on broken ground (Fig. 6.1), and steering using the tangent point (Fig. 7.5). It is not entirely clear whether the whole of the 1 s delay is taken up with the machinery of translating input into output or whether the input is held in memory during this process. If memory is involved, its contents are dumped or overwritten continuously as more input arrives, and the question of whether the memory 'fades' does not arise. In tasks such as tea-making objects are fixated about 0.6 s before manipulation starts, and sub-tasks continue for about 0.6 s after gaze has moved on to the next object (Fig. 5.4). This implies that the visually derived information is held in a store for about 0.6 s before influencing action. Similarly, if cues for steering on a driving simulator are suddenly removed, normal steering continues for about 0.85 s, implying that visually derived information remains available for that period (Land, 1998). In copying tasks some feature of the object to be copied is acquired and then transferred to the copy less than a second later (e.g. Figs 4.9 and 4.12b). The information survives one or two saccades, although here again it is being processed into a motor action. In the view of Tchalenko and Miall (2009), a segment of the original is translated into a visuo-motor mapping while looking at the original and then to a motor command when gaze reaches the copy; there is no requirement to store a 'mental image'. Whether the short-term storage involved in these various activities is best described as short-term memory, working memory, a short-term store, or a sensory or motor buffer is not at all clear.

A very short-term store that resembles more conventional memory with a decay time in the region of a second was demonstrated by Hayhoe et al. (1992). They showed that a pattern of dots presented briefly at different times during different fixations could be integrated in such a way that the precise angles between the dots could be estimated. The precision of the judgments fell off as the interval between the dot presentations increased from 0 to 800 ms. A similar very precise short-term memory is seen when piano players look down to the keys and then back to the score, apparently with no loss of position provided the return is immediate (Fig. 4.6b).

Short-term memory, although of longer duration, is involved in look-ahead fixations. These are glances in which an object is briefly fixated before being acted upon at some time in the future and are a common feature of many tasks (Chapter 5). Pelz and Canoza (2001) found that during a hand-washing task, as subjects approached the wash basin they fixated the tap, soap, and paper towels in sequence, before returning to the tap to guide the hand to grasp it. In a model assembly task, Mennie et al. (2007) found that the typical interval between a look-ahead fixation and the action to which it later contributed was about 3 s, although informally Land et al. (1999) had noted that previously observed objects could be targeted quite accurately and without search up to a minute after the original fixation. There is little doubt that these look-ahead fixations serve to mark the locations of objects to facilitate future fixations or reaches.

Another particularly interesting example of learning taking place over a matter of minutes concerns the adjustment of patterns of gaze to the changing probabilities of external events (adaptive gaze control). In Chapter 6 we discussed the study by Jovancevic-Misic and Hayhoe (in press) of encounters by subjects and oncoming walkers (actors) whose behaviour showed varying degrees of unpredictability and aggression. Subjects rapidly learnt which actors to avoid and who to ignore, spending much longer fixating the most aggressive ('rogue') walker. Changing the roles of the actors, so that the 'rogue' walkers became 'safe', and vice versa, caused a reversal of these fixation patterns but took another 12 encounters for the change to become complete. This demonstrates that patterns of gaze are sensitive to the changing statistics of events in the environment, with learning occurring over a relatively brief period. It implies that the subjects are building up a predictive model of the behaviour of other agents that allows them to act pro-actively. It also shows, once again, that gaze behaviour towards a stimulus is less determined by the stimulus itself and rather by the behavioural context in which it occurs.

The involvement of long-term memory in visually guided behaviour takes many forms. After a number of visits we become familiar with the layout of a room, a building or a whole neighbourhood so that navigating around it requires no conscious effort. Such memories can last months or years. Memories for familiar objects and especially faces can last for decades. The scripts of particular tasks – the schema sequences – are similarly robust; even in patients with dementia the ability to make a cup of tea is retained when many other faculties have been lost. Patterns of sensory-motor coordination, involved for example in playing a musical instrument, or a sport like tennis or squash, may take a very long time to acquire, but once acquired can last a lifetime. An explicit example of the quite complex calibration that a batsman has to learn to hit a scoring shot in cricket is shown in Fig 8.12; these surfaces, which relate observations made up to the bounce point to the co-ordinates needed to make the strike, are acquired over many years of practice on the field and in the nets. They represent components of an internal model that relates the behaviour of cricket balls to the neuromuscular machinery available to hit them effectively.

Sensory-motor learning
How are gaze patterns learned?

Learning to act effectively in the world takes a long time. Children will be 5 or 6 before they can catch a slow ball reliably and about 10 years before they have all the skills to make a cup of tea. In former times apprentices would not be taken on until they were 14 years old, reflecting the age at which basic manipulative skills had been mastered and could then be built on. There is indeed a great deal to learn. In an act as apparently straightforward as making a cup of tea, learning must have taken place in four domains: schema control, gaze control, vision, and motor control. A list of requirements for completing the task, all of which must have been learned at some stage, would include the following. At the 'executive' level, responsible for the schema controlling each action, the sequence in which each of the objects is required for the task – cups, kettle, teabags, milk, and so on – must have been developed. The visual system must have learnt to identify each component as it is needed. The gaze control system must know the likely whereabouts of each item, and for each component of the task the motor control system must have acquired the knowledge of how to perform the appropriate action or actions (Hayhoe et al., 2007).

This rather formidable catalogue does not all have to be learnt at the same time. Some elements, such as picking up an object, are very basic and acquired in the first year or two of life. Others, filling a kettle, for example, are interchangeable with other tasks, which could have been acquired in other, simpler contexts. It probably takes a child about 10 years to perfect the whole tea-making sequence. Little if any of this learning is by explicit instruction. Like most actions, the learning is implicit or 'procedural'. There is very little knowledge of how it comes about.

In contrast to the very slow process of initial skill acquisition, existing motor skills can adapt to new circumstances very rapidly. In an experiment where subjects caught a tennis ball bouncing off the floor, Hayhoe et al. (2005) cryptically substituted a more elastic ball for the original one, resulting in a higher bounce. As in cricket (Chapter 8) subjects initially looked at the hands of the thrower, then down to the position just above the bounce point, anticipating the bounce by about 50 ms. They then followed the ball with smooth pursuit movements. The principal effect of changing the ball to a bouncier one was to disrupt pursuit after the bounce, and a series of saccades was made in place of pursuit. Arrival time at the bounce point was also advanced by about 100 ms, presumably to take account of the uncertainty of the new trajectory. However, accuracy of pursuit returned to normal after only three bounces of the new ball, indicating that the subjects had updated their internal model of the ball's likely trajectory.

Learning eye–hand coordination

It has been pointed out repeatedly that each type of action has its own associated regime of eye movements and that fixations on objects tend to precede actions upon them by up to a second. This is what we observe once an action has been learned, but does this pattern hold during the period while the skill is being acquired? A study by Sailer et al. (2005), the first of its kind, has clearly demonstrated that the answer is no.

Sailer et al. devised a task that involved learning how to use a novel mouse-like tool to control the position of a cursor on a screen to hit a series of consecutively appearing target boxes. The tool consisted of a freely held box with a handle at each end. Applying opposite rotational torque to the two handles moved the cursor up and down the screen, whereas pushing the handles towards or away from each other moved the cursor laterally (in fact the system was isometric, and the handles did not move). Making oblique cursor movements with the tool was evidently quite difficult and took some time to learn. The gaze movements and cursor movements of the subjects were monitored as they learned how to use the tool, and measures of success such as hit rate and path length to target were also measured. The learning process took a total of about 20 minutes.

The most interesting result was that, for most subjects, learning proceeded in three distinct stages: an exploratory phase in which the hit rate remained low, a skill acquisition stage in which the hit rate increased rapidly, and a skill refinement stage in which the rate increased more slowly. The three phases were characterized by very different patterns of both motor control (as shown by the cursor movements) and gaze movements. During the exploratory phase most cursor movements and gaze movements were either horizontal or vertical as the subjects learned to cope with one or other control dimension of the tool (Fig. 12.2a). Gaze generally followed the cursor, with occasional glances to the target, and gaze saccades were generally small, 3° to 4°. At this stage it typically took about 20 s for the cursor to reach the target. During the skill acquisition stage, the subjects slowly learned to move the cursor obliquely, and the hit rate increased to about one target every 2 s (Fig. 12.2b). At the beginning of this second period the eyes continued to track the cursor, although the pattern changed from gaze lagging behind the cursor to leading it by up to 0.3 s: gaze thus began to anticipate cursor position. At the same time gaze saccades became larger, increasing from about 4° to 12°, as more were directed towards the target (successive targets were 18° apart). During the skill refinement stage gaze no longer tracked the cursor but went straight to the next target, with either a single saccade, or with one large and one smaller saccade (Fig. 12.2c). Hit rates increased slightly to just below 1 s^{-1}.

The role of gaze clearly changes as learning progresses. To begin with the eyes follow the movements of the cursor. At this stage vision is being used to check on the effects of the rather inexpert control operations, and learning proceeds by associating particular manipulations with their visual consequences. During the skill refinement stage gaze begins to anticipate cursor movements and, as manipulation becomes more secure, vision is used to provide a series of local goals for cursor movements. Finally, with control of cursor direction established, it is sufficient for gaze to mark the target, that is, the end point of the cursor movement.

The description of the evolution of eye–hand co-ordination in this particular skill, with a gradual transition from a monitoring to an anticipatory role for the eyes, sits well with ideas about skill acquisition in other contexts. Many activities we learn after early childhood have components that require the visual calibration of a manual activity – how much to turn the steering wheel of a car, or the effects of a tennis stroke on a ball's trajectory. These imply a period when vision is mainly concerned with checking consequences, corresponding to the first two phases of the scheme proposed by Sailer et al. (2005). Equally, once the calibration has been established, vision is freed up to look ahead – to the next bend or the intended target of the next stroke (Fig. 7.16, of the learner driver, is relevant here). Vision comes to adopt a feed-forward rather than a feedback role.

It has long been recognized that skill acquisition proceeds in stages. Psychologists distinguish the early attention-demanding stages in learning a new skill, from the later stages in which actions are automatized, and require little or no conscious intervention (Norman and Shallice, 1986; Underwood and Everatt, 1996). There are theoretical models of the internal processes involved in motor control that allow for learning by comparing intended actions with sensory feedback and lead to predictive behaviour

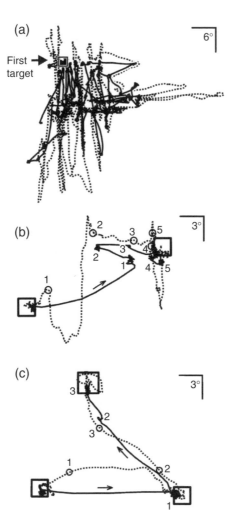

Fig. 12.2 Three stages in learning to use a device in which movement of a cursor on a screen (dotted line) is achieved by moving two bars in and out (horizontal movements) or counter-rotating them (vertical movements). The aim is to move the cursor from one target to the next as it appears. During the first 6 minutes (a) the subjects can only make vertical or horizontal movements. The direction of gaze (full line) lags behind the cursor. During the next 6 minutes (b) oblique cursor movements are still not possible, but the path is much faster and more direct, and gaze is approximately level with the cursor (from 2 onwards). In the final consolidation phase (c) gaze goes directly to the next target, ahead of the cursor, which follows on a rapid, more or less oblique, course. Modified from Sailer et al. (2005).

(see below). These 'forward models' seem to be the kinds of mechanism that are at work during motor learning. We will consider these in the next section.

Internal models of motor control

Visual information from the eyes takes about 100 ms to reach the cortex. During that time a car travelling at 30 mph (= 48.3 kph = 14.4 ms^{-1}) will have moved 1.44 m, and a fast baseball will be a quarter of the way down the pitch. If we were to take the perceived position of objects as their real positions it would be impossible to drive safely or play ball games. Effective action control mechanisms therefore have to have anticipation built into them. From the mid-1990s the idea that the brain has access to internal models, which mimic aspects of the external world and the workings of the body's effector systems, was introduced from robotic engineering into cognitive science (Miall and Wolpert, 1996; Wolpert et al., 1995). These models were of two kinds: *predictors* (or forward models), which estimate the sensory consequences of motor commands and can thereby be used to improve motor performance, and *controllers* (or inverse models), which manage the relationship between the desired goal and the motor commands required to achieve that goal.

Before considering internal models, however, it will be worth spending a little time discussing earlier ideas of action control. The use of feedback loops to control the output of motor systems arguably goes back to James Watt's governor of 1787, which controlled the speed of an engine by automatically adjusting the flow of steam. The idea has been used in biology for well over a century to explain homeostasis in general, the accurate adjustment of muscle force to load, and various visual behaviours such as the optokinetic reflex and smooth pursuit. In essence the output of a system is measured by a sensor, this is compared with the desired output, and it is the resulting difference between desired and actual state (the error) that forms the input to the motor controller, and hence determines the strength of the resulting action (Fig. 12.3). The main problem with feedback loops in their most basic form is that they are slow to respond, partly because of the time taken by the sensors and transmission delays and also because of the time for the musculature to respond. Thus responses to unpredictable disturbances in visual tracking tasks have overall delays in excess of 200 ms. Feedback loops deal very well with slowly changing loads, but when the time course of changes are comparable with or shorter than the delay time of the loop the system is liable to become ineffective or unstable.

One way to improve the performance of a system is to employ feed-forward information. That is, information that anticipates events or disturbances before they occur. Feed-forward systems estimate what is about to happen and are therefore faster than feedback loops, but they are not self-correcting. If they are not correctly calibrated, the response will be inappropriate. For this reason both feed-forward and feedback are often employed in real systems, which then have the benefit of both speed and accuracy (Fig. 12.3). A well-known example is the control of gaze fixation between saccades, where two reflexes – the vestibulo-ocular reflex (feed-forward) and the optokinetic reflex (feedback) – combine to prevent gaze slipping relative to the surroundings, despite movements of the head. Another example of a dual system is steering control, where the distant road regions (especially the tangent point) provide feed-forward information about future road curvature, but the road closer to the car provides feedback about position in lane (Fig. 7.8).

Predictors

In the two examples just mentioned, control of the output (gaze rotation and the car's track curvature) is determined directly by the input variables. There is no need to postulate that the nervous system is operating via internal predictive models because external feed-forward information is available. When, then, is it necessary to invoke internal predictors? One important function of a predictor is to provide the motor controller with accurate ontime feedback about its output, so that corrections for fast disturbances can be made without causing instability. A particularly clear example of this was given by Mehta and Schaal (2002), who got their subjects to balance a vertical 1 m pole on a ping-pong bat. This is a demanding task that relies entirely on visual feedback (it cannot be done blindfold) and is essentially unpredictable because the equilibrium is unstable. By briefly touching the tip of the pole (invisibly) while it was being balanced, Mehta and Schaal found that the visuomotor delay time for an unexpected disturbance was 220 ms. This was compared with the maximum permissible delay for normal balancing, based on a stability analysis, of 160 ms. They concluded that uncorrected feedback (Fig. 12.3) was inadequate and that an internal predictor of some kind was being used. They considered various possible types of predictor and came down in favour of a predictive forward model in the sensory processing stage of motor control. The reason for choosing this, rather than the alternative, a 'tapped delay line' in the motor controller, was that the sensory predictor could cope with 'blank-out periods' when visual feedback was temporarily removed, whereas the tapped delay line could not. They found that their subjects could tolerate blank-outs of 500 to 600 ms.

Mehta and Schaal (2002) suggested that the predictor contains a Kalman filter (Wolpert et al., 1995 had used a Kalman filter as a predictor in a different context). This computational device compares the raw delayed visual feedback with a copy of the actual output to the muscles (efference copy) and combines the information via an iterative process to produce an optimized prediction of the consequences of the current motor action. This prediction can then be used in place of raw feedback to

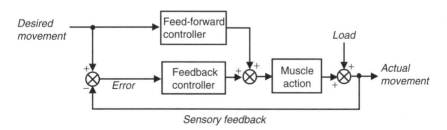

Fig. 12.3 A system incorporating both feed-forward control and a follow-up feedback loop. See text for details.

generate the next input to the motor controller (Fig. 12.4). In the absence of new feed-back information the current prediction holds into the future (although obviously with decreasing reliability), hence the ability of the system to survive brief interruptions of sensory input.

In pole balancing the only available information for control comes from visual feed-back, and so an internal predictor is particularly valuable. Arguably, however, most visually controlled activity is not of this nature. Gaze typically seeks out sources of information about the future by looking ahead to places where action is about to take place. For example, gaze visits the spot where a mug is to be set down about half a sec-ond before this happens (Fig. 5.4). In more complex cases, such as catching or hitting a bouncing ball, gaze visits the anticipated bounce point to obtain timing and future position information (Figs 8.6 and 8.9). Clearly in these examples the brain has built up information about where to look and when, and in that sense it has an internal model containing information about the world and the physical behaviour of objects in it. But this model is not a predictor in the sense used above; it is rather a mechanism for pro-viding feed-forward input to the motor controllers. This is not to say that predictors are not involved at all in the control of actions such as reaching for a mug. For example, the muscular actions that accomplish the reach almost certainly involve forward models that combine efference copy and proprioceptive inflow to produce accurate feedback for the control of arm trajectory (Desmurget and Grafton, 2000). The visual input, however, appears limited to specifying the location of the target.

Controllers

Controllers produce the motor commands that generate particular desired outcomes. If we wish to pick up a cup, the controllers must plan and execute the trajectory of the

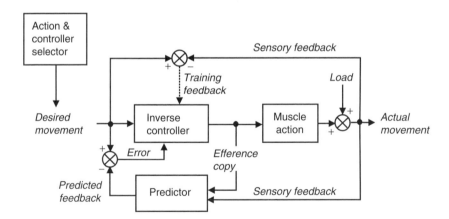

Fig. 12.4 An action system containing an inverse controller in the feed-forward pathway that perfects the task by comparing the desired outcome with the sensory consequences of its behaviour and a predictor in the feedback loop that provides delay-free feedback. Modified from the 'motor control system based on engineering principles' of Frith et al. (2000), which has been redrawn so that it is in similar format to Fig. 12.3.

hand needed to reach the cup, the manipulations required to grasp it, and the force needed to lift it. This involves many muscles contracting by controlled amounts in a precise sequence. Visual input is needed to determine the location of the cup, the orientation of its handle, and to estimate its likely weight (which depends on how full it is). Proprioceptive input from the muscles and joints is also available but in its raw form it is likely to be delayed. How does the brain manage to orchestrate all this to produce an accurate and fluent performance?

It takes several years of our early life to perfect the co-ordination required to pick up a cup competently. Presumably what is occurring during this time is that the brain tunes up its controllers so that the motor commands they issue to the muscles produce actions that give increasingly good matches to the desired result. To do this they must have the ability to learn from errors in their performance. Such controllers are known as *inverse models* – 'inverse' because what they have to do is to transform the desired sensory consequences of an action back into the motor commands that will produce those consequences. This contrasts with, for example, a simple feedback loop which can correct performance online but does not have the ability to acquire and shape the form of the action in the first place. The signal that an inverse controller needs to improve its performance is a measure of the mismatch between the desired and actual sensory consequences of the actions it produces. Learning could then proceed by simple reinforcement, in which case the input would just be a 'did I get it right' statement, or by 'supervised' learning using optimization routines based on the variety of sensory inputs available at the time of task execution. The various possibilities are discussed in detail by Jordan and Wolpert (1999).

Initially a controller will function more or less by trial and error, with a heavy use of error feedback to improve its performance. However, once a controller has acquired the ability to produce the appropriate pattern of motor output the error (training) signal fades away, and the controller now operates in an open loop way, requiring only the 'desired result' instruction as its input. A beautiful example of this transition from learning to open loop execution is the task devised by Sailer et al. (2005), discussed above (Fig. 12.2). Initially, when the mouse-like device is unfamiliar and its operation uncertain, gaze is used to monitor the motor output (the cursor movement on the screen) and, presumably, to train the internal controller. After about 12 minutes the motor action is more or less competent, and gaze behaviour changes from a 'supervisory' role to one in which the next target is fixated ahead of the cursor. Gaze is now used to fix the location of the next 'desired result'.

It is important to be able to match the appropriate motor controller to the task being undertaken, and this may require rapid switching of controllers, based on the immediate circumstances of the action. Wolpert and Flanagan (2001) called this 'context estimation', although J.J. Gibson's word 'affordance' is appropriate too. Consider the case of a batsman facing a fast bowler (Chapter 8, Figs 8.8 and 8.9). His initial decision, made on the basis of the first 100 ms of the ball's flight after it leaves the bowler's hands, is whether to move forward (for full length deliveries) or back (for short deliveries). Somewhere before or shortly after the bounce he has to decide what stroke to make, based on his judgement of the ball's trajectory. There are about 12 different recognized cricket strokes, each involving a distinctly different motor pattern and hence presumably a different motor controller. The controller has to then compute the exact timing of the stroke and position of the bat, based on the feed-forward information available at the time of the bounce (Figs 8.11 and 8.12) and execute the action. As all this takes place in about half a second, all of the decision making and adjustment has to be automatic, acquired over years of practice in the nets and on the field.

A general model

The model of motor control in Fig. 12.4 (based on Frith et al., 2000) incorporates both a predictor to sharpen up the feedback produced by the receptors that monitor output and an inverse controller that allows the system to learn its task from its errors. One should probably imagine that the motor systems of the brain contain a large number of such controllers, with somewhat overlapping roles. Picking up a mug and lifting the lid from a saucepan are different actions, but they use much of the same musculature, so presumably their controllers also share components. How this overlap might be organized is far from clear.

Anatomically, controllers like that envisaged in Fig. 12.4 are likely to have components in a number of brain locations. If we accept the model of Rizzolatti and Lupino (2001, see Chapter 11), then the parietal AIP region would provide 'affordances' (equivalent to the context estimators of Wolpert and Flanagan, 2001), and the premotor cortex would contain 'motor prototypes' (the inverse controllers). The location of predictors could well be the cerebellum, which has long been implicated in aspects motor control involving timing (Miall and Wolpert, 1996). The basal ganglia are known to have a role in motor learning, but it is unclear exactly what this is (Graybiel, 2005).

Frith et al. (2000) pointed out that a model like that in Fig. 12.4 can encompass more than just the control of motor actions. It can also explain how the perceptual distinction is made between self-produced action and external action. They also discussed the use of such models in relation to the awareness of motor actions and the involvement of mental practice in improving performance, and they used the model to discuss which components are likely to be at fault in abnormalities of motor control such as optic ataxia. These considerations are beyond the scope of this chapter, but they do suggest that the model in Fig. 12.4 may be valuable in relating the internal mechanisms of motor control to both the sensory experiences associated with action, and to the underlying physiological mechanisms.

Future directions

Throughout this book we have discussed the possible principles that might underlie the selection of gaze targets. We have dismissed pure image salience in the context of natural behaviour and favoured a higher level of selection, with gaze being directed to objects and locations that are maximally informative in relation to the current behavioural goals. The studies we have reviewed support this principle of selection. Recent evidence from search paradigms also suggests that a good description of human eye movement behaviour can be derived from an optimal observer model that maximizes local information and thereby reduces uncertainty (Najemnik and Geisler, 2005,

2008). We now need an understanding of how 'informativeness' is operationalized in the visual system. In other words, how the schema system is able to instruct the early visual system to recognize objects and other information-bearing regions. It certainly appears that we do indeed look at 'interesting' and 'relevant' locations, but these terms remain hard to define in practice. We have argued that one situation in which salience (in its broad sense) might intrude upon gaze control is when stimuli are unexpected or surprising. Although work is underway to define how we might compute surprise (Itti and Baldi, 2006), current implementations fail to capture surprise within the context of ongoing behaviour: an identical event may be more surprising in one situation than in another.

Many activities involve multitasking and task switching. Consider a football (soccer) player attempting to score a goal. He must attend to the player who is passing the ball to him, the opponent(s) trying to rob him of it, the ball itself and, of course, the goal he is aiming at. We still know little about the ways appropriate patterns of attention switching are achieved within complex tasks. One promising line of work in this respect is that begun by Ballard, Hayhoe and their colleagues. Using virtual and real walking environments they have considered how gaze is allocated between three concurrent tasks: staying within the bounds of a path, avoiding obstacles, and picking up 'litter' (Rothkopf et al., 2007; Sprague et al., 2007). These authors have constructed a model in which switching between tasks is based on minimizing the uncertainty within each task. Attending to a task reduces the uncertainty of quantities relevant to that particular task (e.g. where the obstacles are with respect to the virtual walker's current position for the 'avoid obstacles' task). However, uncertainty increases over time for unattended tasks. The model decides which of the three tasks to attend to based on the current uncertainty for each task. This model produces task-switching behaviour rather like the gaze behaviour observed in a human undertaking the same set of tasks in a virtual walking environment. This approach of task switching based on uncertainty minimization seems a promising direction for future research.

In much of our discussion we have emphasized the role of the schema system: this is where selection of the appropriate actions takes place, and this in turn dictates the behaviourally relevant locations in the world to which gaze must be targeted, and from which information of various kinds must be obtained. We therefore feel that future work will need to consider a range of issues related to schemas. As we have emphasized, a schema is a complex entity that specifies not only the action to be performed but also where to look and what to monitor during the action. How are the associations between these three functions acquired? It would certainly be fruitful to study how adults learn new tasks, and here the study by Sailer et al. (2005), discussed earlier in the chapter, provides an admirable model. It would be even more interesting to investigate how children learn new skills, although this is likely to be harder because the time scale involved is generally much longer. A second question concerns the way schemas are organized in relation to the 'scripts' of extended tasks. It is clear that such scripts are not simple schema lists. In some tasks the ordering of actions within a particular behaviour is fairly fixed, but in most complex behaviours there is a larger degree of flexibility in the organization and ordering of the component actions: the number of ways that one can make a cup of tea is potentially vast! It is thus important for individuals to learn not only the components of individual schemas but also the rules that govern the flexibility of their deployment within each schema sequence.

We have emphasized in this chapter the need to introduce new ideas derived from engineering to account for the ability of the visual and motor systems to operate in an almost delay-free manner. Simple feedback control cannot account for the speed and accuracy achieved in many activities, particularly ball sports. However, it remains unclear how, or even where, entities such as predictors, Kalman filters and forward controllers might operate within the regions of the brain responsible for the control of action. It will certainly be a challenge for anatomists and physiologists to work out what the biological equivalents of these devices look like, and how they function.

Finally, there is a growing consensus that vision and action need to be studied as intricately linked components of natural behaviour, rather than as separate processes. We hope to have shown in this book that some of the principles that emerge from this approach are new and interesting. There is much more to be learned: about the ways that vision is deployed in the control of motor action, the hierarchical organization of complex actions, the physiology of the ascending and descending control pathways, and the nature of the learning processes by which patterns of coordination are acquired.

References

Abrams, R.A., Meyer, D., & Kornblum, S. (1990). Eye-hand coordination: oculomotor control in rapid aimed limb movements. *J. Exptl. Psychol: Human Perc. & Perf.* **16**, 248–267.

Aginsky, V. & Tarr, M.J. (2000). How are different properties of a scene encoded in visual memory? *Visual Cognition* **7**, 147–162.

Aivar, M.P., Hayhoe, M.M., Chizk, C.L., & Mruczek, R.E.B. (2005). Spatial memory and saccadic targeting in a natural task. *J. Vision* **5**, 177–193.

Allport, D.A. (1989). Visual attention. In: Posner, M.I. (Ed.). *Foundations of Cognitive Science.* pp. 631–682.Cambridge, MA: MIT Press.

Altmann, G.T.M. (2004). Language-mediated eye movements in the absence of a visual world: the 'blank screen paradigm'. *Cognition* **93**, B79–B87.

Altmann, G.T.M. & Kamide, Y. (1999). Incremental interpretation at verbs: restricting the domain of subsequent reference. *Cognition* **73**, 247–264.

Altmann, G.T.M. & Kamide, Y. (2007). The real-time mediation of visual attention by language and world knowledge: linking anticipatory (and other) eye movements to linguistic processing. *J. Memory & Language* **57**, 502–518.

Anstis, S.M., Mayhew, J.W., & Morley, T. (1969). The perception of where a face or television portrait is looking. *Amer. J. Psychol.* **82**, 474–489.

Antes, J.R. (1974). The time course of picture viewing. *J. Exptl. Psych.* **103**, 62–70.

Argyle, M. (1988). *Bodily Communication* (2nd ed.). London: Methuen.

Argyle, M. & Dean, J. (1965). Eye-contact, distance and affiliation. *Sociometry* **28**, 289–304.

Armstrong, K.M., Fitzgerald, J.K., & Moore, T. (2006). Changes in visual receptive fields with microstimulation of frontal cortex. *Neuron* **50**, 791–798.

Ashwin, C., Baron-Cohen, S., Wheelwright, S., O'Riordan, M., & Bullmore, E.T. (2007). Differential activation of the amygdala and the 'social brain' during fearful face-processing in Asperger Syndrome. *Neuropsychologia* **45**, 2–14.

Baddeley, A. (2007). *Working Memory, Thought and Action.* Oxford: Oxford University Press.

Baddeley, A. & Hitch, G. (1974). Working memory. In: Bower G.A. (Ed.). *The Psychology of Learning and Motivation.* pp. 48–79. London: Academic Press.

Baddeley, R. & Tatler, B.W. (2006). High frequency edges (but not contrast) predict where we fixate: A Bayesian system identification analysis. *Vision Res.* **46**, 2824–2833.

Bahill, A.T. & Baldwin, D.G. (2004). The rising fastball, and other perceptual illusions of batters. In Hung, G., & Pallis, J. (Eds) *Biomedical Engineering Principles in Sports.* pp. 257–287. New York: Kluwer Academic.

Bahill, A.T. & LaRitz, T. (1984). Why can't batters keep their eyes on the ball? *American Scientist* **72**, 249–253.

Ballard, D.H., Hayhoe, M.M., Li, F., & Whitehead, S.D. (1992). Hand-eye coordination during sequential tasks. *Phil. Trans. Roy. Soc. London B* **337**, 331–339.

Ballard, D.H., Hayhoe, M.M., & Pelz, J.B. (1995). Memory representations in natural tasks. *J. Cogn. Neurosci.* **7**, 66–80.

Bargh, J.A. & Ferguson, M.J. (2000). Beyond behaviorism: on the automaticity of higher mental processes. *Psychol. Bull.* **126**, 925–945.

Baron-Cohen, S. (1995). *Mindblindness: An Essay on Autism and Theory of Mind.* Cambridge, MA: MIT Press.

Batista, A.P. & Newsome, W.T. (2000). Visuo-motor control: giving the brain a hand. *Curr. Biol.* **10**, R145–R148.

Beall, A.C. & Loomis, J.M. (1996). Visual control of steering without course information. *Perception* **25**, 481–494.

Becker, W. (1991). Saccades. In: Carpenter, R.H.S. (Ed.). *Vision and Visual Dysfunction. Vol 8: Eye Movements.* pp. 95–137. Basingstoke: Macmillan.

Beldan, G.W. & Fry, C.B. (1905) *Great Batsmen, Their Methods at a Glance.* London: Macmillan.

Berkeley, G. (1709). An essay towards a new theory of vision. In: Lindsay, A.D. (Ed.) (1910). *A New Theory of Vision and Other Writings.* London: Dent.

Biederman, I. (1981). On the semantics of a glance at a scene. In: Kubovy, M., & Pomerantz, J.R. (Eds), *Perceptual Organization.* pp. 213–253. Hillsdale, NJ: Lawrence Erlbaum Associates.

Biederman, I. (1987) Recognition by components: a theory of human image understanding. *Psych. Rev.* **94**, 115–45.

Biguer, B., Prablanc, C., & Jeannerod, M. (1984). The contribution of coordinated eye and head movements in hand pointing accuracy. *Exp. Brain Res.* **55**, 462–469.

Blair, D.J.R., Morris, J.S., Frith, C.D., Perrett, D.I., & Dolan, R.J. (1999). Dissociable neural responses to facial expressions of sadness and anger. *Brain* **122**, 883–893.

Bock, S.W., Dicke, P., & Thier, P. (2008). How precise is gaze following in humans? *Vision Res.* **48**, 946–957.

Bootsma, R.J. & van Wieringen, P.C.W. (1990). Timing an attacking forehand drive in table tennis. *J. Exptl. Psychol.: Human Perc. & Perf.* **16**, 21–29.

Botvinick, M.M., Braver, T.S., Barch, D.M., Carter, C.S., & Cohen, J.D. (2001). Conflict monitoring and cognitive control. *Psych. Rev.* **108**, 624–652.

Bradley, M.M., Miccoli, L., Escrig, M.A., & Lang, P.J. (2008). The pupil as a measure of emotional arousal and autonomic activation. *Psychophysiology* **45**, 602–607.

Brandt, S.A. & Stark, L.W. (1997). Spontaneous eye movements during visual imagery reflect the content of the visual scene. *J. Cognit. Neurosci.* **9**, 27–38.

Breitmeyer, B.G & Ogmen, H. (2000). Recent models and findings in visual backward masking: a comparison, review, and update. *Perception & Psychophysics*, **62**, 1572–95.

Bridgeman, B., Hendry, D., & Stark, L. (1975). Failure to detect displacement of the visual world during saccadic eye movements. *Vision Res.* **15**, 719–722.

Brochier, T. & Umiltà, M.A. (2007). Cortical control of grasp in non-human primates. *Curr. Opin. Neurobiol.* **17**, 637–643.

Brockmole, J.R. (Ed.) (2008). *The Visual World in Memory.* Hove, UK: Psychology Press.

Brouwer, A. & Knill, D. (2007). The role of memory in visually guided reaching. *J. Vision* **7**(5), 6, 1–12.

Burr, D.C. & Morrone, M.C. (2003). Visual perception during saccades. In: Chalupa, L.M, & Werner, J.S.(Eds). *The Visual Neurosciences Vol. 2.* pp. 1391–1401. Cambridge: MIT Press.

Burr D.C., Morrone, M.C., & Ross, J. (1994) .Selective suppression of the magnocellular visual pathway during saccadic eye movements. *Nature* **371**, 511–513.

Buswell, G.T. (1920). An experimental study of the eye-voice span in reading. *Supplementary Educational Monographs* No. 17. Chicago: Chicago University Press.

Buswell, G.T. (1935). *How People Look at Pictures: A Study of the Psychology of Perception in Art.* Chicago: Chicago University Press.

Butsch, R.L.C. (1932). Eye movements and the eye-hand span in typewriting. *J. Educational Psychology* **23**, 104–121.

Call, J. & Tomasello, M. (2008). Does the chimpanzee have a theory of mind? 30 years later. *Trends Cognit. Sci.* **12**, 187–192.

Campbell, J. (1993). The role of physical objects in spatial thinking. In Eilan, N., McCarthy, R., Brewer,B. (Eds). *Spatial Representation: Problems in Philosophy and Psychology.* pp. 65–95. Oxford: Blackwell.

Carmi, R. & Itti, L. (2006). Visual causes versus correlates of attentional selection in dynamic scenes. *Vision Research* **46**, 4333–4345.

Carpenter, R.H.S. (1988). *Movements of the Eyes.* London: Pion.

Carpenter, R.H.S. (1991) The visual origins of ocular motility. In: Carpenter R.H.S. (Ed.). *Vision and Visual Dysfunction. v.8. Eye movements.* pp.1–10. London: Macmillan.

Carter, C.S., Braver, T.S., Barch, D.M., Botvinick, M.M., Noll, D., & Cohen, J.D. (1998). Anterior cingulate cortex, error detection, and the online monitoring of performance. *Science* **280**, 747–749.

Castet, E. & Masson, G.S. (2000). Motion perception during saccadic eye movements. *Nature Neurosci.* **3**, 177–183.

Cattell, J.M. (1900) Vision with the moving eye. *Psychol. Rev.* **7**, 507–508.

Chalupa, L.M., Werner, J.S. (Eds) (2003) *The Visual Neurosciences Vol. 2.* Cambridge: MIT Press.

Chapman, S. (1968). Catching a baseball. *Amer. J. Physics* **36**, 868–870.

Chattington, M., Wilson, M., Ashford, D., & Marple-Horvat, D.E. (2007). Eye-steering coordination in natural driving. *Exp. Brain Res.* **180**, 1–14.

Chen, X., & Zelinsky, G.J. (2006). Real-world visual search is dominated by top-down guidance. *Vision Res.* **46**, 4118–4133.

Cline, M.G. (1967). Perception of where a person is looking. *Amer. J. Psychol.* **80**, 41–80.

Colby, C.L., Duhamel, J.R., & Goldberg, M.E. (1996). Visual, presaccadic, and cognitive activation of single neurons in monkey lateral parietal area. *J. Neurophysiol.* **76**, 2841–2852.

Colby, C.L, Goldberg, M.E. (1999). Space and attention in parietal cortex. *Ann. Rev. Neurosci.* **22**, 319–349.

Collewijn, H., Martins, A.J., & Steinman, R.M (1981) Natural retinal image motion: origin and change. *Ann. N.Y. Acad. Sci.* **374**, 312–329.

Collewijn, H. & Tamminga, E.P. (1984). Human smooth pursuit and saccadic eye movements during voluntary pursuit of different target motions on different backgrounds. *J. Physiol. (London)* **351**, 217–250.

Cooper, R.P. (2002). Order and disorder in everyday action: the roles of contention scheduling and supervisory attention. *Neurocase* **8**, 61–79.

Cooper, R.P. & Shallice, T. (2000). Contention scheduling and the control of routine activities. *Cognit. Neuropsych.* **17**, 297–338.

Corbetta, M., Akbudak, E., Conturo, T.E., Snyder, A.Z., Ollinger, J.M., Drury, H.A., et al. (1998). A common network of functional areas for attention and eye movements. *Neuron* **21**, 761–773.

Crundall, D. (2005). The integration of top-down and bottom-up factors in visual search during driving. In: Underwood, G. (Ed). *Cognitive Processes in Eye Guidance.* pp. 283–302. Oxford: Oxford University Press.

Crundall, D., Underwood, G., & Chapman., P. (1998). How much do novice drivers see? The effects of demand on visual search strategies in novice and experienced drivers. In: Underwood, G. (Ed.). *Eye Guidance in Reading and Scene Perception.* pp. 395–417. Amsterdam: Elsevier.

Culham, J.C. & Valyear, K.F. (2006). Human parietal cortex in action. *Curr. Opin. Neurobiol.* **16**, 205–212.

Day, B.L., & Reynolds, R.F. (2005). Vestibular reafference shapes voluntary movement. *Current Biology* **15**, 1390–1394.

Deaner, R.O. & Platt, M.L. (2003). Reflexive social attention in monkeys and humans. *Current Biology* **13**, 1609–1613.

Dehaene, S., Posner, M.I., & Tucker, D.M. (1994). Localization of a neural system for error-detection and compensation. *Psychological Science* **5**, 303–305,

Dennett, D.C. (1991). *Consciousness Explained.* Boston MA: Little, Brown & Co.

Desimone, R. & Duncan, J. (1995). Neural mechanisms of selective attention. *Annu. Rev. Neurosci.* **18**, 193–222.

Desmurget, M. & Grafton, S. (2000). Forward modelling allows feedback control for fast reaching movements. *Trends Cognit. Sci.* **4**, 423–431.

Deubel, H. & Schneider, W.X. (1996). Saccade target selection and object recognition: evidence for a common attentional mechanism. *Vision Research* **36**, 1812–1837.

Diamond, M.R., Ross, J., & Morrone, M.C. (2000). Extraretinal control of saccadic suppression. *J. Neurosci.* **20**, 3449–3455.

Dobie, T.G., May, J.G., & Flanagan, M.B. (2003). The influence of visual reference on stance and walking on a moving surface. *Aviation, Space and Environmental Medicine* **74**, 838–845.

Dodge, R. (1900). Visual perception during eye movement. *Psychol. Rev.* **7**, 454–465.

Dodge, R. & Cline, T.S. (1901). The angle velocity of eye movements. *Psychol. Rev.* **8**, 145–157.

Doherty-Sneddon, G., & Phelps, F.G. (2005). Gaze aversion: a response to cognitive or social difficulty? *Memory & Cognition* **33**, 727–733.

Donges, E. (1978). A two-level model of driver steering behavior. *Human Factors* **20**, 691–707.

Drieghe, D., Desmet, T., & Brysbaert, M. (2007). How important are linguistic factors in word skipping during reading? *Brit. J. Psychol.* **98**, 157–171.

Droll, J. & Hayhoe, M. (2007) Trade-offs between working memory and gaze. *J. Exptl. Psychol.: Human Perc. & Perf.* **33**, 1352–1365.

Droll, J.A., Hayhoe, M.M., Triesch , J., & Sullivan, B.T. (2005). Task demands control acquisition and storage of visual information. *J. Exp. Psychol.: Human Perc. & Perf.* **31**, 1416–1438.

Duchowski, A.T. (2003) *Eye Tracking Methodology: Theory and Practice.* Berlin: Springer.

Duhamel, J-R., Colby, C.L., & Goldberg, M.E. (1992). The updating of the representation of visual space in parietal cortex by intended eye movements. *Science* **255**, 90–92.

Ehinger, K., Hidalgo-Sotelo, B., Torralba, A., & Oliva, A. (in press). Modeling search for people in 90 scenes: a combined source model for eye guidance. *Visual Cognition.*

Einhäuser, W., Rutishauser, U., & Koch, C. (2008). Task-demands can immediately reverse the effects of sensory-driven saliency in complex visual stimuli. *J. Vision* **8**(2), 2, 1–19.

Einhäuser, W., Spain, M., & Perona, P. (2008). Objects predict fixations better than early saliency. *J. Vision,* **8**(14), 18, 11–26.

Ekstrom, L.B., Roelfsema, P.R., Arsenault, J.T., Bonmassar, G., & Vanduffel, W. (2008). Bottom-up dependent gating of frontal signals in early visual cortex. *Science* **321**, 414–417.

Elazary, L. & Itti, L. (2008). Interesting objects are visually salient. *J. Vision* **8**(3), 3, 1–15.

Engbert, R., Nuthmann, A., Richter, E.M., & Kliegl, R. (2005). SWIFT: A dynamical model of saccade generation during reading. *Psychol. Rev.* **112**, 777–813.

Epelboim, J., Steinman, R.M., Kowler, E., Pizlo, Z., Erlekens, C.J., & Collewijn, H. (1995). The function of visual search and memory in two kinds of sequential looking task. *Vision Res.* **35**, 3401–3422.

Epelboim, J., Steinman, R.M., Kowler, E., Pizlo, Z., Erlekens, C.J., & Collewijn, H. (1997). Gaze-shift dynamics in two kinds of sequential looking task. *Vision Res.* **37**, 2579–2607.

Epstein, R.A. (2008). Parahippocampal and retrosplenial contributions to human spatial navigation. *Trends Cogn. Sci.* **12**, 388–396.

Erdmann, B. & Dodge, R. (1898). *Psychologische Untersuchungen über das Lesen auf experimenteller Grundlage.* Halle: Niemeyer.

Erikson, C.W. & St James, J.D. (1986). Visual attention within and around the field of focal attention: a zoom lens model. *Perception & Psychophysics* **70**, 225–240.

Fajen, B.R. (2005). Perceiving possibilities for action: on the necessity of calibration and perceptual learning for the visual guidance of action. *Perception* **34**, 717–740.

Fajen, B.R. & Warren, W.H. (2003). Behavioral dynamics of steering, obstacle avoidance, and route selection. *J. Exp.Psychol.: Human Perc. & Perf.* **29**, 343–262.

Fajen, B.R. & Warren, W.H. (2004). Visual guidance of intercepting a moving target on foot. *Perception* **33**, 689–715.

Falkenstein, M., Hohnsbein, J., & Hoormann, J. (1995). Event related potential correlates of errors in reaction tasks. In: Karmos, G., Molnar, M., Csepi, V., Czigler, I., Desmedt, J.E. (Eds). *Perspectives of event-related potentials research.* pp. 287–296. Amsterdam: Elsevier.

Fecteau, J.H. & Munoz, D.P. (2006). Salience, relevance, and firing: a priority map for target selection. *Trends Cogn. Sci.* **10**, 382–390.

Ferreira, F., Apel, J., & Henderson, J.M. (2008) Taking a new look at nothing. *Trends Cognit. Sci.* **12**, 405–420.

Findlay, J.M. & Gilchrist, I.D. (2003). *Active Vision.* Oxford: Oxford University Press.

Findlay, J.M., & Walker, R. (1999). A model of saccade generation based on parallel processing and competitive inhibition. *Behav. Brain Sci.* **22**, 661–721.

Fleischer, A.G. (1986). Control of eye movements by working memory load. *Biol. Cybernetics* **55**, 227–238.

Fogassi, L., Ferrari, P.F., Gesierich, B., Rozzi, S., Chersi, F., & Rizzolatti, G. (2005). Parietal lobe: from action organization to intention understanding. *Science* **308**, 662–667.

Fogassi, L., & Lupino, G. (2005). Motor functions of the parietal lobe. *Curr. Opin. Neurobiol.* **15**, 625–632.

Foulsham, T. & Underwood, G. (2008). What can saliency models predict about eye movements? Spatial and sequential aspects of fixations during encoding and recognition. *Journal of Vision* **8**(2), 6, 1–17.

Friedburg , C., Allen, C.P., Mason, P.J., & Lamb, T.D. (2004). Contribution of cone photoreceptors and postreceptoral mechanisms to the human photopic electroretinogram. *J. Physiol. (Lond)* **556**, 819–843.

Friesen, C.K. & Kingstone, A., (1998). The eyes have it! Reflexive orienting is triggered by nonpredictive gaze. *Psychonomic Bulletin and Review* **5**, 490–495.

Frith, C.D., Blakemore, S-J., & Wolpert, D.M. (2000). Abnormalities in the awareness of and control of action. *Phil. Trans. R. Soc. Lond. B* **355**, 1771–1788.

Frost, D. & Pöppel, E. (1976). Different programming modes of human saccadic eye-movements as a function of stimulus eccentricity: indications of a functional subdivision of visual field. *Biol. Cybernetics* **23**, 39–48.

Fuchs, A.F. (1967) Saccadic and smooth pursuit eye movements in the monkey. *J. Physiol. (London)* **191**, 609–631

Furneaux, S. (1996). *The Role of Eye Movements during Music Reading.* D.Phil Thesis. University of Sussex. UK.

Furneaux, S. & Land, M.F. (1999). The effects of skill on the eye-hand span during musical sight-reading. *Proc. Roy. Soc. London B* **266**, 2453–2440.

Fuster, J.M. (1995) Temporal processing. In: Grafman, J., Holyoak, K.J., & Boller, F. (Eds). *Structure and Functions of the Human Prefrontal Cortex. Annals N. Y. Acad. Sci.* **769**, 173–181.

Fuster, J.M. (2002). Physiology of executive functions. In: Stuss, D.T., & Knight, R.T. (Eds). *Principles of Frontal Lobe Function.* pp. 96–108. Oxford: Oxford University Press.

Gallese, V., Fadiga, L., Fogassi, L., & Rizzolatti, G. (1996). Action recognition in the premotor cortex. *Brain* **119**, 593–609.

Gandhi, N.J. & Sparks, D.L. (2003). Changing views of the role of superior colliculus in the control of gaze. In: Chalupa, L.M., Werner, J.S. (Eds). *The Visual Neurosciences.* pp. 1449–1465. Cambridge: MIT Press.

Geruschat, D.R., Hassan, S.E., & Turano, K.A. (2003). Gaze behavior while crossing complex intersections. *Optometry and Vision Science* **80**, 515–528.

Gibson, J.J. (1958). Visually controlled locomotion and visual orientation in animals. *Brit. J. Psychol.* **49**, 182–194.

Gibson, J.J. (1966). *The Senses Considered as Perceptual Systems.* New York: Appleton-Century-Crofts.

Gibson, J.J. (1979). *The Ecological Approach to Visual Perception.* Boston: Houghton Mifflin.

Gibson, J.J. & Crooks L.R. (1938). A theoretical field-analysis of automobile driving. *Amer. J. Psychol.* **51**, 453–471.

Gibson, J.J. & Pick, A.D. (1963). Perception of another person's looking behavior. *Amer. J. Psychol.* **76**, 386–394.

Gilbert, S.J. & Burgess, P.W. (2008). Executive function. *Current Biology* **18**, R110–R114.

Glickstein, M. (2000). How are visual areas of the brain connected to motor areas for the sensory guidance of movement? *Trends Neurosci.* **23**, 613–617.

Goldman-Rakic, P.S. (1995) Architecture of the prefrontal cortex and the central executive. In: Grafman, J., Holyoak, K.J., & Boller, F. (Eds). *Structure and Functions of the Human Prefrontal Cortex. Annals N. Y. Acad. Sci.* **769**, 71–83.

Goossens, B.M.A., Dekleva, M., Reader, S.M., Sterck, E.H.M., &.Bolhuis, J.J. (2008). Gaze following in monkeys is modulated by observed facial expressions. *Anim. Behav.* **75**, 1673–1681.

Goossens, H.H.L.M. & van Opsal, A.J. (1997). Human eye-head coordination in two dimensions under different sensorimotor conditions. *Exp. Brain Res.* **114**, 542–560.

Gottlieb, J.P., Kusunoki, M., & Goldberg, M.E. (1998). The representation of visual salience in monkey parietal cortex. *Nature* **391**, 481–484.

Grasso, R., Prevost, P., Ivanenko, Y.P., & Berthoz, A. (1998). Eye-head coordination for the steering of locomotion in humans: an anticipatory synergy. *Neurosci. Lett.* **253**, 115–118.

Gray, R. & Regan, D. (1998). Accuracy of estimating time to collision using binocular and monocular information. *Vision Res.* **38**, 499–512.

Graybiel, A.M. (2005). The basal ganglia: learning new tricks and loving it. *Curr. Opin. Neurobiol.* **15**, 623–625.

Graziano, M. (2006). The organization of behavioral repertoire in motor cortex. *Ann. Rev. Neurosci.* **29**, 105–134.

Grimes, J. (1996). On the failure to detect changes in scenes across saccades. In: Atkins, K. (Ed.). *Perception: Vancouver Studies in Cognitive Science, Vol.2*. pp. 89–110. New York: Oxford University Press.

Guitton, D. (1991). Control of saccadic eye and gaze movements by the superior colliculus and basal ganglia. In: Carpenter, R.H.S. (Ed.). *Vision and Visual Dysfunction vol 8: Eye Movements*, pp. 244–276. Basingstoke: Macmillan Press.

Guitton, D. (1992) Control of eye-head coordination during orienting gaze shifts. *Trends in Neurosciences* **15**, 174–179.

Guitton, D., Bergeron, A., Choi, W.Y., & Matsuo, S. (2003). On the feedback control of orienting gaze shifts made with eye and head movements. *Prog. Brain Res.* **142**, 55–68.

Guitton, D, Kearney, R.E., Wereley, N., & Peterson, B.W. (1986). Visual, vestibular and voluntary contributions to human head stabilization. *Exp. Brain Res.* **64**, 59–69.

Guitton, D. & Volle, M. (1987) Gaze control in humans: eye-head coordination during orienting movements to targets within and beyond the oculomotor range. *J. Neurophysiol.* **58**, 427–459.

Gullberg, M. (2002). Eye movements and gestures in human interaction. In: Hyönä, J., Radach, R., & Deubel, H. (Eds). *The Mind's Eyes: Cognitive and Applied Aspects of Eye Movements.* pp. 685–703. Oxford: Elsevier.

Haenny, P.E., Maunsell, J.H., & Schiller, P.H. (1988). State dependent activity in monkey visual cortex. II. Retinal and extraretinal factors in V4. *Exp. Brain Res.* **69**, 245–259.

Hallett, P.E. (1978). Primary and secondary saccades to goals defined by instructions. *Vision Res.* **18**, 1279–1296.

Hayhoe, M. (2000). Vision using routines: a functional account of vision. *Visual Cognition* **7**, 43–64.

Hayhoe, M. (2008). Visual memory in motor planning and action. In: Brockmole, J.R. (Ed.). *The Visual World in Memory.* pp. 117–139. Hove, UK: Psychology Press.

Hayhoe, M. & Ballard, D. (2005) Eye movements in natural behavior. *Trends Cogn. Sci.* **9**, 188–194.

Hayhoe, M., Droll, J., & Mennie, N. (2007). Learning where to look. In: Van Gompel, R.P.G., Fischer, M.H., Murray, W.S., & Hill, R.L. (Eds) *Eye Movements: A Window on Mind and Brain.* pp. 641–660. Oxford: Elsevier.

Hayhoe, M., Mennie, N., Sullivan, B., & Gorgos, K. (2005). The role of internal models and prediction in catching balls. *Proc. Amer. Assn. Artif. Intel.* Fall 2005.

Hayhoe, M.M., Lachter, J., & Moeller, P. (1992). Spatial memory and integration across saccadic eye movements. In: Rayner K. (Ed.). *Eye Movements and Visual Cognition: Scene Perception and Reading.* pp. 130–145. New York: Springer.

Hayhoe, M.M., Srivastava, A., Mruczec, R., & Pelz, J.B. (2003). Visual memory and motor planning in a natural task. *J. Vision* **3**, 49–63

Haynes, J.D., Sakai, K., Rees, G., Gilbert, S., Frith, C., & Passingham, R.E. (2007). Reading hidden intentions in the human brain. *Current Biology* **17**, 323–328.

Henderson, J.M. (1992). Object identification in context – the visual processing of natural scenes. *Canad. J. Psychol – Rev. Canad. de Psychol.* **46**, 319–341.

Henderson, J.M., Brockmole, J.R., Castelhano, M.S., & Mack, M.L. (2007). Visual saliency does not account for eye movements during search in real-world scenes. In: van Gompel, R.P.G., Fischer, M.H., Murray, W.S., Hill, R.L. (Eds). *Eye Movements: A Window on Mind and Brain.* pp. 537–562. Oxford: Elsevier.

Hering, E. (1879). Der Raumsinn und die Bewegungen des Auges. In: Herman, L. (Ed.). *Handbuch der Physiologie Vol. 3, Part 1: Physiologie des Gesichtsinnes.* pp. 343–601. Leipzig: Vogel.

Hershler, O., Hochstein, S. (2005). At first sight: a high-level pop out effect for faces, *Vision Res.* **45**, 1707–1724.

Hess, E.H. & Polt, J.M. (1960). Pupil size as related to interest value of visual stimuli. *Science* **132**, 349–350.

Hess, E.H. & Polt, J.M. (1964). Pupil size in relation to mental activity during simple problem solving. *Science* **143**, 1190–1192.

Hildreth, E.C., Beusmans, J.M.H., Boer, E.R., & Royden, C.S. (2000). From vision to action: experiments and models of steering control during driving. *J. Exp. Psychol.: Hum. Perc. & Perf.* **26**, 1106–1132.

Hochberg, J. (1968). In the mind's eye. In: Haber, R.N. (Ed.). *Contemporary Theory and Research in Visual Perception.* pp. 309–331. New York: Holt.

Hoffman, J.E. & Subramaniam, B. (1995). The role of visual attention in saccadic eye movements. *Percept. Psychophys.* **57**, 787–795.

Hollands, M.A. & Marple-Horvat, D.E. (1996). Visually guided stepping under conditions of step cycle-related denial of visual information. *Exp. Brain Res.* **109**, 343–356.

Hollands, M.A., Patla, A.E., & Vickers, J.N. (2002). "Look where you're going!": gaze behaviour associated with maintaining and changing the direction of locomotion. *Exp. Brain Res.* **143**, 221–231.

Hollingworth, A. (2006). Scene and position specificity in visual memory for objects. *J. Exptl. Psycho.: Learning Memory & Cognition* **32**, 58–69.

Hollingworth, A. & Henderson, J.M. (2002). Accurate visual memory for previously attended objects in natural scenes. *J. Exptl. Psychol.: Human Perc. & Perf.* **28**, 113–136.

Holsanova, J., Hedberg, B., & Nilsson, N. (1999). Visual and verbal focus patterns when describing pictures. In: Becker, W., Deubel, H., & Mergner, T. (Eds). *Current Oculomotor Research: Physiological and Psychological Aspects,* pp. 303–304. New York, Kluwer Academic & Plenum Publishers.

Hooge, I.T.C., Over, E.A.B., van Wezel, R.J.A., & Frens, M.A. (2005). Inhibition of return is not a foraging facilitator in saccadic search and free viewing. *Vision Res.* **45**, 1901–1908.

Hoyle, F. (1957). *The Black Cloud.* Harmondsworth: Penguin Books.

Humphrey, K. & Underwood, G. (2008). Fixation sequences in imagery and in recognition during the processing of pictures of real-world scenes. *J. Eye Movement Res.* **2**(2), 3, 1–15.

Hunter, J. (1786). *Observations on Certain Parts of the Animal Oeconomy.* Sold at: 13 Castle Street, Leicester Square, London.

Imai, T., Moore, S.T., Raphan, T., & Cohen, B. (2001). Interaction of the body, head, and eyes during walking and turning. *Exp. Brain Res.* **136**, 1–18.

Inhoff, A.W. & Rayner, K. (1986). Parafoveal word processing during eye fixations in reading: effects of word frequency. *Perception & Psychophysics* **40**, 431–439.

Inhoff, A.W. & Wang, J. (1992). Encoding of text, manual movement planning, and eye-hand coordination during copy-typing. *J. Exp. Psychol.: Human Perc. & Perf.* **18**, 437–448.

Intraub, H. (1980). Presentation rate and the representation of briefly glimpsed pictures in memory. *J. Exptl. Psychol.: Human Learning and Memory* **6**, 1–12.

Intraub, H. (1981). Identification and processing of briefly glimpsed visual scenes. In: Fisher D.F., Monty, R.A., & Senders, J.W. (Eds). *Eye Movements: Cognition and Visual Perception.* pp. 181–190. Hillsdale, NJ: Lawrence Erlbaum Associates.

Irwin, D.E. (1992). Memory for position and identity across eye-movements. *J. Exptl. Psychol.: Learning Memory & Cognition* **18**, 307–317.

Irwin, D.E. & Andrews, R. (1996). Integration and accumulation of information across saccadic eye movements. In: T. Inui, T., McClelland, J.L. (Eds). *Attention and Performance XVI: Information Integration in Perception and Communication.* pp. 125–155. Cambridge: MIT Press .

Irwin, D.E. & Zelinsky, G.J. (2002). Eye movements and scene perception: memory for things observed. *Perception & Psychophysics* **64**, 882–895.

Itti, L. & Baldi, P. (2006). Bayesian surprise attracts human attention. *Advances in Neural Information Systems 19.* pp. 547–554. Cambridge: MIT Press .

Itti, L. & Koch, C. (2000). A saliency-based search mechanism for overt and covert shifts of visual attention. *Vision Res.* **40**, 1489–1506.

Itti, L. & Koch, C. (2001). Computational modelling of visual attention. *Nature Rev. Neurosci.* **2**, 194–203.

James, W. (1890). *The Principles of Psychology.* New York: Henry Holt & Co.

Javal, L.É. (1878). Essai sur la physiologie de la lecture. *Annales d'Oculistique* **80**, 240–274.

Javal, L.É. (1879). Essai sur la physiologie de la lecture. *Annales d'Oculistique* **82**, 242–253.

Jeannerod, M. (1997) *The Cognitive Neuroscience of Action.* Oxford: Blackwell.

Johansson, R., Holsanova, J., & Holmqvist, K. (2006). Pictures and spoken descriptions elicit similar eye movements during mental imagery, both in light and in complete darkness. *Cognit. Sci.* **30**, 1053–1079.

Johansson, R.S., Westling, G., Bäckström, A., & Flanagan, J.R. (2001). Eye-hand coordination in object manipulation. *J. Neuroscience* **21**, 6917–6932.

Johnson-Frey, S.H. (2004). The neural bases of complex tool use in humans. *Trends Cogn. Sci.* **8**, 71–77.

Jordan, M.I. & Wolpert, D.M., 1999. Computational motor control. In: Gazzaniga, M. (Ed.). *The Cognitive Neurosciences.* pp. 601–620. Cambridge: MIT Press .

Jost, T., Ouerhani, N., von Wartburg, R., Muri, R., & Hugli, H. (2005). Assessing the contribution of color in visual attention. *Computer Vision and Image Understanding,* **100**, 107–123.

Jovancevic, J., Sullivan, B., & Hayhoe, M. (2006). Control of attention and gaze in complex environments. *J. Vision* **6**, 1431–1450.

Jovancevic-Misic, J. & Hayhoe, M. (in press). Adaptive gaze control in natural environments. *J. Neurosci.*

Jovancevic-Misic, J., Sullivan, B., Chajka, K., & Hayhoe, M. (2007). Control of gaze when walking in a real environment. *J. Vision* **7**(9), 1000, 1000a.

Judd, C.H. (1905). The Müller-Lyer illusion. *Psychological Monographs* **7**, 55–81.

Kahneman, D. & Treisman, A. (1984). Changing views of attention and automaticity. In: Parasuraman, R., Davies, D.R. (Eds). *Varieties of Attention.* pp. 29–61. New York: Academic Press.

Kanan, C., Tong, M.H., Zhang, L., & Cottrell, G.W. (2009). SUN: Top-down saliency using natural statistics. *Visual Cognition.* (doi 10.1080/13506280902771138).

Kandil, F.I., Rotter, A., & Lappe, M. (2009). Driving is smoother and more stable when using the tangent point. *J. Vision* 9(1), 11, 1–11.

Kappé, B. (2005). *Driving simulators for driver training: state of the art.* www. esafetysupport. org/download/research_and_development/HumanistA_02Driving.pdf

Kawagoe, R., Takikawa, Y., & Hikosaka, O. (1998). Expectation of reward modulates cognitive signals in the basal ganglia. *Nature Neurosci.* 1, 411–416.

Kemeny, A. & Panerai, F. (2003). Evaluating perception in driving simulation experiments. *Trends Cogn. Sci.* 7, 31–37.

Kennedy, A. & Pynte, J. (2008). The consequences of violations to reading order: an eye movement analysis. *Vision Res.* 48, 2309–2320.

Kennedy, A. Pynte, J., & Ducrot, S. (2002). Parafoveal-on-foveal interactions in word recognition. *Quart. J. Exp. Psychol.: Human Experimental Psychology* 55, 1307–1337.

Kingstone, A., Smilek, D., Ristic, J., Friesen, C.K., & Eastwood, J.D. (2003). Attention, researchers! It is time to take a look at the real world. *Current Directions in Psychological Science* 12, 176–180.

Klatzky, R.L. (1998). Allocentric and egocentric spatial representations: definitions, distinctions, and interconnections. In: Freska, C., Habel, C., Wender, K.F. (Eds). *Spatial Cognition – An Interdisciplinary Approach to Representation and Processing of Spatial Knowledge (Lecture Notes in Artificial Intelligence 1404).* pp. 1–17. Berlin: .Springer-Verlag.

Klein, R.M. (1980). Does oculomotor readiness mediate cognitive control of visual attention? In: R.S. Nickerson (Ed.). *Attention and Performance VIII.* pp. 259–276. Hillsdale, NJ: Lawrence Erlbaum.

Klein, R.M. (2000). Inhibition of return. *Trends Cogn. Sci.* 4, 138–147.

Kleinke, C.L. (1986). Gaze and eye contact: a research review. *Psychol. Bull.* 100, 78–100.

Klin A., Jones, W., Schultz, R., Volkmar, F., & Cohen, D. (2002). Visual fixation patterns during viewing of naturalistic social situations as predictors of social competence in individuals with autism. *Arch. Gen. Psychiatry* 59, 809–816.

Knudsen, E.I. (2007). Fundamental components of attention. *Annu. Rev. Neurosci.* 30, 57–78.

Kobayashi, H., Kohshima, S. (1997). Unique morphology of the human eye. *Nature* 387, 767–768.

Koch, C. & Ullman, S. (1985). Shifts in selective visual attention: towards the underlying neural circuitry. *Human Neurobiol.* 4, 219–227.

Koechlin, E., Ody, C., & Kouneiher, F. (2003). The architecture of cognitive control in the human prefrontal cortex. *Science* 302, 1181–1185.

Kowler E. (1991). The stability of gaze and its implications for vision. In: Carpenter, R.H.S. (Ed.). *Vision and Visual Dysfunction. Vol. 8. Eye Movements.* pp. 71–92. London: Macmillan.

Kuhn, G. & Benson, V. (2007). The influence of eye-gaze and arrow pointing distractor cues on voluntary eye movements. *Perception & Psychophysics* 69, 966–971.

Kuhn G. & Land, M.F. (2006). There's more to magic than meet the eye. *Current Biology* 16, R950–R251.

Kuhn G. & Tatler, B.W. (2005) Magic and fixation: now you see it, now you don't. *Perception* **34**, 1153–1161.

Kuhn, G., Tatler, B.W., Findlay, J.M., & Cole, G.G. (2008). Misdirection in magic: implications for the relationship between eye gaze and attention. *Visual Cognition* **16**, 391–405.

Kustov, A.A. & Robinson, D.L. (1996). Shared neural control of attention shifts and eye movements. *Nature* **384**, 74–77.

Laeng, B. & Teodorescu, D.S. (2002). Eye scanpaths during visual imagery reenact those of perception of the same visual scene. *Cognit. Sci.* **26**, 207–231.

Lamare, M. (1892). Des mouvements des yeux dans la lecture. *Bulletins et Mémoires de la Société Française d'Ophthalmologie* **10**, 354–364.

Land, M.F. (1998). The visual control of steering. In: Harris, L.R., & Jenkin, M. (Eds). *Vision and Action.* pp. 163–180. Cambridge: Cambridge University Press.

Land, M.F. (1999) Motion and vision: why animals move their eyes. *J. Comp. Physiol. A* **185**, 341–352.

Land, M.F. (2004). The coordination of rotations of eyes, head and trunk in saccadic turns produced in natural situations. *Exp. Brain Res.* **159**, 151–160.

Land, M.F. (2006). Eye movements and the control of actions in everyday life. *Prog. Retinal & Eye Res.* **25**, 296–324.

Land, M.F. (2009). Vision, eye movements, and natural behavior. *Visual Neurosci.* **26**, 51–62.

Land, M.F. & Furneaux, S. (1997). The knowledge base of the oculomotor system. *Phil. Trans. Roy. Soc. London B* **352**, 1231–1239.

Land, M.F. & Hayhoe, M. (2001). In what ways do eye movements contribute to everyday activities? *Vision Res.* **41**, 3559–3565.

Land, M.F. & Horwood, J. (1995). Which parts of the road guide steering? *Nature* **377**, 339–340.

Land, M.F. & Lee, D.N. (1994). Where we look when we steer. *Nature* **369**, 742–744.

Land, M.F. & McLeod, P. (2000). From eye movements to actions: how batsmen hit the ball. *Nature Neurosci.* **3**, 1340–1345.

Land M.F. & Nilsson, D-E. (2002). *Animal Eyes.* Oxford: Oxford University Press.

Land, M.F. & Tatler, B.W. (2001). Steering with the head: the visual strategy of a racing driver. *Current Biology* **11**, 1215–1220.

Land, M.F., Furneaux, S.M., & Gilchrist, I.D. (2001). The organization of visually mediated actions in a subject without eye movements. *Neurocase* **8**, 80–87.

Land, M.F., Mennie, N., & Rusted, J. (1999). The roles of vision and eye movements in the control of activities of daily living. *Perception* **28**, 1311–1328.

Langton, S.R.H., Watt, R.J., & Bruce, V. (2000). Do the eyes have it? Cues to the direction of social attention. *Trends in Cognit. Sci.* **4**, 50–58.

Lee, D.S. (1976). A theory of visual control of braking based on information about time to collision. *Perception* **5**, 437–459.

Lee, D.N. & Lishman ,R. (1977). Visual control of locomotion. *Scand. J. Psychol.* **18**, 224–230.

Leekham, S., Baron-Cohen, S., Perrett, D.I., Milders, M., & Brown, S. (1997). Eye-direction detection: a dissociation between geometric and joint attention skills in autism. *Brit. J. Dev. Psychol.* **15**, 77–95.

Levin, D.T. & Simons, D.J. (1997). Failure to detect changes to attended objects in motion pictures. *Psychonomic Bulletin & Review* **4**, 501–506.

Li, L. & Warren, W.H. (2000). Perception of heading during rotation: sufficiency of dense motion parallax and reference objects. *Vision Res.* **40**, 3873–3894.

Li, Z.P. (2002). A saliency map in primary visual cortex. *Trends Cogn. Sci.* **6**, 9–16.

Loomis, J.M., Beall, A., Macuga, K.L., Kelly. J.W., & Smith, R.S. (2006). Visual control of action without retinal optic flow. *Psychol. Sci.* **17**, 214–221.

López Moliner, J., Field, D.T., & Wann, J.P. (2007). Interceptive timing: prior knowledge matters. *J. Vision* 7(13), 11, 1–8.

MacKay, D.M. (1973). Visual stability and voluntary eye movements. In: Jung, R. (Ed.). *Handbook of Sensory Physiology*, Vol. VIII / 3A. pp. 307–331. Berlin: Springer.

Macknik, S.L., King, M., Randi, J, Robbins, A., Teller, Thompson, J., & Martinez-Conde, S. (2008). Attention and awareness in stage magic: turning tricks into research. *Nature Rev. Neurosci.* **9**, 871–879.

Mackworth, N.H., & Morandi, A.J. (1967). The gaze selects informative detail within pictures. *Percept. Psychophys.* **2**, 547–552.

Mackworth, N.H., & Thomas, E.L. (1962) Head-mounted eye-movement camera. *J. Opt. Soc. America* **52**, 713–716.

Macuga, K.L., Beall, A.C., Kelly, J.W., Smith, R.S., & Loomis, J.M. (2006). Changing lanes: inertial information facilitates performance when visual feedback is removed. *Exp. Brain Res.* **178**, 141–150.

Malcolm, G.L., Lanyon, L.J., Fugard, A.J.B., & Barton, J.J.S. (2008). Scan patterns during the processing of facial expressions versus identity: an exploration of task-driven and stimulus-driven events. *J. Vision* 8(8), 2, 1–9.

Marigold, D.S. & Patla, A.E. (2008). Visual information from the lower visual field is important for walking across multi-surface terrain. *Exp. Brain Res.* **188**, 23–31.

Marple-Horvat, D.E., Chattington, M., Anglesea, M., Ashford, D.G., Wilson, M., & Keil., D. (2005). Prevention of coordinated eye movements and steering impairs driving performance. *Exp. Brain. Res.* **163**, 411–420.

Marr, D. (1982). *Vision*. San Francisco: W.H. Freeman.

Mars, F. (2008). Driving around bends with manipulated eye-steering coordination. *J. Vision* 8(11), 10, 1–11.

Matelli, M., Luppino, G., & Rizzolatti, G. (1991). Architecture of superior and mesial area 6 and the adjacent cingulate cortex. *J. Comp. Neurol.* **311**, 445–462.

Maunsell, J.H. & Treue, S. (2006). Feature-based attention in visual cortex. *Trends Neurosci.* **29**, 317–322.

Mays, L.E. (2003). Neural control of vergence eye movements. In: Chalupa, L.M., & Werner, J.S. (Eds). *The Visual Neurosciences*. pp. 1415–1427. Cambridge: MIT Press .

Mazer, J.A. & Gallant, J.L. (2003). Goal-related activity in V4 during free viewing visual search: Evidence for a ventral stream visual salience map. *Neuron* **40**, 1241–1250.

McBeath, M.K., Shaffer, D.M., & Kaiser, M.K. (1995). How baseball fielders determine where to run to catch fly balls. *Science* **268**, 569–573.

McBeath, M.K., Shaffer, D.M., Roy, W.L., & Krauchunas, S.M. (2003). A linear optical trajectory informs the fielder where to run to the side to catch fly balls. *J. Exptl. Psych.: Human Perc. and Perf.* **29**, 1244–1250.

McConkie, G.W., & Rayner, K. (1975). The span of the effective stimulus during a fixation in reading. *Perception & Psychophysics* **17**, 578–586.

McConkie, G.W. & Rayner, K. (1976). Identifying the span of the effective stimulus in reading: literature review and theories of reading. In: Singer, H., & Ruddell, R.B. (Eds). *Theoretical Models and Processes of Reading*. pp. 137–162. Newark, NJ: International Reading Association.

McConkie, G.W., Kerr, P.W., Reddix, M.D., & Zola, D. (1988). Eye movement control during reading: I. The location of initial eye fixations in words. *Vision Res.* **28**, 1107–1118.

McConkie, G.W., & Zola, D. (1979). Is visual information integrated across successive fixations in reading? *Perception and Psychophysics* **25**, 221–224.

McKinney, T., Chajka, K., & Hayhoe, M. (2008). Pro-active gaze control in squash. *J. Vision* **8**(6), 111, 111a.

McLeod, P. (1987). Visual reaction time and high-speed ball games. *Perception* **16**, 49–59.

McLeod, P. & Dienes, Z. (1966). Do fielders know where to go to catch the ball or only how to get there? *J. Exptl. Psych.: Human Perc. & Perf.* **22**, 531–543.

McLeod, P., Dienes, Z., & Reed, N. (2006). The generalized optic acceleration cancellation theory of catching. *J. Exp.. Psychol.: Human Perc. & Perf.* **32**, 139–148.

McPeek, R.M. & Keller, E.L. (2002). Superior colliculus activity related to concurrent processing of saccade goals in a visual search task. *J. Neurophysiol.* **87**, 1805–1815.

Mehta, B. & Schaal, S. (2002). Forward models in visuomotor control. *J. Neurophysiol.* **88**, 942–953.

Melcher, D. (2001). Persistence of visual memory for scenes – A medium-term memory may help us to keep track of objects during visual tasks. *Nature* **412**, 401–401.

Melcher, D. (2006). Accumulation and persistence of memory for natural scenes. *J. Vision* **6**, 8–17.

Mennie, N., Hayhoe, M., & Sullivan, B. (2007). Look-ahead fixations: anticipatory eye movements in natural tasks. *Exp. Brain Res.* **179**, 427–442.

Miall, R.C. & Tchalenko, J. (2001). A painter's eye movements: a study of eye and hand movement during portrait drawing. *Leonardo: Int. J. Arts & Sciences* **34**, 35–40

Miall, R.C. & Wolpert, D.M. (1996). Forward models for physiological motor control. *Neural Networks* **9**, 1265–1279.

Miall, R.C., Gowan, E., & Tchalenko, J. (2009). Drawing cartoon faces – a functional imaging study of the cognitive neuroscience of drawing. *Cortex* **45** (3), 394–406.

Michaels, C.F. & Oudejans R.R.D. (1992). The optics and actions of catching fly balls: zeroing out optical acceleration. *Ecological Psychology* **4**, 199–222.

Miller, E.K. & Cohen, J.D. (2001). An integrative theory of prefrontal cortex function. *Ann. Rev. Neurosci.* **24**, 167–202.

Milner, A.D. & Goodale, M.A. (1995). The *Visual Brain in Action*. Oxford: Oxford University Press.

Miura, T. (1987). Behavior oriented vision: functional field of view and processing resources. In: O'Regan , J.K., & Lévy-Schoen, A., (Eds). *Eye Movements: from Physiology to Cognition*. pp. 563–572. Amsterdam: North-Holland .

Mokler, A. & Fischer, B. (1999). The recognition and correction of involuntary prosaccades in an antisaccade task. *Exp. Brain Res.* **125**, 511–516.

Montello, D.R. (1993). Scale and multiple psychologies of space. In: Frank, A.U., & Campari, I. (Eds). *Spatial Information Theory: A Theoretical Basis for GIS*. pp. 312–321. Berlin: Springer-Verlag.

Moore, T. & Armstrong, K.M. (2003). Selective gating of visual signals by microstimulation of frontal cortex, *Nature* **421**, 370–373.

Moran, J. & Desimone, R. (1985). Selective attention gates visual processing in extrastriate cortex. *Science* **229**, 782–784.

Morasso, R., Bizzi, E., & Dichgans, J. (1973). Adjustments of saccade characteristics during head movements. *Exp. Brain Res.* **16**, 492–500.

Morrison, R.E. (1984). Manipulation of stimulus onset delay in reading: evidence for parallel programming of saccades. *J. Exp. Psychol.: Human Perc. & Perf.* **10**, 667–682.

Moscovitch, M., Rosenbaum, R.S., Gilboa, A., Addis, G.R., Westmacott, R., Grady, C., et al. (2005). Functional neuroanatomy of remote episodic, semantic and spatial memory: a unified account based on multiple trace theory. *J. Anat.* **207**, 35–66.

Moser, E.I., Kropff, E., & Moser, M-B. (2008). Place cells, grid cells and the brain's spatial representation system. *Annu. Rev. Neurosci.* **31**, 69–89.

Motter, B.C. & Belky, E.J. (1998). The guidance of eye movements during active visual search. *Vision Research* **38**, 1805–1815.

Mourant, R.R. & Rockwell, T.H. (1970). Mapping eye-movement patterns to the visual scene in driving: an exploratory study. *Human Factors* **12**, 81–87.

Mourant, R.R. & Rockwell, T.H. (1972). Strategies of visual search by novice and experienced drivers. *Human Factors* **14**, 325–335.

Müller, S. & Abernethy, B. (2006). Batting with occluded visionL an in situ examination of the information pick-up and interceptive skills of high- and low-skilled cricket batsmen. *J. Science & Medicine in Sport* **9**, 446–458.

Murray, D.W., Reid, I.D., & Davison, A.J. (1996). Steering and navigation behaviours using fixation. In: Fisher, R.B., Trucco, E. (Eds). *Proc. 7th Brit. Machine Vision Conf. Vol.2.* pp. 635–644. University of Edinburgh: BMVA Press.

Najemnik, J. & Geisler, W.S. (2005). Optimal eye movement strategies in visual search. *Nature* **434**, 387–391.

Najemnik, J. & Geisler, W.S. (2008). Eye movement statistics in humans are consistent with an optimal search strategy. *Journal of Vision* **8**(3), 4, 1–14.

Nakayama, K. (1981). Differential motion hyperacuity under conditions of common image motion. *Vision Research* **21**, 1475–1482.

Navalpakkam, V. & Itti, L. (2005). Modelling the influence of task on attention. *Vision Res.* **45**, 205–231.

Nelson, W.W., & Loftus, G.R. (1980). The functional visual field during picture viewing. *J. Exp. Psych.: Human Learning and Memory* **6**, 391–319.

Neumann, O. (1966). Theories of attention. In: Neumann, O., & Sanders, A.F. (Eds). *Handbook of Perception and Action, Vol. 3.* pp. 389–446. London: Academic Press.

Nieuwenhuis, S., Ridderinkhof, K.R., Blom, J.,B and, G.P.H., & Kok, A. (2001). Error-related brain potentials are differentially related to awareness of response errors: Evidence from an antisaccade task. *Psychophysiology* **38**, 752–760.

Nobe S., Hayamizu, S., Hasegawa, O., & Takahashi, H. (2000). Hand gestures of an anthropo-morphic agent: Listeners' eye fixation and comprehension. *Bull. Jap. Cognit. Sci. Soc.* **7**, 86–92.

Norman, D.A. & Shallice, T. (1986). Attention to action: willed and automatic control of behavior. In: Davidson, R.J., Schwarts, G.E., & Shapiro, D. (Eds). *Consciousness and Self-regulation. Advances in Research and Theory. Vol. 4.* pp. 1–18. New York: Plenum.

Noton, D. & Stark, L. (1971). Scanpaths in eye movements during pattern perception. *Science* **171**, 308–311.

Nystrom, M. & Holmqvist, K. (2008). Semantic override of low-level features in image viewing – both initially and overall. *J. Eye Movement Res.* **2**(2), 2, 1–11.

Oliva, A. & Torralba, A. (2006). Building the gist of a scene: the role of global image features in recognition. *Prog. Brain Res.* **155**, 23–36.

O'Keefe. J. & Nadel, L. (1978). *The Hippocampus as a Cognitive Map*. Oxford: Oxford University Press.

O'Regan, J.K. (1990). Eye movements and reading. In: Kowler E. (Ed.). *Eye Movements and Their Role in Visual and Cognitive Processes.* pp. 395–453. Amsterdam: Elsevier.

O'Regan, J.K. (1992). Solving the real mysteries of visual perception – the world as an outside memory. *Canad. J. Psychol.-Revue Canad. de Psychol.* **46**, 461–488.

O'Regan, J.K., Deubel, H., Clark, J.J., & Rensink, R.A. (2000). Picture changes during blinks: looking without seeing and seeing without looking. *Visual Cognition* **7**, 191–211.

O'Regan, J.K. & Lévy-Schoen, A. (1983). Integrating visual information from successive fixations – does trans-saccadic fusion exist? *Vision Res.* **23**, 765–768.

O'Regan, J.K. & Noë, A. (2001). A sensorimotor account of vision and visual consciousness. *Behav. and Brain Sci.* **24**, 939–973; discussion 973–1031.

Oudejans, R.R.D., Michaels, C.F., Bakker, F.C., & Davids, K. (1999). Shedding some light on catching in the dark: perceptual mechanisms for catching fly balls. *J. Exp. Psychol.: Human Perc. & Perf.* **25**, 531–542.

Oudejans, R.R.D., van de Langenberg, R.W., & Hutter, R.I. (2002). Aiming at a far target under different viewing conditions: visual control in basketball jump shooting. *Human Movement Sci.* **21**, 457–480.

Outerbridge, J.S. & Melville Jones, G. (1971). Reflex vestibular control of head movements in man. *Aerospace Med.* **42**, 935–940.

Panchuk, D. & Vickers, J.N. (2006). Gaze behaviors of goaltenders under spatial-temporal constraints. *Human Movement Sci.* **25**, 733–752.

Pardo, J.V., Pardo, P.J., Janer, K.W., & Raichle, M.E. (1990). The anterior cingulate cortex mediates processing selection in the stroop attentional conflict paradigm. *Proc. Nat. Acad. Sci. USA.* **87**, 256–259.

Parkhurst, D.J., Law, K., & Niebur, E. (2002). Modeling the role of salience in the allocation of overt visual attention. *Vision Res.* **42**, 107–123.

Parkhurst, D.J. & Niebur, E. (2003). Scene content selected by active vision. *Spatial Vision* **16**, 125–154.

Passingham, R.E. (1993). *The Frontal Lobes and Voluntary Action*. Oxford: Oxford University Press.

Passingham, R.E., Rowe, J.B., & Sakai, K. (2005). Prefrontal cortex and attention to action. In: Humphreys, G.W., & Riddoch, M.J. (Eds). *Attention in Action: Advances from Cognitive Science.* pp. 263–286. Hove, UK: Psychology Press.

Patla, A.E. (2004). Gaze behaviors during adaptive human locomotion: insights into how vision is used to regulate locomotion. In: Vaina, L.M., Beardsley, S.A., & Rushton, S.K. (Eds). *Optic Flow and Beyond.* pp. 383–399. Norwell, MA: Kluwer.

Patla, A.E., Prentice, S.D., Rietdyk, S., Allard, F., & Martin, C. (1999). What guides the selection of alternate foot placement during locomotion in humans. *Exp. Brain Res.* **128**, 441–450.

Patla, A.E. & Vickers, J.N. (2003). How far ahead do we look when required to step on specific locations in the travel path during locomotion. *Exp. Brain Res.* **148**, 133–138.

Pelz, J.B. & Canoza, R. (2001). Oculomotor behavior and perceptual categories in complex tasks. *Vision Res.* **41**, 3587–3596.

Perrett, D.I., Harries, M.H., Bevan, R., Thomas, S., Benson, P.J., Mistlin, A.J., et al. (1989). Frameworks of analysis for the neural representation of animate objects and actions. *J. Exp. Biol.* **146**, 87–113.

Perrett, D.I., Hietanen, J.K., Oram, M.W., Benson, P.J., & Rolls, E.T. (1994). Organization and functions of cells responsive to faces in the temporal cortex. *Phil. Trans. R. Soc. Lond. B* **335**, 23–30.

Peterson, B.W. & Boyle, R.D. (2004). Vestibulocollic reflexes. In: Highstein, S.M., Fay, R.R., & Popper, A.N.(Eds). *The Vestibular System. Springer Handbook of Auditory Research Vol. 19.* pp. 343–374. Berlin: Springer.

Petersen, S.E., Fox, P.T., Posner, M.I., Mintun, M., & Raichle, M.E. (1988). Positron emission tomographic studies of the cortical anatomy of single word processing. *Nature* **331**,585–589.

Petrides, M. & Pandya, D.N. (2002). Association pathways of the prefrontal cortex and functional observations. In: Stuss, D.T., & Knight, R.T. (Eds). *Principles of Frontal Lobe Function*, pp. 31–50. Oxford: Oxford University Press.

Pola, J. & Wyatt, H.J. (1991). Smooth pursuit: response characteristics, stimuli and mechanisms. In: Carpenter R.H.S. (Ed.). *Vision and Visual Dysfunction. Vol.8. Eye movements.* pp. 138–156. London: Macmillan.

Pollatsek, A., Reichle, E.D., & Rayner, K. (2006). Attention to one word at a time in reading is still a viable hypothesis: Rejoinder to Inhoff, Radach, and Eiter (2006). *J. Exp. Psychol. Human Perc.& Perf.* **32**, 1496–1500.

Posner, M.I. (1980). Orienting of attention. *Quart. J. Exp. Psychol.* **32**, 3–25.

Posner, M.I. & DiGirolamo, G.J. (1998). Executive attention: conflict, target detection and cognitive control. In: Parasuraman, R. (Ed.). *The attentive brain.* pp. 401–423. Cambridge: MIT Press.

Posner, M.I., Nissen, M.J., & Ogden, W.C. (1978). Attended and unattended processing modes: the role of set for spatial location. In: Pick, H.L., & Saltzman, I.J. (Eds). *Modes of Perceiving and Processing Information.* pp. 137–157. Hillsdale, NJ: Lawrence Erlbaum.

Pynte, J., Kennedy, A., & Ducrot, S. (2004). The influence of parafoveal typographical errors on eye movements in reading. *Europ. J. Cognit. Psychol.* **16**, 178–202.

Radach, R., Kennedy, A., & Rayner, K. (2004). *Eye Movements and Information Processing during Reading.* Hove, UK: Psychology Press.

Ramachandran,V.S., & Oberman, L.M. (2006). Broken mirrors: a theory of autism. *Scient. Amer.* **295**(5), 62–69.

Rao, R.P.N., Zelinski, G.J., Hayhoe, M.M., & Ballard, D.H., (2002). Eye movements in iconic visual search. *Vision Res.* **42**, 1447–1463.

Rayner, K., (1998). Eye movements in reading and information processing: 20 years of research. *Psychol. Bull.* **124**, 372–422.

Rayner, K., & Pollatsek, A. (1989). *The Psychology of Reading.* Englewood Cliffs, NJ: Prentice-Hall.

Regan, D. (1992). Visual judgments and misjudgments in cricket, and the art of flight. *Perception* **21**, 91–115.

Regan, D. & Beverley, K.I. (1982). How do we avoid confounding the direction we are moving with the direction we are looking? *Science* **215**, 194–196.

Regan, D. & Gray, R. (2000). Visually guided collision avoidance and collision achievement. *Trends Cogn. Sci.* **4**, 99–107.

Reichle, E.D., Pollatsek, A., Fisher, D.L., & Rayner, K. (1998). Towards a model of eye movement control in reading. *Psychol. Rev.* **105**, 125–157.

Reichle, E.D., Pollatsek, A., & Rayner, K. (2006). E-Z Reader: a cognitive-control, serial-attention model of eye-movement behavior during reading. *Cognitive Systems Research* **7**, 4–22.

Reinagel, P. & Zador, A.M. (1999). Natural scene statistics at the centre of gaze. *Network-Computation in Neural Systems* **10**, 341–350.

Remington, R.W. (1980). Attention and saccadic eye movements. *J. Exp. Psychol.: Human Perc. & Perf.* **6**, 726–744.

Renninger, L.W., Coughlan, J., & Vergheese, P. (2005). An information maximization model of eye movements. In Saul, L.K., Weiss, Y., & Bottou, L. (Eds). *Advances in Neural Information Processing Systems* (Vol. 17), pp. 1121–1128. Cambridge: MIT Press .

Rensink, R.A. (2000). The dynamic representation of scenes. *Visual Cognition* **7**, 17–42.

Rensink, R.A. (2002). Change detection. *Annu. Rev. Psychol.* **53**, 245–277.

Rensink, R.A., O'Regan, J.K., & Clark, J.J. (1997). To see or not to see: the need for attention to perceive changes in scenes. *Psychol. Sci.* **8**, 368–373.

Reynolds, J.H. & Chelazzi, L. (2004). Attentional modulation of visual processing. *Annu. Rev. Neurosci.* **27**, 611–647.

Ribot, T. (1906). *Psychologie de l'Attention.* Paris: Felix Alcan.

Ricciardelli, P., Bricolo, E., Aglioti, S.M., & Chelazzi, L. (2002). My eyes want to look where your eyes are looking: exploring the tendency to imitate another individual's gaze. *Neuroreport* **13**, 2259–2264.

Richardson, D.C. & Spivey, M.J. (2000). Representation, space and Hollywood Squares: looking at things that aren't there anymore. *Cognition* **76**, 269–295.

Richardson, D.C., Altmann, G.T.M., Spivey, M.J., & Hoover, M.A. (in press). Much ado about nothing. *Trends in Cognitive Sciences.*

Riemersma, J.B.J. (1981). Visual control during straight road driving. *Acta Psychologica* **48**, 215–225.

Ripoll, H., Fleurance, P., & Caseneuve, D. (1987). Analysis of visual patterns of table tennis players. In: O'Regan, J.K., Levy-Schoen, A. (Eds). *Eye Movements: from Physiology to Cognition.* pp. 616–617. Amsterdam: North-Holland.

Ristic, J., Friesen, C.K., & Kingstone, A. (2002). Are eyes special? It depends on how you look at it. *Psychonomic Bulletin & Review* **9**, 507–513.

Rizzolatti, G. & Arbib, M. (1998). Language within our grasp. *Trends Neurosci.* **21**, 188–194.

Rizzolatti, G. & Craighero, L. (2004). The mirror-neuron system. *Ann. Rev. Neurosci.* **27**, 169–192.

Rizzolatti, G. & Luppino, G. (2001). The cortical motor system. *Neuron* **31**, 889–901.

Rizzolatti, G., Riggio, L., Dascola, I., & Umiltà, C. (1987). Reorienting attention across the horizontal and vertical meridians – evidence in favor of a premotor theory of attention. *Neuropsychologia* **25**, 31–40.

Robertshaw, K.D., & Wilkie, R.M. (2008) Does gaze influence steering around a bend? *J. Vision* **8**(4), 18, 1–13.

Robinson, D.A. (1964) The mechanics of human saccadic eye movements. *J. Physiol. (London)* **174**, 245–264.

Robinson, D.L. & Petersen, S.E. (1992). The pulvinar and visual salience. *Trends Neurosci.* **15**, 127–132.

Rock, P.B., & Harris, M.G. (2006). Tau-dot as a potential variable for visually guided braking. *J. Exp. Psychol: Human Perc. & Perf.* **32**, 251–267.

Roelfsema, P.R., Lamme, V.A.F., & Spekreijse, H. (1998). Object-based attention in the primary visual cortex of the macaque monkey. *Nature* **395**, 376–381.

Rothkopf, C.A., & Ballard, D.H., & Hayhoe, M.M. (2007). Task and context determine where you look. *J. Vision* **7**(14), 16, 1–20.

Rushton, S.K. & Wann. J.P. (1999). Weighted combination of size and disparity: a computational model for timing a ball catch. *Nature Neurosci.* **2**, 186–190.

Rushton, S.K., Harris, J.M., Lloyd, M.R., & Wann, J.P. (1998). Guidance of locomotion on foot uses perceived target location rather than optic flow. *Current Biology* **8**, 1191–1194.

Sailer, U., Flanagan, J.R., & Johansson R.S. (2005). Eye-hand coordination during learning of a novel visuomotor task. *J. Neurosci.* **25**, 8833–8842.

Salvucci, D.D. & Gray, R. (2004). A two-point control model of steering. *Perception* **33**, 1233–248.

Salvucci, D.D. & Liu, A. (2002). The time course of a lane change: driver control and eye movement behavior. *Transportation Res.* **F 5**: 123–132.

Savelsbergh, G.J.P. & Whiting, H.T.A. (1996). Catching: a motor learning and developmental perspective. In: Heuer, H., & Keele, S.W. (Eds). *Handbook of Perception and Action. Vol. 2. Motor Skills.* pp. 461–501. London: Academic Press.

Savelsbergh, G.J., Williams, A.M., van der Kamp, J., & Ward, P. (2002). Visual search, anticipation and expertise in soccer goalkeepers. *J. Sports Sci.* **20**, 279–287.

Savelsbergh, G.J., Williams, A.M., van der Kamp, J., & Ward, P. (2005). Anticipation and visual search behaviour in expert soccer goalkeepers. *Ergonomics* **48**, 1686–1697.

Scherberger, H. & Andersen, R.A. (2003). Sensorimotor transformations in the posterior parietal cortex. In: Chalupa, L.M., & Werner, J.S. (Eds). *The Visual Neurosciences.* pp. 1324–1336. Cambridge: MIT Press.

Schwartz, M.F. (2006). The cognitive neuropsychology of everyday action and planning. *Cogn. Neuropsych.* **23**, 202–221.

Schwartz, M.F., Reed, E.S., Montgomery M.W., Palmer, C., & Mayer, N.H. (1991). The quantitative description of action disorganisation after brain damage: a case study. *Cogn. Neuropsych.* **8**, 381–414.

Senju, A. & Csibra, G. (2008). Gaze following in human infants depends on communicative signals. *Current Biology* **18**, 668–671.

Serences, J.T. & Yantis, S. (2006). Selective visual attention and perceptual coherence. *Trends Cogn. Sci.* **10**, 38–45.

Shaffer, D.M., McBeath, M.K., Roy, W.L., & Krauchunas, S.M. (2003). A linear optical trajectory informs the fielder where to run to the side to catch fly balls. *J. Exp. Psychol: Human Perc. & Perf.* **29**, 1244–1250.

Shallice, T. (2002). Fractionation of the supervisory system. In: Stuss, D.T., & Knight, R.T., (Eds). *Principles of Frontal Lobe Function.* pp. 261–277. Oxford: Oxford University Press.

Shallice, T. & Burgess, P.W. (1996). Domains of supervisory control and the temporal organisation of behaviour. *Phil. Trans. R. Soc. B* **351**, 1405–1412.

Shepherd, M., Findlay, J.M., & Hockey, R.J. (1986). The relationship between eye-movements and spatial attention. *Quart. J. Exp. Psychol. A – Human Exp. Psychol.* **38**, 475–491.

Shinoda, H., Hayhoe, M.M., & Shrivastava, A. (2001). What controls attention in natural environments? *Vision Res.* **41**, 3535–3545.

Simons, D.J. (1996). In sight, out of mind: when object representations fail. *Psychol. Sci.* **7**, 301–305.

Simons, D.J. & Rensink, R.A. (2005). Change blindness: past, present and future. *Trends Cogn. Sci.* **9**, 16–20.

Smilek, D., Birmingham, E., Cameron, D., Bischof, W., & Kingstone, A. (2006). Cognitive ethology and exploring attention in real-world scenes. *Brain Res.* **1080**, 101–119.

Smith, T.J. & Henderson, J.M. (2008). Edit blindness: the relationship between attention and global change blindness in dynamic scenes. *J. Eye Movement Res.* **2**(2), 6, 1–17.

Smith, T.J. & Henderson, J.M. (2009). Facilitation of return during scene viewing. *Visual Cognition.* doi 10.1080/13506280902771138).

Snowden, R., Thompson, P., & Troscianko, T. (2006). *Basic Vision.* Oxford: Oxford University Press.

Sommer, M.A. & Wurtz, R.H. (2003). The dialogue between cerebral cortex and superior colliculus: implications for target selection and corollary discharge. In: Chalupa, L.M., & Werner, J.S. (Eds). *The Visual Neurosciences.* pp. 1466–1484. Cambridge: MIT Press .

Sommer, M.A. & Wurtz R.H. (2008). Brain circuits for the internal monitoring of movements. *Annu. Rev. Neurosci.* **31**, 317–318.

Sprague, N., Ballard, D.H., & Robinson, A. (2007). Modeling embodied visual behaviors. In: *ACM Transactions on Applied Perception Vol. 4 (2).* http://doi.acm.org/10.1145/1265957.1265960.

Stark, M., Lies, P., Zillich, M., Wyatt, J., & Schiele, B. (2008). Functional object class detection based on learned affordance cues. In: Gasteratos, A., Vincze, M., Tsotsos, J.K. (Eds). *Computer Vision Systems: 6th International Conference (ICVS 2008).* pp. 435–444. Berlin: Springer-Verlag.

Steinman, R.M. (2003). Gaze control under natural conditions. In: Chalupa, L.M., & Werner, J.S. (Eds). *The Visual Neurosciences.* pp. 1339–1356. Cambridge: MIT Press.

Stratton, G.M. (1902). Eye-movements and the aesthetics of visual form. *Philosophische Studien* **20**, 336–359.

Stratton, G.M. (1906). Symmetry, linear illusions and the movements of the eye. *Psychological Review* **14**, 82–96.

Stroop, J.R. (1935). Studies of interference in serial verbal reactions. *J. Exp. Psychol.* **18**, 643–662.

Stuss, D.T., Shallice, T., Alexander, M.P., & Picton, T.W. (1995). A multidisciplinary approach to anterior attentional functions. In Grafman, J., Holyoak, K.J., & Boller, F. (Eds). *Structure and Functions of the Human Prefrontal Cortex. Annals N Y Acad Sci* **769**, 191–211.

Summala, H. (1998). Forced peripheral vision driving paradigm: evidence for the hypothesis that car drivers learn to keep in lane with peripheral vision. In: Gale, A.G. (Ed.). *Vision in Vehicles VI.* pp. 51–60. Amsterdam: Elsevier.

Summala, H., Nieminen, T., & Punto, M. (1996). Maintaining lane position with peripheral vision during in-vehicle tasks. *Human Factors* **38**, 442–451.

Symons, L.A., Lee, K., Cedrone, C.C., & Nisimura, M. (2004). What are you looking at? Acuity for triadic eye gaze. *J. Gen. Psychol.* **131**, 451–469.

Tanenhaus, M.K., Spivey-Knowlton, M.J., Eberhard, K M., & Sedivy, J.C. (1995). Integration of visual and linguistic information in spoken language comprehension. *Science* **268**, 1632–1634.

Tatler, B.W. (2001) Characterising the visual buffer: real-world evidence for overwriting early in each fixation. *Perception* **30**, 993–1006.

Tatler, B.W. (2007). The central fixation bias in scene viewing: selecting an optimal viewing position independently of motor biases and image feature distributions. *J. Vision* 7(14), 4, 1–17.

Tatler, B.W. (Ed.) (in press). Eye guidance and natural scenes. *Visual Cognition*. Also available as: Tatler, B.W. (Ed.) (2009). *Eye Guidance in Natural Scenes*. Hove: Psychology Press.

Tatler, B.W., Baddeley, R.J., & Gilchrist, I.D. (2005). Visual correlates of fixation selection: effects of scale and time. *Vision Res.* **45**, 643–659.

Tatler, B.W., Baddeley, R.J., & Vincent, B.T. (2006). The long and the short of it: spatial statistics at fixation vary with saccade amplitude and task. *Vision Res.* **46**, 1857–1862.

Tatler, B.W., Gilchrist, I.D., & Land, M.F. (2005). Visual memory for objects in natural scenes: from fixations to object files. *Quart. J. Exp. Psych. Section A: Human Exp. Psychol.* **58**, 931–960.

Tatler, B.W., Gilchrist, I.D., & Rusted, J. (2003). The time course of abstract visual representation. *Perception* **32**, 579–592.

Tatler, B.W. & Kuhn, G. (2007). Don't look now: the misdirection of magic. In: van Gompel, R., Fischer, M., Murray, W., & Hill, R. (Eds). *Eye Movement Research: Insights into Mind and Brain*. pp. 697–714. Amsterdam: Elsevier.

Tatler, B.W. & Melcher, D. (2007). Pictures in mind: initial encoding of object properties varies with the realism of the scene stimulus. *Perception* **36**, 1715–1729.

Tatler, B.W. & Troscianko, T. (2002). A rare glimpse of the eye in motion. *Perception* **31**, 1403–1406.

Tatler, B.W. & Vincent, B.T. (2009). Systematic tendencies in scene viewing. *J. Eye Movement Res.* **2**(2), 5, 1–18. (doi 10.1080/13506280902764539).

Tatler, B.W. & Vincent, B.T. (in press). The prominence of behavioural biases in eye guidance. *Visual Cognition*.

Tatler, B.W. & Wade, N.J. (2003). On nystagmus, saccades and fixations. *Perception* **32**, 167–184.

Tchalenko, J., Dempere-Marco, L., Hu, X.P., & Yang, G.Z. (2003). Eye movement and voluntary control in portrait drawing. In: Hyönä, J.R., & Deubel, H. (Eds). *The Mind's Eye: Cognitive and Applied Aspects of Eye Movement Research*. pp. 705–727. Amsterdam: Elsevier.

Tchalenko, J.S. (2007). Eye movements in drawing simple lines. *Perception* **36**, 1152–1167.

Tchalenko, J.S. & Miall, C. (2009). Eye-hand strategies in copying complex lines. *Cortex* **45**, 368–376.

Thomas, E.L. (1968). Movements of the eye. *Scient. Amer.* **219**(2), 88–95.

Thompson, K.G. & Bichot, N.P. (2005). A visual salience map in the primate frontal eye field. *Prog. Brain Res.* **147**, 251–262.

Tipples, J. (2002). Eye gaze is not unique: automatic orienting in response to uninformative arrows. *Psychonomic Bulletin & Review* **9**, 314–318.

Torralba, A. & Oliva, A. (2003). Statistics of natural image categories. *Network-Computation in Neural Systems* **14**, 391–412.

Torralba, A., Oliva, A., Castelhano, M.S., & Henderson, J.M. (2006). Contextual guidance of eye movements and attention in real-world scenes: the role of global features in object search. *Psych. Rev.* **113**, 766–786.

Triesch, J., Ballard, D.H., Hayhoe, M.M., & Sullivan B.T. (2003). What you see is what you need. *J. Vision* **3**, 86–94.

Treisman, A. (1988). Features and objects. *Quart. J. Exp. Psychol.* **40A**, 201–237.

Treisman, A. & Gelade, G. (1980). A feature integration theory of attention. *Cogn. Psychol.* **12**, 97–136.

Tresilian, J. (1995). Study of a servo-control strategy for projectile interception. *Quart. J. Exptl. Psych.: Human Exptl. Psych.* **48A**, 688–715.

Turano, K.A., Geruschat, D.R., & Baker, F.H. (2003). Oculomotor strategies for the direction of gaze tested with a real-world activity. *Vision Res.* **43**, 333–346.

Underwood, G., Chapman, P., Crundall, D., Cooper, S., & Wallén, R. (1999). The visual control of steering and driving: where do we look when negotiating curves. In Gale, A.G. (Ed.). *Vision in Vehicles VII*. pp. 245–252. Amsterdam: Elsevier.

Underwood, G. & Everatt, J. (1996). Automatic and controlled information processing: the role of attention in the processing of novelty. In: Neumann, O., & Sauders, A.F. (Eds). *Handbook of Perception and Action. Vol.3. Attention.* pp. 185–227. London: Academic Press.

Underwood, G. & Foulsham, T. (2006). Visual saliency and semantic incongruency influence eye movements when inspecting pictures. *Quart. J. Exp. Psychol.* **59**, 1931–1949.

Underwood, G., Foulsham, T., van Loon, E., Humphreys, L., & Bloyce, J. (2006). Eye movements during scene inspection: a test of the saliency map hypothesis. *Europ. J. Cognit. Psychol.* **18**, 321–342.

Unema, P.J.A., Pannasch, S., Joos, M., & Velichkovsky, B.M. (2005). Time course of information processing during scene perception: the relationship between saccade amplitude and fixation duration. *Visual Cognition* **12**, 473–494.

Ungerleider, L.G. & Pasternak, T. (2003). Ventral and dorsal processing streams. In: Chalupa, L.M., & Werner, J.S. (Eds). *The Visual Neurosciences.* pp. 541–562. Cambridge: MIT Press.

Van Essen, D.C. (2003). Organization of visual pathways in macaque and human cerebral cortex. In: Chalupa, L.M., & Werner, J.S. (Eds). *The Visual Neurosciences.* pp. 507–521. Cambridge: MIT Press.

Van Gompel, R.P.C., Fischer, M.H., Murray, W.S., & Hill, R.L. (Eds) (2007). *Eye Movements: A Window on Mind and Brain.* Amsterdam: Elsevier.

Velichkovsky, B.M., Joos, M., Helmert, J.R., & Pannasch, S. (2005). Two visual systems and their eye movements: evidence from static and dynamic scene perception. In: Bara, B.G., Barsalou, L., & Bucciarelli, M. (Eds), *Proceedings of the XXVII Conference of the Cognitive Science Society.* pp. 2283–2288. Mahwah, NJ: Lawrence Erlbaum.

Vickers, J.N. (1996). Visual control when aiming at a far target. *J. Exptl. Psychol: Human Perc. & Perf.* **22**, 342–354.

Vickers, J.N. (2002). On the ball: *Science Hotline: Scientific American Frontiers.* www.pbs.org/saf/1206/hotline/hvickers.htm

Vincent, B.T., Troscianko, T., & Gilchrist, I.D. (2007). Investigating a space-variant weighted salience account of visual selection. *Vision Res.* **47**, 1809–1820.

Wade, N.J. & Tatler, B.W. (2005). *The Moving Tablet of the Eye: The Origins of Modern Eye Movement Research.* Oxford: Oxford University Press.

Wallis, G. & Bülthoff, H. (2000). What's scene and not seen: influences of movement and task upon what we see. *Visual Cognition* **7**, 175–190.

Wallis, G., Chatziastros, A., & Bülthoff, H. (2002). An unexpected role for visual feedback in vehicle steering control. *Current Biology* **12**, 295–299.

Walls, G.L. (1962). The evolutionary history of eye movements. *Vision Res.* **2**, 69–80.

Wann, J.P. & Land, M.F. (2000). Steering with or without the flow. Is the retrieval of heading necessary? *Trends Cogn. Sci.* **4**, 319–324.

Wann, J.P. & Wilkie, R.M. (2004). How do we control high speed steering? In: Vaina, L.M., Beardsley, S.A., & Rushton ,S.K. (Eds). *Optic Flow and Beyond.* pp. 371–389. Dordrecht: Kluwer Academic Publishers.

Warren, W.H. & Hannon, D.J. (1988). Direction of self-motion is perceived from optical flow. *Nature* **336**, 162–163.

Warren, W.H., Kay, B.A., Zosh, W.D., Duchon, A.P., & Sahuc, S. (2001). Optic flow is used to control human walking. *Nature Neurosci.* **4**, 213–216.

Wartburg, R. von, Wurtz, P., Pflugshaupt, T., Nyffeler, T., Lüthi, M., & Müri, R.M. (2007). Size matters: saccades during scene perception. *Perception* **36**, 355–365.

Watts, R.G. & Bahill, A.T. (1990). *Keep Your Eye on the Ball. The Science and Folklore of Baseball.* New York: W.H. Freeman.

Weaver, H.E. (1943). A study of visual processes in reading differently constructed musical selections. *Psychological Monographs* **55**, 1–30.

Westheimer, G.A. & McKee, S. (1975). Visual acuity in the presence of retinal image motion. *J. Opt. Soc. Am.* **65**, 847–850.

White, S.J. & Liversedge, S.P. (2004). Orthographic familiarity influences initial eye fixation positions in reading. *Europ. J. Cognit. Psychol.* **16**, 52–78.

Williams, A.M., Singer, R.N., & Frehlich, S.G. (2002). Quiet eye duration, expertise, and task complexity in near and far aiming tasks. *J. Mot. Behav.* **34**, 197–207.

Wise, S.P., Boussaoud, D., Johnson, P.B., & Caminiti, R. (1997). Premotor and parietal cortex: corticocortical connectivity and combinatorial combinations. *Ann. Rev. Neurosci.* **20**, 25–42.

Wiseman, R. (2008). *Quirkology: The Curious Science of Everyday Lives.* London: PanMacmillan.

Wittmann, M., Kiss, M., Gugg, P., Alexander, S., Fink, M., Pöppel, E., et al. (2006). Effects of display position of a visual in-vehicle task on simulated driving. *Applied Ergonomics* **37**, 187–199.

Wolfe, J.M. (1994). Guided search 2.0: A revised model of visual search. *Psychonomic Bull. Rev.* **1**, 202–238.

Wolfe, J. M.(1998). What can 1 million trials tell us about visual search? *Psychological Science* **9**, 33–39.

Wolfe, J.M. (2003). Moving towards solutions of some enduring controversies in visual search. *Trends Cogn. Sci.* **7**, 70–76.

Wolpert, D.M. & Flanagan, J.R. (2001). Motor prediction. *Current Biology* **11**, R729–R732.

Wolpert. D.M., Ghahramani, Z., & Jordan, M.I. (1995). An internal model for sensorimotor integration. *Science* **269**, 1880–1882.

Wollaston, W.H. (1824). On the apparent direction of eyes in a portrait. *Phil. Trans. R. Soc.* **114**, 247–256.

Yang, S.N. & McConkie, G.W. (2001). Eye movements during reading: a theory of saccade initiation times. *Vision Res.* **41**, 3567–3585.

Yarbus, A. (1967). *Eye Movements and Vision.* New York: Plenum Press.

Yilmaz, E.R. & Nakayama, K. (1995). Fluctuation of attention levels during driving, *Invest. Ophthal. Vis. Sci.* **36**, S940.

Yilmaz, E.R. & Warren, W.H. (1995). Visual control of braking: a test of the tau-dot hypothesis. *J. Exp. Psychol.: Human Perc. & Perf.* **21**, 996–1014.

Zangemeister, W.H., Jones, A., & Stark, L. (1981). Dynamics of head movement trajectories: main sequence relationship. *Exp. Neurol.* **71**, 76–91.

Zwahlen, H.T. (1993). Eye scanning rules for drivers: how do they compare with actual observed eye-scanning behavior? *Transportation Research Record* **1403**, 14–22.

Index